Regulation of Chemokine-Receptor Interactions and Functions

Special Issue Editor
Martin J. Stone

MDPI • Basel • Beijing • Wuhan • Barcelona • Belgrade

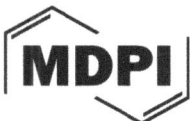

MDPI

Special Issue Editor
Martin J. Stone
Monash University
Australia

Editorial Office
MDPI AG
St. Alban-Anlage 66
Basel, Switzerland

This edition is a reprint of the Special Issue published online in the open access journal *International Journal of Molecular Sciences* (ISSN 1422-0067) in 2017 (available at:
http://www.mdpi.com/journal/ijms/special_issues/chemokine_receptor_2016).

For citation purposes, cite each article independently as indicated on the article page online and as indicated below:

Lastname, F.M.; Lastname, F.M. Article title. *Journal Name.* **Year.** *Article number, page range.*

First Edition 2018

ISBN 978-3-03842-728-5 (Pbk)
ISBN 978-3-03842-727-8 (PDF)

Cover image: Neutrophil chemotaxis in mouse postcapillary venules, visualised by intravital imaging. Cover photo courtesy of Professor Michael Hickey, Monash University, VIC, Australia.

Table of Contents

About the Special Issue Editor

Martin J. Stone is a researcher and teacher in the Monash University Department of Biochemistry and Molecular Biology and the Monash Biomedicine Discovery Institute, Melbourne, Australia. He received his BSc and MSc(Hons) degrees from the University of Auckland (New Zealand) and his PhD from the University of Cambridge (UK). He was a postdoctoral research fellow at the Scripps Research Institute in (San Diego, USA) and a faculty member at Indiana University (Bloomington, USA) before moving to Monash in 2007. Associate Professor Stone's research focuses on the biochemistry and pharmacology of chemokines and their receptors, which are critical in directing migration of leukocytes in inflammatory responses. Recently, his lab has made important contributions to understanding the influence of receptor tyrosine sulfation on chemokine recognition, the structural basis by which chemokines differentially activate a shared receptor, and the discovery of tick proteins that suppress chemokine-mediated host defenses.

International Journal of
Molecular Sciences

MDPI

Editorial

Regulation of Chemokine–Receptor Interactions and Functions

Martin J. Stone

Infection and Immunity Program, Monash Biomedicine Discovery Institute and Department of Biochemistry and Molecular Biology, Monash University, Clayton VIC 3800, Australia; martin.stone@monash.edu; Tel.: +61-3-9902-9246

Received: 6 November 2017; Accepted: 10 November 2017; Published: 14 November 2017

Inflammation is the body's response to injury or infection. As early as 2000 years ago, the Roman encyclopaedist Aulus Cornelius Celsus recognised four cardinal signs of this response—redness, heat, swelling and pain; a fifth sign is loss of function. The underlying cause of these common symptoms remained a mystery until the 19th century, when Rudolf Virchow "claim(ed) for the leukocyte a place in the field of pathology" [1]. It is now widely recognised that all inflammatory responses involve migration of leukocytes (white blood cells) to the affected tissues, where they accumulate and carry out a plethora of functions including elimination of pathogens, regulation of immunity and tissue repair.

While leukocyte recruitment is a beneficial response to pathogen invasion, we are all too familiar with the detrimental roles it can play in numerous diseases. As an example, in allergic asthma, the recruited leukocytes include eosinophils, which can then undergo degranulation, releasing toxic proteins that induce airway constriction and difficulty breathing [2]. In this case, the inflammatory response causes more damage than the initial stimulus (the allergen), so it would be beneficial to suppress the leukocyte recruitment. The same is true in many other inflammatory diseases, such as atherosclerosis, rheumatoid arthritis, multiple sclerosis, dermatitis, etc. However, it is essential that such a therapeutic strategy should not suppress inflammation so much as to make the patient susceptible to infections. To successfully achieve the right balance between the "yin and yang" of inflammation, we need to understand the biochemical mechanisms underlying leukocyte recruitment.

Enter chemokines and chemokine receptors. Over a period of about 20 years beginning in the late 1980s, researchers discovered a family of related proteins that are secreted by various cell types as an early response to tissue damage and attract leukocytes towards the affected tissues. These proteins were named chemokines (chemotactic cytokines) due to their ability to induce chemotaxis, which is migration of cells towards a chemical stimulus. They elicit this function by activating chemokine receptors, a family of G protein-coupled receptors expressed on the surfaces of leukocytes. Importantly, different types of leukocytes express different chemokine receptors, so much of the selectivity of leukocyte responses, i.e., which types of leukocytes are recruited in a given situation, arises from the complementarity between the specific chemokines expressed in the affected tissues and the specific receptors expressed on the different leukocytes. The chemokine–receptor network was clearly an attractive target to suppress unwanted inflammation while still enabling appropriate responses to pathogens.

Following the discovery of chemokines and their receptors, there has been an enormous body of research exploring their roles in normal physiology and inflammatory diseases as well as the mechanistic basis of their activity. Indeed, a PubMed search for "chemokine" now gives almost 150,000 hits. Pick an inflammatory disease of interest and there is a good chance you will be able to find analyses of affected tissues showing the types of leukocytes recruited and elevated concentrations of the chemokines responsible. In many cases, knockout mice or pharmacological inhibition studies have shown that eliminating the relevant chemokine–receptor interactions significantly reduces inflammatory symptoms. These results have emboldened drug companies to develop small molecules or biologics that target chemokine receptors (or occasionally chemokines) and to test them in clinical trials against a wide range of inflammatory diseases [3].

However, despite much hope and the investment of billions of dollars, the results have been disappointing and most trials have failed. The reasons are complex and varied but commonly the tested drugs do not show the same efficacy or target selectivity in humans as they did in animal models. Perhaps this should not be surprising as the chemokine–receptor networks differ between species, and drugs that exhibit high specificity in one species could easily have off-target effects in another. Moreover, even in a single species, inhibition of one receptor may not be sufficient to block a response if alternative, compensatory receptors are still active.

Clearly, much of the difficulty in successfully targeting chemokines and their receptors arises from the complexity of their biology. Not only are these protein families extensive and promiscuous but there are numerous mechanisms known by which their activities are modulated. Despite a substantial body of basic research, our understanding of these mechanisms remains incomplete and more work is needed. Fortunately, chemokines and their receptors have caught the attention of many basic researchers who continue to explore their structures, biochemical functions, modes of interaction, pharmacology and mechanisms of regulation. This Special Issue highlights a variety of approaches being taken to elucidate these aspects of chemokine–receptor function.

As an introduction to this Special Issue, my colleagues and I have reviewed the variety of mechanisms by which chemokines and their receptors can be regulated [4], summarized schematically in Figure 1 of this review. We give an overview of the two protein families, and their network of selective interactions and we discuss what is known about the structural basis of these interactions. We highlight the variation of chemokine and receptor primary sequences through polymorphisms, mutations, splice variants and proteolytic modifications and we describe a variety of other post-translational modifications that can enhance or reduce their functions, either directly or by altering their stability or localization. In addition, we explore the complexity of downstream cellular signals stimulated by chemokines acting upon their receptors and give a brief overview of natural and synthetic inhibition approaches.

Our review also touches on the oligomerization of both chemokines and chemokine receptors and the interactions of chemokine oligomers with glycosaminoglycans (GAGs), which affects biological activity by enabling the formation of chemokine gradients that promote leukocyte chemotaxis. These latter two topics are discussed in more detail in two other review articles in this issue. Miller and Mayo provide an in-depth analysis of the tertiary and quaternary structures of chemokines, and their functional consequences, with a particular focus on the phenomenon of heterodimerization [5]. Considering that most chemokines homodimerize and the dimerization interfaces are largely conserved within each of the two major subfamilies of chemokines (CC and CXC), it makes sense that different chemokines from the same subfamily can form heterodimers with each other. This greatly increases the number of dimeric species that could be present within the biological milieu, binding to GAGs and swapping chemokine protomers with each other. As discussed by Thompson et al. [6], the situation is further complicated by the variety of different GAG structures, the influence of GAGs on chemokine oligomers and the effects of the tissue microenvironment.

The interplay between chemokine heterodimerzation and GAG binding is evident in the two articles by Brown et al. in this Special Issue [7,8]. First, they show that the chemokine CXCL7, which exists in equilibrium between monomeric and dimeric forms, is able to bind to GAGs even in its monomeric state [7], although structural modeling suggests that dissociation from GAGs is a prerequisite for receptor binding. Second, they demonstrate that CXCL7 heterodimerizes with several other CXC chemokines and they use a trapped heterodimer to show that the GAG interactions of the heterodimer are distinct from those of the CXCL7 monomer [8].

In addition to their heterogeneity of three-dimensional structure and GAG-binding, chemokines can also vary substantially in their covalent molecular structures due to heterogeneous post-translational modifications. One common modification is limited proteolysis, which commonly alters the functionally important N-terminal regions of chemokines. Illustrating this effect, Metzemaekers et al. show that three chemokine ligands of the receptor CXCR3 are all inactivated by N-terminal cleavage but that GAGs protect the chemokines from this cleavage while also competing with the receptor for chemokine binding [9]. Another post-translational modification of chemokines is the nitration of various amino acid side chain groups by reactive nitrogen species. In their review article, Thompson et al. [6] discuss this modification and its consequences for recognition of both chemokine receptors and GAGs. An additional modification, investigated by Nguyen et al. [10], is the cyclization of an N-terminal glutamine residue to yield pyroglutamate. Considering the importance of the chemokine N-terminus for function, this modification has the potential to influence receptor interactions. However, the authors show that pyroglutamate formation (and other N-terminal modifications) do not substantially affect the potency of 5P12-RANTES, a variant of RANTES/CCL5 that inhibits HIV entry via the chemokine receptor CCR5. They also define the kinetics of N-terminal cyclization, which may influence the functions of other chemokines such as the monocyte chemoattractant proteins (MCPs).

Just as chemokines may be post-translationally modified, so too can their receptors. One important modification is the sulfation of tyrosine residues in the N-terminal regions of the receptors, thought to be the initial site of chemokine interaction. A number of previous studies have demonstrated that tyrosine sulfation enhances chemokine binding affinity and, in some cases, can alter chemokine binding selectivity [11]. In this Special Issue, Moussouras et al. provide a new example of the latter effect [12]. They demonstrate the application of computational solvent mapping to identification of sulfotyrosine-binding hot spots on the surfaces of several CXC chemokines and experimentally validate their prediction that sulfotyrosine would bind specifically to some chemokines but not others.

Studies of tyrosine sulfation of chemokine receptors (and other proteins) have been challenging due to the difficulties generating sufficient quantities of homogeneously sulfated receptors or receptor fragments. In spite of recent progress in these methods [13], sulfated proteins and peptides will always suffer from marginal and variable stability. Therefore, it may be advantageous to use sulfotyrosine analogues with enhanced stability. To this end, Phillips et al. present a comparison of CCR7-derived peptides containing sulfotyrosine and the more stable analogue phosphotyrosine [14]. Importantly, they show that the phosphorylated peptides retain the same binding site specificity as the sulfated peptides, thus supporting their future utility as sulfopeptide surrogates.

It is well established that cells expressing chemokine receptors exhibit a variety of signaling responses to the cognate chemokine ligands of those receptors. In this Special Issue, Adamski et al. report a remarkable variation on this paradigm, showing that cells expressing the chemokine CXCL16 can also respond to the corresponding receptor CXCR6 [15]. This "reverse signaling" effect is only possible because the chemokine domain of CXCL16 is linked, via a long mucin stalk, to a transmembrane helix and a short cytoplasmic domain. The authors demonstrate that the reverse signaling is reliant on the cytoplasmic domain of CXCL16. Moreover, their finding that CXCL16 expression was increased in fast-migrating glioblastoma cells suggests that the observed reverse signaling may have important consequences for tumor cell migration (metastasis).

In searching for effective strategies to inhibit chemokines and their receptors, researchers have explored a wide variety of approaches. One approach is to use proteins naturally produced by pathogens to suppress chemokine-mediated inflammation during infection. To this end, Nguyen et al. describe their biophysical studies of two poxvirus proteins, one of which broadly inhibits mammalian chemokines while the other inhibits chemokine receptors [16]. They find that these two proteins bind extremely tightly to each other and propose a structural basis for the high affinity interaction. This study may help to guide the development of protein-based therapeutics but also raises questions about the balance between these proteins binding to each other versus inhibiting host inflammation during viral infection.

Although inhibition of chemokines or their receptors is an attractive strategy against inflammation and tumor metastasis, a confounding factor is that some chemokine–receptor interactions have important homeostatic or protective functions. An example is described by Sakumoto et al., who report that the expression levels of several chemokines and chemokine receptors are elevated in the endometrium of cows during pregnancy [17]. The increase in some of these proteins appears to be regulated by interferon τ, which acts as a bovine reproductive hormone, leading the authors to suggest that the chemokines and receptors may contribute to the maintenance of normal endometrial function during pregnancy.

The articles in this Special Issue emphasize the remarkable range of mechanisms by which the chemokine–receptor network is regulated in nature and can potentially be controlled therapeutically. The diversity of these mechanisms underlines the ongoing evolutionary battle between pathogens and their hosts and the subtle balance between beneficial and detrimental biological outcomes. While much remains to be learned, fundamental mechanistic studies, such as those described herein, will continue to provide invaluable guidance in the development of effective pharmaceutical interventions for many inflammatory diseases.

Acknowledgments: This work was supported by Australian Research Council Discovery Grant DP130101984 and ANZ Trustees Grant 12-3831.

Conflicts of Interest: The author declares no conflict of interest.

References

1. Lin, J.I. Rudolf Virchow: Creator of Cellular Pathology. *Lab. Med.* **1983**, *1983*, 791–794. [CrossRef]
2. Rothenberg, M.E.; Zimmermann, N.; Mishra, A.; Brandt, E.; Birkenberger, L.A.; Hogan, S.P.; Foster, P.S. Chemokines and chemokine receptors: Their role in allergic airway disease. *J. Clin. Immunol.* **1999**, *19*, 250–265. [CrossRef] [PubMed]
3. Proudfoot, A.E. Chemokine receptors: Multifaceted therapeutic targets. *Nat. Rev. Immunol.* **2002**, *2*, 106–115 [CrossRef] [PubMed]
4. Stone, M.J.; Hayward, J.A.; Huang, C.; Huma, Z.E.; Sanchez, J. Mechanisms of Regulation of the Chemokine-Receptor Network. *Int. J. Mol. Sci.* **2017**, *18*, 342. [CrossRef] [PubMed]
5. Miller, M.C.; Mayo, K.H. Chemokines from a Structural Perspective. *Int. J. Mol. Sci.* **2017**, *18*, 2088. [CrossRef] [PubMed]
6. Thompson, S.; Martinez-Burgo, B.; Sepuru, K.M.; Rajarathnam, K.; Kirby, J.A.; Sheerin, N.S.; Ali, S. Regulation of Chemokine Function: The Roles of GAG-Binding and Post-Translational Nitration. *Int. J. Mol. Sci.* **2017**, *18*, 1692. [CrossRef] [PubMed]
7. Brown, A.J.; Sepuru, K.M.; Rajarathnam, K. Structural Basis of Native CXCL7 Monomer Binding to CXCR2 Receptor N-Domain and Glycosaminoglycan Heparin. *Int. J. Mol. Sci.* **2017**, *18*, 508. [CrossRef] [PubMed]
8. Brown, A.J.; Joseph, P.R.; Sawant, K.V.; Rajarathnam, K. Chemokine CXCL7 Heterodimers: Structural Insights, CXCR2 Receptor Function, and Glycosaminoglycan Interactions. *Int. J. Mol. Sci.* **2017**, *18*, 748. [CrossRef] [PubMed]
9. Metzemaekers, M.; Mortier, A.; Janssens, R.; Boff, D.; Vanbrabant, L.; Lamoen, N.; Van Damme, J.; Teixeira, M.M.; De Meester, I.; Amaral, F.A.; et al. Glycosaminoglycans Regulate CXCR3 Ligands at Distinct Levels: Protection against Processing by Dipeptidyl Peptidase IV/CD26 and Interference with Receptor Signaling. *Int. J. Mol. Sci.* **2017**, *18*, 1513. [CrossRef] [PubMed]
10. Nguyen, A.F.; Schill, M.S.; Jian, M.; LiWang, P.J. The Effect of N-Terminal Cyclization on the Function of the HIV Entry Inhibitor 5P12-RANTES. *Int. J. Mol. Sci.* **2017**, *18*, 1575. [CrossRef] [PubMed]
11. Ludeman, J.P.; Stone, M.J. The structural role of receptor tyrosine sulfation in chemokine recognition. *Br. J. Pharmacol.* **2014**, *171*, 1167–1179. [CrossRef] [PubMed]
12. Moussouras, N.A.; Getschman, A.E.; Lackner, E.R.; Veldkamp, C.T.; Dwinell, M.B.; Volkman, B.F. Differences in Sulfotyrosine Binding amongst CXCR1 and CXCR2 Chemokine Ligands. *Int. J. Mol. Sci.* **2017**, *18*, 1894. [CrossRef] [PubMed]

13. Stone, M.J.; Payne, R.J. Homogeneous sulfopeptides and sulfoproteins: Synthetic approaches and applications to characterize the effects of trosine sulfation on biochemical function. *Acc. Chem. Res.* **2015**, *48*, 2251–2261. [CrossRef] [PubMed]

14. Phillips, A.J.; Taleski, D.; Koplinski, C.A.; Getschman, A.E.; Moussouras, N.A.; Richard, A.M.; Peterson, F.C.; Dwinell, M.B.; Volkman, B.F.; Payne, R.J.; et al. CCR7 Sulfotyrosine Enhances CCL21 Binding. *Int. J. Mol. Sci.* **2017**, *18*, 1857. [CrossRef] [PubMed]

15. Adamski, V.; Mentlein, R.; Lucius, R.; Synowitz, M.; Held-Feindt, J.; Hattermann, K. The Chemokine Receptor CXCR6 Evokes Reverse Signaling via the Transmembrane Chemokine CXCL16. *Int. J. Mol. Sci.* **2017**, *18*, 1468. [CrossRef] [PubMed]

16. Nguyen, A.F.; Kuo, N.W.; Showalter, L.J.; Ramos, R.; Dupureur, C.M.; Colvin, M.E.; LiWang, P.J. Biophysical and Computational Studies of the vCCI:vMIP-II Complex. *Int. J. Mol. Sci.* **2017**, *18*, 1778. [CrossRef] [PubMed]

17. Sakumoto, R.; Hayashi, K.G.; Fujii, S.; Kanahara, H.; Hosoe, M.; Furusawa, T.; Kizaki, K. Possible Roles of CC- and CXC-Chemokines in Regulating Bovine Endometrial Function during Early Pregnancy. *Int. J. Mol. Sci.* **2017**, *18*, 742. [CrossRef] [PubMed]

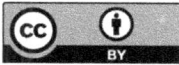

International Journal of
Molecular Sciences

MDPI

Review

Mechanisms of Regulation of the Chemokine-Receptor Network

Martin J. Stone [1,2,*], **Jenni A. Hayward** [1,2], **Cheng Huang** [1,2], **Zil E. Huma** [1,2] **and Julie Sanchez** [1,2]

1   Infection and Immunity Program, Monash Biomedicine Discovery Institute, Monash University, Clayton, VIC 3800, Australia; jenni.hayward@monash.edu (J.A.H.); cheng.huang@monash.edu (C.H.); zil.huma@monash.edu (Z.E.H.); julie.sanchez@monash.edu (J.S.)
2   Department of Biochemistry and Molecular Biology, Monash University, Clayton, VIC 3800, Australia
*   Correspondence: martin.stone@monash.edu; Tel.: +61-3-9902-9246

Academic Editor: Elisabetta Tanzi
Received: 21 December 2016; Accepted: 26 January 2017; Published: 7 February 2017

Abstract: The interactions of chemokines with their G protein-coupled receptors promote the migration of leukocytes during normal immune function and as a key aspect of the inflammatory response to tissue injury or infection. This review summarizes the major cellular and biochemical mechanisms by which the interactions of chemokines with chemokine receptors are regulated, including: selective and competitive binding interactions; genetic polymorphisms; mRNA splice variation; variation of expression, degradation and localization; down-regulation by atypical (decoy) receptors; interactions with cell-surface glycosaminoglycans; post-translational modifications; oligomerization; alternative signaling responses; and binding to natural or pharmacological inhibitors.

Keywords: chemokine; chemokine receptor; regulation; binding; expression; glycosaminoglycan; post-translational modification; oligomerization; signaling; inhibitor

1. Introduction

It has long been recognized that a hallmark feature of the inflammatory response is the accumulation of leukocytes (white blood cells) in injured or infected tissues, where they remove pathogens and necrotic tissue by phagocytosis and proteolytic degradation. A major advance in our understanding of the molecular mechanisms underlying leukocyte migration (trafficking) was the discovery of the chemokines and chemokine receptors [1–3]. Chemokines are small proteins expressed in tissues during normal immune surveillance or in response to injury or infection. They subsequently bind and activate chemokine receptors, G protein-coupled receptors (GPCRs) imbedded in the cell membranes of leukocytes, thereby inducing leukocyte adhesion to the vessel wall, morphological changes, extravasation into the inflamed tissue, and chemotaxis along the chemokine gradient to the site of injury or infection [1].

In addition to their roles in leukocyte trafficking, chemokine activation of chemokine receptors can give rise to a variety of additional cellular and tissue responses, including proliferation, activation, differentiation, extracellular matrix remodeling, angiogenesis, and tumor metastasis [4–7]. Moreover, two major pathogens (HIV-1 and the malarial parasite *Plasmodium vivax*) have evolved mechanisms to utilize chemokine receptors to invade host cells [8,9], and other viruses or parasites produce proteins that inhibit chemokines or their receptors so as to suppress the host immune response. Due to their central roles in inflammation, many chemokine receptors (and to a lesser extent chemokines) have been identified as potential therapeutic targets in a wide range of inflammatory diseases [10].

Considering the importance of chemokine-receptor interactions in responding to environmental threats but the potential risks of excessive leukocyte recruitment, it is perhaps not surprising that numerous mechanisms (summarized in Figure 1) have evolved to regulate the activities of both chemokines and their receptors. These mechanisms may involve modulation of the concentrations of these proteins in specific tissues, changes in their molecular structures, or alteration of their interactions, all of which will influence leukocyte trafficking. This Special Issue of the *International Journal of Molecular Sciences* focuses on the natural and pharmacological mechanisms by which the activities of chemokines and their receptors can be regulated. In this review article, we provide an overview and highlight illustrative examples of these biochemical and cellular mechanisms.

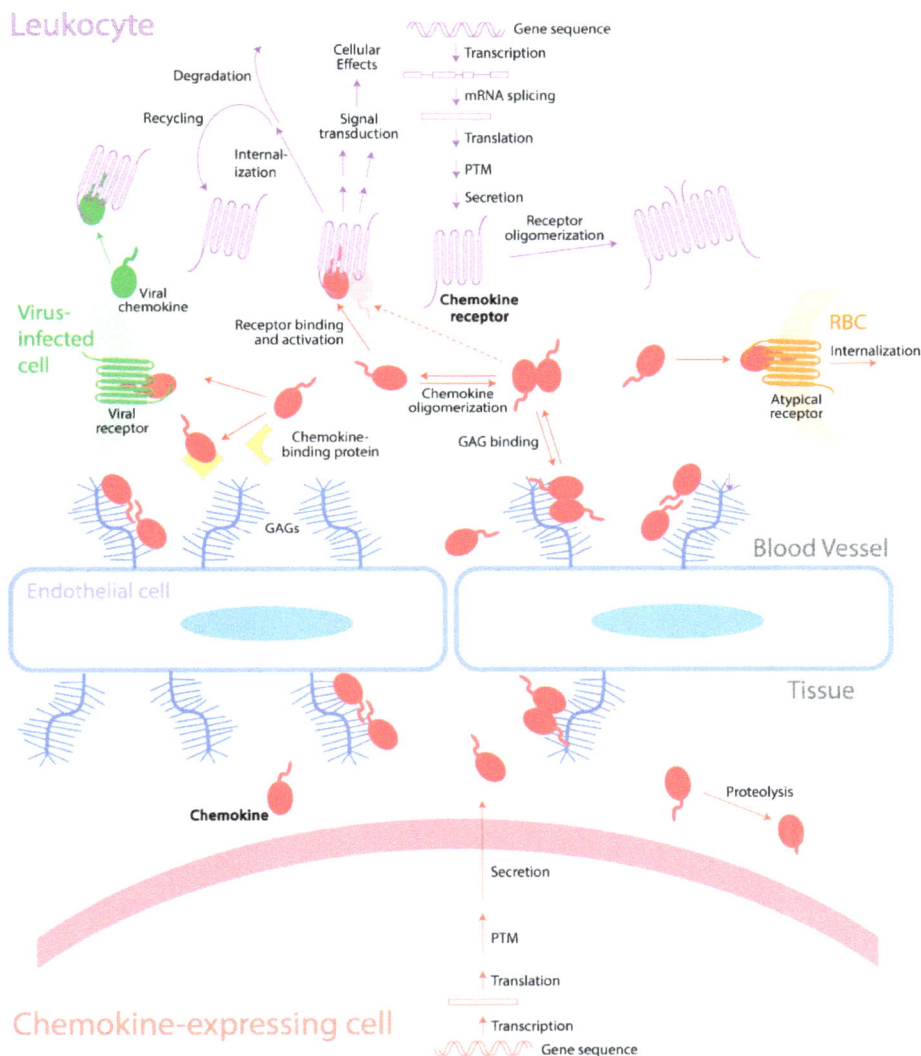

Figure 1. Schematic overview of regulation mechanisms of the chemokine-receptor network. Abbreviations: PTM: post-translational modification; RBC: red blood cell. Arrows in red, purple, green and orange indicate processes involving chemokines, chemokine receptors, viral chemokines and atypical receptors, respectively.

2. The Chemokine and Chemokine Receptor Protein Families

2.1. The Chemokine Protein Family

Chemokines are small proteins (usually ~70–80 amino acid residues) with conserved sequence and structural features. The human genome and other mammalian genomes each encodes approximately 50 different chemokines (Figure 2), which are classified into two major subfamilies (CC and CXC) and two minor subfamilies (CX3C and XC) based on the spacing of conserved cysteine residues approximately 10 residues from the N-terminal end of the peptide chain. In the CC, CXC, and CX3C subfamilies, the two Cys residues (which form disulfide bonds to other conserved Cys residues within the chemokine) are separated by 0, 1, and 3 residues, respectively, whereas in the XC subfamily the second Cys (and its disulfide bond partner) are absent from the sequence. Chemokines are designated according to their subfamily classification by systematic names composed of a prefix (CCL, CXCL, CX3CL, or XCL; "L" signifies a ligand as opposed to a receptor) followed by an identifying number. However, most chemokines also have common or historical names relating to their earliest characterized functions. Herein we use the systematic names but also give the common name (or abbreviation) of each chemokine when it is first mentioned.

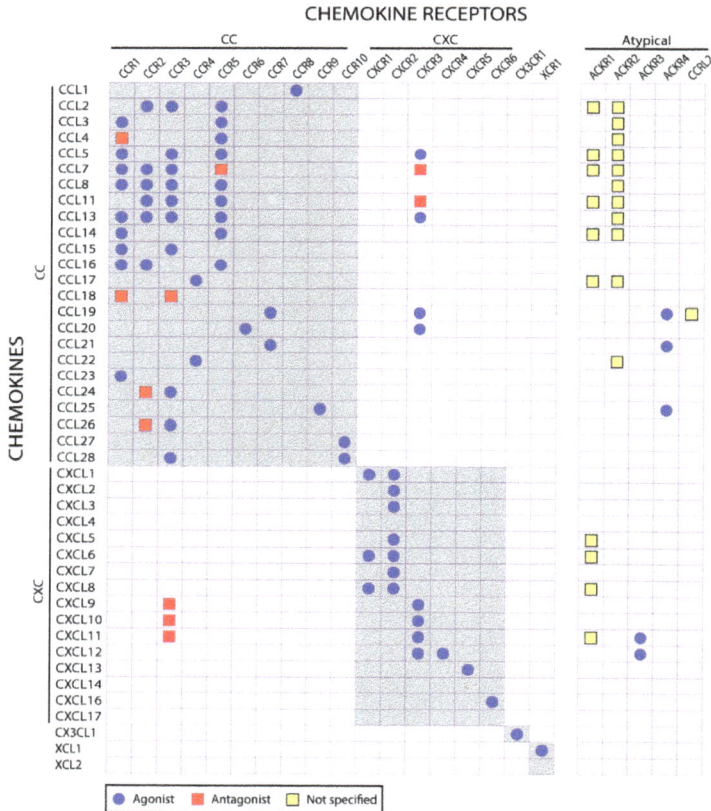

Figure 2. The human chemokine-receptor network. Human chemokines and receptors are listed with symbols indicating whether they are specified as agonists or antagonists (or not specified) in the IUPHAR database. Note that, although CXCL1 is listed as a CXCR1 agonist in IUPHAR, the database reference suggests that it is actually an antagonist [11].

In addition to the sequence classification, chemokines have also been categorized based on their biological roles. Whereas most chemokines are considered proinflammatory because their expression is induced in response to tissue damage, a small subset are classified as constitutive as they are expressed in healthy tissue and play roles in maintaining normal immune functions such as lymphocyte homing to the bone marrow.

2.2. The Chemokine Receptor Protein Family

Chemokine receptors are GPCRs—integral membrane proteins composed of seven transmembrane helical segments. Different subsets of leukocytes express different arrays of chemokine receptors enabling them to respond to the appropriate ligands. Upon binding to their cognate chemokine ligands, the receptors undergo conformational changes giving rise to activation of intracellular effectors (G proteins or β-arrestins), initiation of signal transduction pathways and, ultimately, cellular responses. As discussed below, some chemokines may bind to receptors without inducing transmembrane signals and a few receptors (known as atypical receptors) are not G protein-coupled but still bind to chemokines.

Mammalian genomes each encode approximately 20 chemokine receptors (Figure 2). Because the receptors were discovered after the chemokines and most of them are selective for members of one chemokine subfamily, they are classified according to the subfamily of chemokines to which most of their ligands belong. Thus, receptors are named using the prefixes CCR, CXCR, CX3CR, and XCR followed by an identifying number.

2.3. Selectivity of Chemokine-Receptor Interactions

Most chemokines bind and activate several receptors. Similarly, most chemokine receptors respond to multiple chemokine ligands. This selectivity of recognition is an intrinsic property of the chemokine-receptor pair, i.e., a consequence of their amino acid sequences. However, selectivity can be altered by modification of the proteins (see below). Initially, the existence of multiple ligands for the same receptor was thought to represent biochemical redundancy. However, it is now often argued to be a sophisticated strategy enabling fine tuning of leukocyte responses to different inflammatory stimuli.

Figure 2 illustrates the complexity of chemokine-receptor recognition and selectivity. Notably, others reviews of chemokines and receptors often show similar illustrations, but typically these diagrams all differ from each other in their details, depending on the source of the information. Indeed there are numerous apparent inconsistencies in the literature on chemokine-receptor recognition, indicating that conclusions regarding agonist or antagonist activity are often dependent on such variables as cell type, growth conditions, source of chemokine, and assays used.

An important consequence of multiple ligands activating the same receptor is that, if they are present in the same tissues, they would be expected to compete with each other. Thus, the degree of saturation of a particular receptor by a particular cognate chemokine will depend not only on the available concentrations of receptor and chemokine but also on the available concentrations of other chemokines to which the receptor binds and other receptors to which the chemokine binds. Moreover, in addition to being dependent on the degree of receptor saturation (equilibrium binding), transmembrane signaling may also be influenced by the association and dissociation rates (kinetics) of chemokine-receptor pairs. At present, little is known about such kinetic effects. In summary, even without considering the many additional mechanisms of regulation discussed below, the complexity of the chemokine-receptor network makes it very difficult to draw direct inferences about receptor activation simply from measurements of chemokine concentrations and receptor expression levels.

2.4. Structural Basis of Chemokine-Receptor Recognition

The three-dimensional (3D) structures of many chemokines have been determined by NMR spectroscopy and/or X-ray crystallography [12] and the structures of several chemokine receptors have now been solved, including two with bound chemokines [13,14]. Numerous mutational studies have identified functionally important elements of both chemokines and receptors.

Like other GPCRs, chemokine receptors consist of seven transmembrane helices aligned approximately parallel to each other and packed together in a compact bundle (Figure 3a) [15–17]. The extracellular face of the receptor includes an extended, largely unstructured N-terminal region and three connecting loops (extracellular loops, ECL1, 2, and 3), with conserved disulfide bonds connecting the N-terminus to ECL3 and ECL1 to ECL2; the longest loop, ECL2, contains a β-hairpin structure. The cytoplasmic face of the receptor includes three additional connecting loops (intracellular loops, ICL1, 2, and 3) and the C-terminal region, which is truncated in most structures but is expected to contain an additional helix (helix 8) and the site of attachment for a lipid anchor.

Chemokines fold into a conserved, compact tertiary structure consisting of a 3-stranded antiparallel β-sheet packed against a single α-helix (Figure 3b). The ~20–25 residues preceding the first β-strand consist of: an unstructured N-terminal region (~10 residues), the conserved cysteine-containing motif (CC, CXC, CX3C or C), an irregularly structured loop designated the "N-loop", and a single turn of 3_{10}-helix. The first conserved cysteine residue forms a disulfide bond to the "30s loop", located between the β1- and β2-strands, whereas the second conserved cysteine residue forms a disulfide bond to the β3-strand. Thus, the disulfides are essential for formation of the folded chemokine structure and receptor interactions.

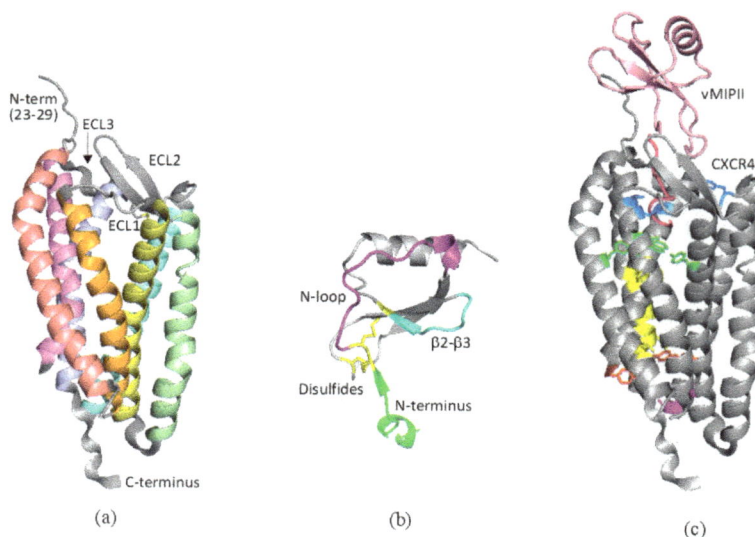

Figure 3. Structural basis of chemokine-receptor recognition. (**a**) One monomer unit of the receptor CXCR4 (PDB code 4RWS [14]) with extracellular regions labeled; transmembrane helices are colored salmon (I), orange (II), yellow (III), green (IV), turquoise (V), violet (VI), and magenta (VII). (**b**) A typical chemokine monomeric unit (CCL2/MCP-1, PDB code 1DOK [18]) highlighting the critical regions for receptor recognition. (**c**) Structure of CXCR4 bound to vMIPII (PDB code 4RWS [14]) showing the chemokine in pink (N-terminal region in hot pink) and the receptor in gray, with residues proposed to be involved in transmembrane signaling [19] colored according to their putative roles: blue, chemokine engagement; green, signal initiation; yellow, signal propagation; red, microswitch residues; magenta, G protein coupling. In panels (**a**,**c**) residues 1-22 are not shown as they were not modeled in the crystal structure.

The recent structures of chemokine-bound receptors [13,14], in addition to several structures of chemokines bound to receptor fragments [20–22], have confirmed two central aspects of the popular "two-site model" for chemokine-receptor interactions [23] (Figure 3c). First, the N-terminal region of the receptor binds to a shallow groove formed by the N-loop and β3-strand of the cognate chemokine. Second, although the chemokine N-terminus is disordered in the free chemokine, it binds to a site buried within the receptor transmembrane helical bundle, thereby undergoing induced fit to the receptor. The two-site model implies that these two aspects of the interaction occur sequentially as two separate steps, representing initial binding and subsequent activation. However, it has now become clear that elaborations of this model are necessary to explain many subtleties of the chemokine-receptor network [24]. Importantly, while structures of a few activated GPCRs have now been described [25], there is no structure for a chemokine-receptor complex in the activated state, so the structural basis of transmembrane signaling remains to be established. Nevertheless, a recent shotgun mutagenesis study of CXCR4 has identified a network of interactions likely to participate in signal transmission during receptor activation (Figure 3c) [19].

3. Genetic and mRNA Splice Variants of Chemokines and Receptors

3.1. Variation Between Species

Chemokine-receptor systems are present in all mammals, as well as some more primitive vertebrates [26,27], but have been most extensively characterized in humans and mice. Most human chemokines and receptors have orthologs in mice and vice versa, allowing mouse experiments to reveal biological functions relevant to human physiology and disease. However, some chemokines (CCL13/MCP-4, CXCL8/IL-8, CCL14/HCC-1, CCL18/DC-CK-1/PARC) are expressed in humans but not mice and, conversely, two chemokines (CCL12/MCP-5 and CXCL15/Lungkine) have been reported in mice but no ortholog has yet been identified in humans [28,29]. Similarly, mice express the chemokine receptor Ccr1-like1 (Ccr1l1), which is not found in humans [29]. Moreover, it should be noted that the selectivity of chemokine-receptor binding and activation, their expression patterns and other mechanisms of functional regulation, may differ between species, so extrapolating the conclusions of animal experiments to humans should be approached with care.

3.2. Polymorphisms in Chemokine Genes

A variety of polymorphisms have been identified in either the coding or non-coding regions of chemokine genes. These have the potential to alter expression levels, stability, and interactions with receptors or other binding partners. Consequently a number of these polymorphisms have been associated with increased or decreased disease progression.

Seven single nucleotide polymorphisms (SNPs) have been reported in the CCL2/MCP-1 gene. Four of these are present in the distal regulatory region, one in the promoter region, one in the first intron and one in the 3' flanking region [30]. Four of these SNPs are associated with increased levels of MCP-1 protein expression [30]. In particular, the SNP −2578 A/G, in the distal regulatory region, increases the level of MCP-1 expression, occurs at higher frequency in individuals with complications of atherosclerosis such as myocardial infarction and stroke [30,31], and has also been associated with systemic sclerosis [32], multiple sclerosis [33], rheumatoid arthritis [34], and Alzheimer's disease [35]. On the other hand, in a large cohort of HIV patients, homozygosity for the MCP-1 −2518 G allele was associated with a 50% reduction in the risk of acquiring HIV-1, although after infection this MCP-1 genotype enhanced disease progression with a 4.7-fold increased risk of HIV-related dementia [36].

Hellier et al. (2003) [37] have reported two polymorphisms in the promoter region of the CCL5/RANTES gene. The −403G→A polymorphism has been found to increase CCL5 expression, thus leading to increased sensitivity to asthma, atopy, and HIV [38]. In contrast, although the chemokine CCL17/TARC is thought to contribute to allergic disorders, the −431 C/T SNP in the gene encoding CCL17 increases chemokine expression without enhancing susceptibility to atopic dermatitis [38].

The chemokine CXCL12/SDF-1 is the ligand for the receptor CXCR4, which also acts as a coreceptor for HIV infection of leukocytes, especially T cells. A SNP has been reported in the 3'-untranslated evolutionarily conserved region of the gene encoding CXCL12 and homozygotes for this SDF1-3'A allele have shown a phenomenal protection against AIDS [39]. One hypothesis is that the polymorphism leads to overexpression of the chemokine thereby binding a high proportion of CXCR4 molecules and preventing their interaction with the viral coat protein [40].

Finally, Hellier et al. [37] have reported a polymorphism in the coding region of CCL8/MCP-2, causing a mutation of Gln-46 to Lys. Although the functional effect of this mutation is currently unknown [37], this mutation occurs in a region of the chemokine known to be involved in electrostatic attraction between the positively charged chemokine and negatively charged receptor, so we speculate that it may influence affinity and potency.

3.3. Polymorphisms in Chemokine Receptor Genes

As noted for chemokine ligands, a number of polymorphisms have also been identified in the genes encoding chemokine receptors. For example, in CCR2, nine SNPs have been observed that are associated with susceptibility to and severity of several diseases, including atherosclerosis, pulmonary disease, multiple sclerosis, HIV and hepatitis C virus infection, and cancer [41–45]. In contrast, the CCR2 polymorphism 190 G/A, which gives rise to a conservative amino acid change from valine to isoleucine in the first transmembrane helix of the receptor, is associated with delayed progression of HIV, apparently because it indirectly reduces the cell surface expression of the HIV-co-receptor CCR5 [46,47].

CCR5 is the co-receptor for infection of macrophages by M-tropic strains of HIV. A 32bp deletion in CCR5 to give the variant CCR5-Δ32bp was first identified in 1996 [48,49]. This 32bp region codes for a region corresponding to the second extracellular loop of CCR5; the deletion causes a frame shift, leading to early termination of translation, resulting in a truncated non-functional protein, which lacks three trans-membrane segments of the receptor [50]. Thus, the CCR5-Δ32bp mutation provides strong protection against HIV-transmission and causes a delay in disease progression [51].

The Duffy antigen receptor for chemokines (DARC) was identified first as the human blood group antigen, but was later determined to be an atypical chemokine receptor (see below) and the cell-surface protein used by the malarial parasite *Plasmodium vivax* to invade red blood cells. A polymorphism (−46C) in the promoter region of the *DARC* gene, if homozygous, disturbs the binding site for the transcription factor GATA-1, thereby reducing DARC expression and yielding protection against *P. vivax* infection [52].

3.4. Chemokine Receptor Splice Variants

In addition to genetically encoded mutations, the amino acid sequences of chemokine receptors can be influenced by alternative splicing of precursor mRNA. For example, CCR2 can exist as two splice variants, CCR2A (360 amino acids) and CCR2B (374 amino acids), which differ from each other in their carboxy terminal regions [53]. Bartoli et al. [54] have shown that these isoforms are expressed in different cell types in idiopathic inflammatory myopathies. As another example, CXCR3, which is found to be involved in cancer metastasis and inflammatory diseases, exists in three differentially spliced forms—CXCR3A, CXCR3B, and CXCR3Alt. CXCR3A and CXCR3B differ only in the lengths of their N-terminal regions; CXCR3B has a longer N-terminus containing two additional potential sulfation sites (see below). However, the third variant CXCR3Alt is a truncated protein working more like an atypical or decoy receptor. It has five transmembrane helices, with a short C-terminal region and lacks the third intracellular loop [55]. These splice variants have been reported to show specific expression in particular cell types leading to different functional characteristics. Recently, it has been shown that these variants activate different signaling pathways and show tissue-specific biased agonism [55].

4. Regulation of Expression, Degradation and Localization

4.1. Expression

Some chemokines and receptors are constitutively expressed in specific tissues and cell types, contributing to homeostatic functions such as T cell development, stem cell migration, and lymphoid organogenesis [56]. Others are induced at sites of injury or infection as part of the inflammatory response. Moreover, a few chemokines and their receptors appear to have both homeostatic and pro-inflammatory functions. Detailed classifications of the homeostatic versus inflammatory chemokines and receptors have been presented previously [29,57,58].

Homeostatic chemokines and receptors tend to be specific for each other, as exemplified by the chemokine CXCL12 and its receptor CXCR4. CXCL12, the only cognate chemokine of CXCR4, is constitutively expressed by bone marrow stromal cells, whereas CXCR4 is expressed on hematopoietic stem cells. Thus, the activation of CXCR4 by CXCL12 promotes homing of hematopoietic stem cells to the bone marrow [59]. Plerixafor (AMD3100), one of the two commercialized chemokine receptor antagonists, can inhibit the interaction between CXCL12 and CXCR4, thereby enhancing the mobilization of hematopoietic stem cells into peripheral blood for stem cell collection and transplantation [60]. A second homeostatic chemokine-receptor pair is CCL25/TECK, which is constitutively strongly expressed in the thymus with relatively low expression in other organs [61], and CCR9, expressed on T cells. Similarly, the homing chemokine CCL19/MIP-3β/exodus-3 is highly expressed in the T cell zone of lymph nodes where it plays a role in T cell recruitment and migration by activation of the receptor CCR7 [62,63].

In contrast to the few homeostatic chemokines and receptors, the majority of chemokines and receptors are upregulated in response to inflammatory stimuli. Indeed there are hundreds (perhaps thousands) of papers reporting increased chemokine and/or receptor levels in diseased tissues compared to healthy controls. Moreover, often numerous chemokines and/or receptors are highly expressed in the same disease tissue, making it difficult to separate the causes and effects of the inflammation. As one example, Iwamoto and co-workers have described the increased expression of six CC chemokines, five CXC chemokines, XCL1, and CX3CL1 in the synovial tissues of rheumatoid [64] arthritis patients, compared to other forms of arthritis or healthy controls [65]. The consequent infiltration of leukocytes into the joints is thought to contribute to fibrosis and cartilage and bone degradation. Overexpression of chemokines is also a common feature of tumors. For example, the expression of CCL5 was increased more than 50-fold in primary breast cancer tissue compared to the normal tissue adjacent to the tumor [66–68].

4.2. Internalization and Recycling or Degradation

After binding and activation by chemokines, chemokine receptors typically undergo internalization, followed by either degradation or recycling to the plasma membrane. The well-studied mechanism of receptor internalization is clathrin-mediated endocytosis [64]. The process starts with receptor activation by the ligand and phosphorylation (mediated by G protein receptor kinases, GRKs) of serine or threonine residues near the C-terminus of the receptor, leading to receptor desensitization. The phosphorylated receptors, containing the "dileucine" motif, facilitate the recruitment of endocytosis-related molecules adaptin 2 (AP2) and β-arrestin [69]. The complex of the receptor with AP2 and β-arrestin further attracts clathrin, leading to internalization of the receptor from the plasma membrane to form clathrin-coated vesicles. The receptor and ligand are then unloaded to endosomes in which the chemokine and receptor can dissociate under the acidic endosomal conditions allowing the receptor to be recycled back to the cell membrane [69]. Alternatively the receptor and ligand can be transported to the lysosome for degradation. Studies of receptors CCR5 and CXCR2 suggest that a PDZ ligand domain at the C-terminus of receptors can direct sorting of the receptors between recycling or degradation pathways [70,71].

There is considerable variability in the susceptibility of different chemokine receptors to lysosomal degradation. Whereas some receptors, such as CCR5 or CCR7, are resistant to degradation in the lysosome, activated CXCR4 undergoes lysosomal degradation through ubiquitination at a lysine residue in the C-terminus by E3 ubiquitin ligase AIP4 [64,72,73]. On the other hand, CXCR7 and CCR7 can be constitutively ubiquitinated. Ligand activation can lead to the de-ubiquitination of CXCR7, resulting in receptor recycling, whereas ligand-induced de-ubiquitination was not observed for CCR7 [74,75]. Further investigation is required to better define the determinants of receptor ubiquitination and degradation.

4.3. Atypical (Decoy) Chemokine Receptors as Chemokine Scavengers

Although the major function of chemokine receptors is to guide the migration of leukocytes in response to chemokines, there are several receptors that can recognize chemokines without eliciting the classical GPCR signaling events or chemotaxis. These receptors, variously referred to as "decoy" or "silent" chemokine receptors, have now been classified as the "atypical" chemokine receptor family (ACKR). The family consists of four major receptors (ACKR1/DARC, ACKR2/D6, ACKR3/CXCR7, and ACKR4/CCX-CKR/CCRL1) with two others (ACKR5/CCRL2 and ACKR6/PITPNM3) under further functional investigation.

The atypical receptors share the seven transmembrane helix domain of chemokine receptors and bind to chemokines, but most of them lack the highly conserved "DRYLAIV" motif in the second intracellular loop, which is involved in G protein activation. Rather than inducing G protein-mediated signals, atypical receptors are able to signal by recruitment of β-arrestin and consequent internalization and degradation of the receptor and bound chemokine. Notably, atypical chemokine receptors tend to display high ligand promiscuity (Figure 2). Thus, the main function of ACKRs is thought to be regulation of the innate and adaptive immune response by acting as a chemokine reservoir or scavenger [76–81]. This role has been demonstrated both in vitro and in vivo for ACKR2/D6, the first receptor to be functionally classified as an atypical chemokine receptor [82,83]. Interestingly, in addition to being an atypical chemokine receptor ACKR1/DARC (Duffy Antigen and Receptor for Chemokines) is the human blood group antigen and is also the receptor for infection of reticulocytes by the malarial parasite *Plasmodium vivax* [8].

4.4. Localization by Binding to Glycosaminoglycans (GAGs)

Chemokines, particularly in their oligomeric forms (see below), bind avidly to glycosaminoglycans (GAGs), polysaccharides expressed on the surfaces of most cells. Based on their repeating disaccharide units, GAGs can be divided into four groups: heparin/heparan sulfate, chondroitin sulfate/dermatan sulfate, keratan sulfate, and hyaluronic acid [84]. The highly sulfated and acidic GAGs bind to basic residues within chemokines through electrostatic interactions. These interactions are thought to help maintain high local concentrations of chemokines near their sites of expression (inflammatory loci), to establish concentration gradients of chemokines that promote leukocyte chemotaxis, and possibly to directly present chemokines to their receptors [85]. The importance of chemokines binding to GAGs has been convincingly demonstrated in vivo; chemokine mutants defective in GAG binding but capable of receptor activation in vitro are severely impaired in their ability to induce leukocyte chemotaxis in animal experiments [86]. Moreover, the effects of such mutations may be tissue-specific. For example, mutation of GAG-binding residues reduces the neutrophil recruitment activity of CXCL8 in the peritoneum but enhances this activity in the lung [87].

In addition to simple localization of chemokines, GAGs may regulate chemokine function by indirect mechanisms. Different cell types (or diseased versus healthy cells) express different arrays of GAGs, which can selectively bind to different chemokines. For example, CCL5 has high affinity for both heparin and dermatan sulfate, whereas CCL2 can bind more strongly to heparin or heparan sulfate than to chondroitin sulfate or dermatan sulfate [88]. Thus, GAGs could influence the relative concentrations of available chemokines and thereby the populations of different leukocytes recruited. Finally, as discussed below, by selectively binding to chemokine oligomers GAGs also promote chemokine oligomerization, which could, in turn, influence their receptor activation and protect them from proteolysis [84].

5. Post-Translational Modifications

5.1. Proteolytic Processing of Chemokines

Chemokines are initially translated with a ~23 amino acid signal sequence, which is cleaved prior to secretion of the mature protein. However, careful biochemical analysis of chemokines isolated from biological samples has shown that they may be further processed by either N-terminal or C-terminal truncation; often both full-length and one or more truncated forms are observed [89,90]. Truncation occurs through the catalytic action of proteases, some of which have been identified [90]. In particular, matrix metalloproteinases can process each of the monocyte-directed CC chemokines near their N- or C-termini [91].

Structure–function studies have highlighted a crucial role for the N-terminal regions of chemokines in receptor activation. Consistent with these observations, natural N-terminal truncation can either increase or decrease the activity of chemokines at their receptors or can alter their selectivity across several receptors. For example, the neutrophil chemoattractant CXCL8 exists in two forms (−2–77 and 1–77) resulting from alternative signal peptide cleavage [92]. These two proteins have different susceptibility to subsequent cleavage by aminopeptidases, giving rise to two additional forms (2–77 and 3–77), which have enhanced affinity for heparin. Moreover, further proteolytic processing catalyzed by the blood coagulation proteases thrombin or plasmin gives a shorter form (6–77) with increased chemotactic activity. Interestingly, CXCL8(6–77) is also formed under the action of a bacterial protease in cultures of the periodontal pathogen *Porphyromonas gingivalis*, apparently a mechanism to elicit an enhanced host response to this pathogen [93]. The complexity of chemokine N-terminal truncation is further demonstrated by the case of CCL14. Full-length CCL14(1–74) is a weak CCR1 agonist but is cleaved by plasmin or urokinase plasminogen activator to give CCL14(9–74), a potent agonist of CCR1 [94]. However, subsequent removal of two additional residues, catalyzed by dipeptidyl peptidase IV (CD26), gives biologically inactive CCL14(11–74) [95]. Interestingly, the most active form, CCL14(9–74), is also most efficiently bound, internalized and degraded by the decoy receptor D6 [96], suggesting that D6 internalization and dipeptidyl peptidase IV cleavage represent two alternative strategies to accomplish the same biological effect.

Truncation of chemokines at their C-termini is much less likely to influence receptor activation as this region of chemokines does not directly interact with chemokine receptors. However, the C-terminal region may be involved in oligomerization and/or GAG binding. Thus, for example, the splice variant of CXCL12 known as SDF-1α undergoes removal of a single C-terminal residue in human serum, thereby reducing its ability to bind to heparin or to cell surfaces and to stimulate cell proliferation and chemotaxis, although the truncation has no effect on receptor activation in vitro [97]. On the other hand, the chemokines MIP-1α and MIP-1β, are cleaved internally ~8–11 residues from their C-termini and then further degraded, thus inactivating these chemokines [98]. Cleavage of these chemokines by the protease cathepsin D is highly selective over other chemokines and is suggested to play a role in reducing the immune response to breast tumors [98].

5.2. Other Post-Translational Modifications of Chemokines

In addition to proteolytic processing, a number of other chemokine post-translational modifications have been observed. N- and O-glycosylation are common modifications of secreted proteins. O-glycosylation has been observed on several chemokines, including CCL2, CCL5, CCL11/eotaxin-1, CCL14, and CX3CL1/fractalkine [99–104]. Although glycosylation has not been shown to directly influence receptor activation by these chemokines, both CCL5 and CCL14 are glycosylated near to their N-termini [102,103] so it seems likely that receptor interactions will be affected. In addition, it is possible that glycosylation may have indirect effects on chemokine function by altering stability, rates of clearance, or localization.

Pyroglutamate is a modified amino acid formed by the dehydration and cyclization of an N-terminal glutamine or glutamate residue in a peptide or protein (Figure 4). This transformation is catalyzed by the enzyme glutaminyl cyclase in vivo but can also occur spontaneously in vitro [105]. Human and some murine chemokines of the monocyte chemoattractant protein family (CCL2, CCL8, CCL7/MCP-3, and CCL13) have N-terminal glutamine residues that undergo pyroglutamate formation [106–108]. There are conflicting reports regarding the influence of this modification on receptor activation by CCL2 [109,110]. However, pyroglutamate has been found to increase the stability of CCL2 to N-terminal degradation by aminopeptidases [109]. Moreover, glutaminyl cyclase contributes to the pathogenesis of both Alzheimer's disease and fatty liver disease and pyroglutamate formation of CCL2 has been suggested as a possible underlying mechanism in both diseases [111].

Citrullination is the deimination of arginine residues of peptides or proteins to yield citrulline residues (Figure 4). This modification is catalyzed by enzymes called peptidylarginine deiminases and is known to occur to several chemokines influencing their activities [112,113]. CXCL8 undergoes citrullination at Arg-5, resulting in slightly higher affinity for CXCR1 and slightly lower affinity for both CXCR2 and heparin in vitro [113]. Curiously, in vivo models gave contrasting results, with citrullinated CXCL8 being less effective at inducing neutrophil extravasation into the peritoneal cavity recruitment [113] but more effective at mobilizing neutrophils from the bone marrow into the bloodstream [114]. For other chemokines studied—CXCL5/ENA-78, CXCL10/IP-10, CXCL11/I-TAC, and CXCL12—citrullination generally decreased receptor binding or activation [115–117].

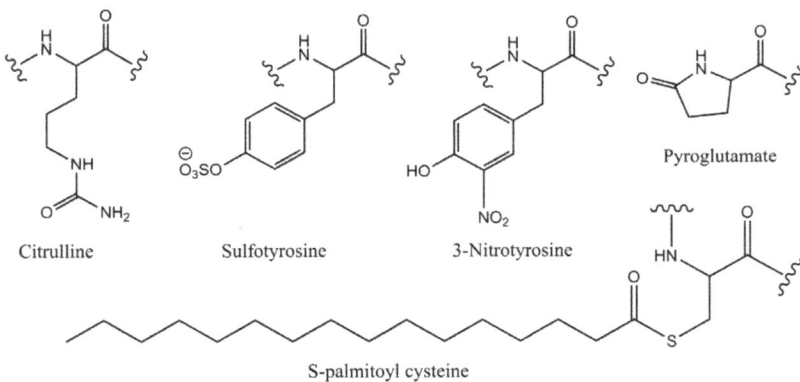

Figure 4. Examples of post-translationally modified amino acid residues found in chemokines and chemokine receptors.

One common feature of inflamed tissues is oxidative stress, the production of reactive oxygen and nitrogen species, which can subsequently modify proteins, influencing many biochemical functions. In particular, some chemokines have been shown to undergo nitration, which typically occurs on tyrosine or tryptophan side chains, as a consequence of reaction with peroxynitrite (Figure 4) [112]. CCL2 underdoes nitration in response to macrophage activation [118] and nitrated CCL2 has reduced monocyte-binding and chemotactic function [118,119]. Similarly nitration of CCL5 attenuates its chemotactic activity [120]. In addition to direct modification of chemokine structure and activity, nitration or nitrosylation (addition of NO rather than NO_2) of other proteins can indirectly influence chemokine or receptor function. For example, nitrosylation of mitogen-activated protein kinase phosphatase 7 deactivates this phosphatase, thereby enabling signaling in response to the chemokine CXCL12 [121] and nitric oxide synthesis can promote expression of the receptor CXCR4 [122].

5.3. Post-Translational Modifications of Chemokine Receptors

Chemokine receptors are also subject to a variety of post-translational modifications, with implications for chemokine recognition and signaling. As is typical for GPCRs, chemokine receptors are reversibly phosphorylated on their cytoplasmic regions, thereby desensitizing them to activation and regulating binding by β-arrestins and consequent internalization [69,123–125]. Palmitoylation (Figure 4) and ubiquitination have also been suggested to influence these receptor functions, as discussed previously [69]. Here, we focus on the two most widely studied modifications of chemokine receptors, glycosylation, and tyrosine sulfation.

Many (or perhaps most) chemokine receptors, including decoy receptors and viral receptor mimics, are heterogeneously *N*- and/or *O*-glycosylated, in some cases influencing receptor function [126–135]. For example, removal of sialic acid moieties from CCR5 significantly reduced the efficacy of signaling by chemokines at this receptor but had little effect on CCR5-mediated HIV-1 infection [134]. On the other hand, *N*-linked glycosylation was found to influence the ability of CXCR4 to support infection by different strains of HIV-1 [133]. Similar to CCR5, CCR7 is polysialylated in its extracellular domain and this modification is required for recognition of the chemokine CCL21/6Ckine/SLC/exodus-2 [136,137]. The importance of this modification in vivo was demonstrated using polysialyltransferase-deficient mice, which lacked the ability to recruit dendritic cells to secondary lymphoid organs in response to inflammatory challenge [137]. Moreover, human dendritic cells were found to further regulate CCR7 activity by secreting enzymes that deglycosylate this receptor [136]. As noted for chemokines, receptor glycosylation can also have secondary effects such as protection from proteolysis, which was observed for CXCR2 [138]. Finally, in a fascinating response to bacterial infection, proteases in the airways of cystic fibrosis patients were found to cleave CXCR1 expressed on neutrophils, releasing glycosylated CXCR1 peptides [139]. These peptides then acted on Toll-like receptors on bronchial epithelial cells to stimulate expression of CXCL8, a major ligand for CXCR1 and CXCR2, apparently a mechanism to promote additional neutrophil recruitment.

Another important post-translational modification of chemokine receptors is tyrosine sulfation, addition of a sulfate group, and a negative charge to the phenolic hydroxyl of a tyrosine side chain (Figure 4). Sulfation is a common modification of secreted proteins mediated by two tyrosylprotein sulfotransferase enzymes, which are localized to the trans-Golgi network [140]. These enzymes are selective for tyrosine residues close in sequence to acidic amino acids, a motif found in the N-terminal (chemokine-binding) regions of most chemokine receptors [141]. Several chemokine receptors have been shown to be sulfated [8,135,142,143]. Mutation of the sulfated residues, or metabolic inhibition of sulfation, tends to reduce chemokine binding affinity and potency of receptor activation [141]. Moreover, many chemokine receptors contain two or more tyrosine residues in their N-terminal regions and the pattern of sulfation could potentially modulate selectivity for different ligands. In support of this mechanism, Choe et al. [8] have found that mutation of Tyr-41 in the decoy receptor DARC suppresses binding of CCL2, CCL5, and CXCL1/GROα/MGSA-α but not CXCL8, whereas mutation of Tyr-30 of DARC suppresses binding of CXCL8 but not the other three chemokines.

We and others have used tyrosine-sulfated peptides derived from the N-terminal regions of chemokine receptors to understand the structural and energetic basis of chemokine recognition [144]. These studies have confirmed that sulfation enhances affinity and selectivity of chemokine binding [145–148] and have also suggested that binding to the sulfated region of the receptor can allosterically modulate chemokine dimerization [147–149]. Moreover, NMR structural studies using these model systems have shown that the sulfotyrosine residues bind into an electropositive groove on the chemokine surface, with distinct orientations for different chemokine-receptor pairs [21,22]. These structures provide insights into the mechanism by which sulfation regulates receptor function.

6. Oligomerization of Chemokines and Chemokine Receptors

6.1. Oligomerization of Chemokines

Most chemokines form dimeric or higher order oligomeric structures [84]. Strikingly, the CXC and CC chemokines generally form distinct dimer structures (Figure 5). CXC chemokines dimerize via their β1-strands, thereby forming a continuous 6-strand antiparallel β-sheet with the α-helices of both protomers adjacent to each other on the same face of the β-sheet (Figure 6). Importantly, this dimer structure leaves the N-terminus, N-loop and β3-strand exposed on the surface of the dimer. Therefore, CXC chemokine dimers can bind and activate chemokine receptors [150–153]. Indeed, trapped forms of the CXCL8 and CXCL12 dimers (i.e., those that cannot dissociate to the monomeric state) displayed distinct receptor activation properties relative to corresponding monomeric chemokines [151,152,154]. In contrast to CXC chemokines, CC chemokines dimerize by formation of an antiparallel β-sheet between the N-terminal regions of the two protomers (Figure 5b). Due to the importance of the N-terminal regions in receptor activation, CC chemokine dimers are inactive [155,156].

In some cases, chemokine dimers can further associate to form tetrameric structures, containing both CXC- and CC-type dimers (Figure 5c) [18,157], or to form high order aggregates [158,159]. Due to the burial of N-terminal and N-loop elements, these higher order structures are also expected to be unable to activate receptors.

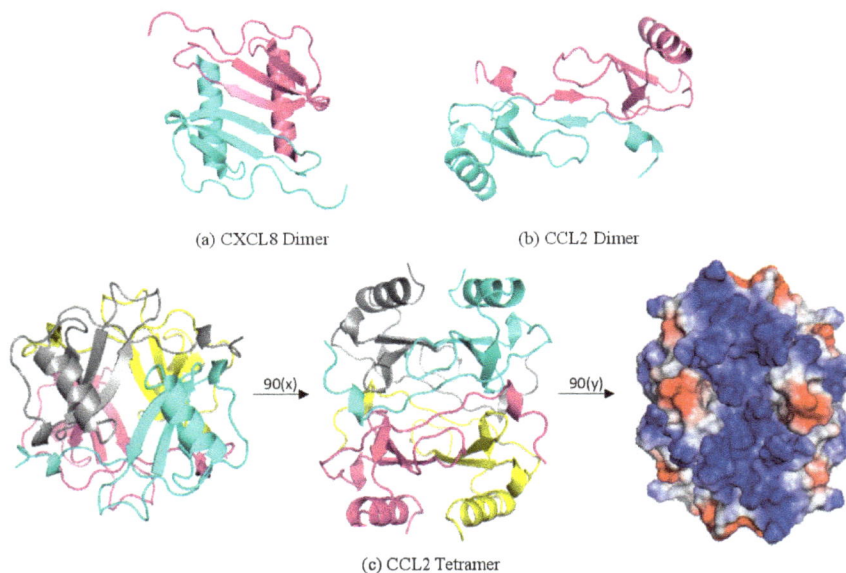

(a) CXCL8 Dimer   (b) CCL2 Dimer

(c) CCL2 Tetramer

Figure 5. Oligomeric structures of chemokines. (**a,b**) Dimer structures of (**a**) CXCL8/IL-8 and (**b**) CCL2/MCP-1, highlighting the distinct dimer interfaces for CXC and CC chemokines, respectively. (**c**) Tetramer structure of CCL2, highlighting: (left) the CXC-type dimer interfaces (cyan to gray and magenta to yellow protomers); (center) the CC-type dimer interfaces (cyan to magenta and yellow to gray protomers); and (right) the highly electropositive (dark blue) surface involved in GAG binding.

Chemokine dimers can readily dissociate into the monomeric forms. Considering that the equilibrium dissociation constants for dimerization are generally in the micromolar to millimolar regime and the physiological concentrations of chemokines are generally expected to be sub-micromolar, oligomerization was initially considered to be a possible artefact of the high concentrations used for structure determination. However, it is now apparent that oligomerization is critical for binding to GAGs and thereby creating the localized chemokine gradients required for effective chemotaxis [84–86,160–162]. Figure 5c highlights the electropositive surface that forms upon tetramerization of CCL2, thereby promoting cooperative binding to GAG polymers.

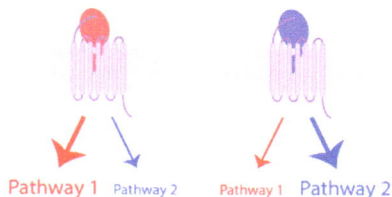

Figure 6. Schematic representation of biased agonism. The red chemokine (**left**) selectively activates pathway 1, whereas the blue chemokine (**right**) selectively activates pathway 2.

Most studies of chemokine dimers have utilized conditions under which a single chemokine is present or dominant. However, physiological circumstances more often involve multiple chemokines being present, raising the possibility that they could form heterodimers (or higher oligomers) and adding a further level of complexity to structural regulation. In support of this possibility, Mayo and coworkers have shown that CXCL4/PF4 and CXCL8 form heterodimers and that the heterodimers have enhanced anti-proliferative and chemotactic activity in comparison to homo-oligomers of either chemokine [163]. Detailed molecular dynamics calculations further predict the formation of heterodimers between other pairs of CXC chemokines, between various CC chemokines and between CXC and CC chemokines [164,165]. Considering that many chemokines exist in multiple post-translationally modified forms, it is also likely that heterodimers can assemble from different forms of the same chemokine. In support of this possibility, a synthetic, N-terminally truncated, inactive form of CCL2 can bind to full-length CCL2, thereby competitively inhibiting receptor activation [166].

Finally, Volkman and colleagues have characterized a remarkable structural transformation of the only XC chemokine XCL1/lymphotactin [167,168]. Monomeric XCL1 has the canonical chemokine fold, is an agonist of receptor XCR1 and does not bind appreciably to GAGS. However, homodimeric XCL1 has a completely different tertiary and quaternary structure from those of other chemokines and is inactive at XCR1 yet binds with high avidity to GAGs. Although interconversion of the two structural forms requires unfolding and refolding of the protein, the two states can interconvert rapidly. Moreover, both states are significantly populated under typical physiological conditions but the equilibrium between them is sensitive to solution conditions such as salt concentration and temperature and is regulated by GAG binding.

6.2. Oligomerization of Chemokine Receptors

A further level of complexity in chemokine-receptor interactions is oligomerization of receptors. GPCRs are generally thought to exist as dimers or possibly higher order oligomeric complexes and most chemokine receptor structures determined to date have been homodimers. Chemokine receptors could potentially self-associate (to form "homomers"), associate with other chemokine receptors (to form "heteromers"), or associate with other non-chemokine GPCRs. Examples of all three have been reported. Moreover, the formation of such oligomers could potentially influence receptor function by a variety of mechanisms, including: modulating interactions with chemokine ligands; modulating interactions with signaling effectors such as G proteins; affecting trafficking to the plasma membrane; affecting localization within the membrane; altering receptor stability; or modulating internalization and/or receptor recycling to the membrane. Many of these potential effects have been investigated for chemokine receptors, as discussed in several detailed reviews [161,169–172].

Chemokine receptors, like other GPCRs, dimerize by approximately parallel association of their transmembrane (TM) helices, although the specific helices involved in the interactions may vary. In crystal structures CXCR4 dimerizes by association of TM4 and TM5 [14,15], whereas CCR5 (in complex with the drug maraviroc) dimerizes by association of TM1 and TM7 [17], although mutational analysis of CCR5 suggested that dimerization involves residues in TM1 and TM4 [173]. Irrespective of the specific TM helices involved in dimerization, it seems reasonable to expect that ligand binding within the TM bundle may affect not only the conformation of the bundle (as required for signaling) but also the structure and/or stability of the dimerization interface. Conversely, formation of different dimers may affect ligand binding.

Evidence for homo- and/or hetero-oligomerization in cells has been reported for numerous CC and CXC chemokine receptors and for the decoy receptor DARC [169]. Generally, these receptor oligomers have been found to exist constitutively, i.e., not to require induction by ligand binding or activation. However, in many cases, activation by chemokines induces a change in the oligomer structure or appears to increase homomer formation [169]. It should be noted that observation of oligomer formation in cells typically requires heterologous expression of receptors modified with tags to facilitate detection by antibodies (typically using co-immunoprecipitation experiments) or by fluorescence or bioluminescence resonance energy transfer (FRET or BRET) techniques. Changes in the signals observed in these experiments may result either from alterations in the populations of multimeric species or from conformational changes within preformed oligomers. Therefore, the results should be interpreted with care. Nevertheless, the extensive body of experimental evidence provides a high level of confidence that chemokine receptors do oligomerize and that the oligomers are sensitive to ligand binding.

The interplay between oligomerization and ligand binding is exemplified by the observations that different ligands can induce distinct alterations in receptor oligomer structure. For example, the chemokines CCL2 and CXCL12 differentially influenced the conformations (measured as maximal BRET signals) of CXCR4 homomers and CCR2/CXCR4 heteromers without affecting the propensity of these oligomers to assemble [174]. Coupling between ligand binding and dimerization has also been inferred by comparing competitive ligand binding measurements for receptors expressed alone or together with a receptor with which it forms heteromers. Thus, for example, the CCR5 ligand CCL4/MIP-1β does not bind directly to CCR2 and therefore cannot displace the cognate chemokine CCL2 from CCR2 when this receptor is expressed alone. However, when CCR2 is co-expressed (and dimerized) with CCR5, CCL4 effectively displaces CCL2 from binding to CCR2 within the heteromer [175]. These data suggested that there can be strong negative allostery for chemokine binding to receptor protomers within a dimer or, taken to its extreme, that only one ligand can bind to a receptor dimer.

A critical question regarding receptor oligomers is whether they simply act as the sum of the two contributing receptors or alternatively synergize to yield more sensitive or different downstream signaling responses. In a seminal study, Mellado et al. [176] have reported that cells co-expressing CCR2 and CCR5 respond cooperatively to ligands of these receptors. Specifically, simultaneous treatment with CCL2 and CCL5 (ligands for CCR2 and CCR5, respectively) induced a Ca^{2+} signal equivalent to treatment with an approximately 10-fold higher concentration of each individual chemokine. The allosteric response to the combination of ligands was supported by cross-linking experiments showing that simultaneous treatment with CCL2 and CCL5 either induced heteromer formation or altered the conformation of existing heteromers. Mellado et al. further examined the effect of the dominant negative CCR2 mutant CCR2B Y13F on cooperative signaling. Remarkably, this mutant was shown to heterodimerize with CCR5 such that CCL5 signaling was inhibited by simultaneous treatment with CCL2. Further experiments indicated that effective signaling via the CCR2-CCR5 heteromer appears to require both receptors to be signaling competent and to form distinct complexes with downstream kinases. Finally, the same study revealed that the Ca^{2+} signal induced by simultaneous treatment with CCL2 and CCL5 was not sensitive to the $G_{\alpha i}$ inhibitor pertussis toxin, whereas

Int. J. Mol. Sci. **2017**, *18*, 342

the Ca^{2+} signals induced by the individual chemokines were inhibited by pertussis toxin. Thus, allosteric signaling at the CCR2-CCR5 heteromer induced a unique downstream signaling pathway in comparison to each individual receptor.

As discussed above, one important aspect of chemokine-receptor regulation is the ability of ligands to induce internalization of their receptors and to be internalized themselves in the process. The decoy receptor DARC utilizes this mechanism to act as a chemokine scavenger. However, it has also been shown that DARC can form heteromers with CCR5 that block CCR5 signaling in response to its ligands but still permit ligand binding and internalization of CCR5 [177]. Thus, DARC reduces the local concentrations of chemokines not only by direct internalization but also by promoting chemokine internalization indirectly via oligomerization with other receptors.

In addition to oligomerizing with themselves or each other, some chemokine receptors have also been found to form heteromers with other members of the GPCR superfamily. In one example, CCR5 has been shown to form heteromers with the complement C5a receptor and C5a-stimulation of this receptor caused cross-phosphorylation as well as internalization of CCR5 [123]. In a second example, Mustafa et al. [178] showed that CXCR2 forms heteromers with the α_{1A}-adrenoceptor (α_{1A}AR), that the α_{1A}AR agonist norepinephrine stimulated recruitment of β-arrestin only in cells co-expressing CXCR2, and that norepinephrine-stimulated β-arrestin recruitment could be inhibited by an allosteric inverse agonist of CXCR2. Finally, several studies have provided evidence for heteromer formation and allosteric regulation between chemokine receptors CCR5, CXCR2, and CXCR4 and various members of the opioid receptor family [179–182]. Considering the vast number of GPCRs and their co-expression in many of the same cell types as chemokine receptors, it is likely that our current knowledge of heteromer formation and their functional consequences barely scratches the surface.

7. Regulation of Signaling Pathways

7.1. Overview of Signaling Pathways—G Proteins and Arrestins

Chemokine receptors are members of the GPCR superfamily, the largest class of membrane receptors in the human proteome. Chemokine binding induces a conformational change in the 7-transmembrane helix domain of the receptor, which can induce a variety of downstream signaling events mediated by either heterotrimeric G proteins or arrestins. These signals typically involve activation of other intracellular effectors such as adenylyl cyclase. The specific signals induced can be regulated by variations in the available signaling machinery in different cellular contexts as well as by differences between the intrinsic structural interactions of chemokine ligands with their receptor.

Upon activation, GPCRs function as guanine nucleotide exchange factors (GEFs), which allows the α subunit of the heterotrimeric G protein to transition from inactive (GDP-bound) to active (GTP-bound) and to dissociate from the βγ subunits. Both parts of the G protein are able to interact with other effectors to generate signal transduction. The Gα proteins are divided into four major classes based on their sequence and function: $G\alpha_q$ activates phospholipase C to upregulate the level of intracellular calcium; $G\alpha_s$ stimulates the production of cAMP; $G\alpha_i$ inhibits the production of cAMP; and $G\alpha_o$ controls other signaling functions [183,184]. The Gβγ dimer can act as a Gα inhibitor when bound to a Gα subunit, because it favors the interaction between Gα and GDP. However, when the Gβγ complex is dissociated from Gα, it can also participate in the signaling cascade. For example, Gβγ can regulate ion channels [185] and is also involved in phosphorylation of the extracellular signal-regulated kinases (ERK 1/2) via the protein kinase C/protein kinase A pathway [186,187].

The arrestin family also includes four subtypes. Arrestin-1 (visual arrestin) and arrestin-4 (cone arrestin) are located exclusively in retinal rods and cones. Arrestin-2 (or β-arrestin 1) and arrestin-3 (or β-arrestin 2) are non-visual arrestins that are expressed in numerous cell types. The affinity of β-arrestins for the non-phosphorylated (inactive) receptor is low which limits any basal activity. When the receptor is activated by an agonist, β-arrestin is able to displace the G protein before it is activated giving rise to G protein-independent β-arrestin signaling. On the other hand, when β-arrestin competes with the G protein after its activation, this leads to G protein-dependent β-arrestin signaling. The latter signaling has been well studied and include ERK phosphorylation, receptor internalization, and desensitization (see above) [188]. G protein-independent β-arrestin mediated signaling is less well characterized, but it has been identified using GPCR mutants unable to bind to G proteins, which are still able to signal through the ERK phosphorylation pathway [189,190].

7.2. Regulation of Signaling in Different Cellular Contexts

Regulation of chemokine receptor (and other GPCR) signaling pathways is a highly complex phenomenon that has to be considered with respect to its cellular context. There are approximately 20 Gα subunits, 5 Gβ subunits, and 12 Gγ subunits [184], resulting in a huge array of possible heterotrimeric G proteins. The expression levels of these various subunits vary between cell types or under different conditions and the different complexes are expected to compete with each other for association with a particular receptor. In addition, the availability of particular G proteins may depend on the presence of other GPCRs in the same cell. Moreover, the ability of a chemokine receptor to signal is also dependent on the presence of other factors such as regulators of G protein signaling (RGS) proteins, which negatively regulate G protein signaling by acceleration of GTP hydrolysis by Gα [191–193], or lipids, such as cholesterol, which can potentially influence receptor oligomerization and conformational changes [194,195].

Considering these potential variations in signaling pathways between cells, perhaps it should not be surprising that the literature describing chemokine-chemokine receptor signaling is full of apparent inconsistencies. As one example, different studies have concluded that CCL11 is a partial agonist and an antagonist of CCR2 [196–198]. Thus, although detailed mechanistic studies of chemokine-receptor interactions typically require carefully controlled experimental conditions using immortalized cell lines, it is important to validate the biological relevance of results using primary cells.

7.3. Partial Agonism

Within a specific cellular context, it is sometimes observed that different chemokines can induce different signals via the same receptor. The simplest type of differential signaling is partial agonism, in which one chemokine (defined as a "full agonist") induces a maximal response whereas another chemokine (a "partial agonist") induces a lower response than the full agonist, even when added at concentrations sufficient to fully saturate the receptor [199]. For example, Berchiche et al. [200] have reported that CCL2 activates CCR2 to induce maximal β-arrestin recruitment, whereas other chemokines induce a lower level of β-arrestin recruitment by activation of CCR2 in the same cell line. It is important to note that partial agonism is most readily detected using non-amplified (proximal) signaling assays such as β-arrestin recruitment or direct measurements of G protein dissociation. For more highly amplified assays (e.g., cAMP levels, Ca^{2+} levels or phosphorylation of downstream effectors), even partial activation of a receptor can give rise to maximal responses. In the latter case, a partial agonist is expected to have lower potency that a full agonist (i.e., a higher concentration will be require to attain the full signal), even if it associates with the receptor with the same affinity as the full agonist. Recently, we have observed this phenomenon for activation of CCR2 by CCL2, CCL7, and CCL8 (unpublished results).

7.4. Biased Agonism

Biased agonism, also known as functional selectivity or agonist-selective signaling, is an increasingly developed concept based on the idea that agonists acting at the same receptor can have different abilities to activate different signaling pathways, as shown schematically in Figure 6. This phenomenon has been observed for a variety of GPCRs and is believed to be due, at least in part, to the ability of receptors to adopt multiple active conformations, each leading to a different balance of signaling outcomes and each differentially stabilized by different ligands [201]. The phenomenon is of particular interest when designing therapeutic agents [202]. For example, if several agonists of one receptor have been selected for a desired function, it might be possible to minimize undesirable side effects by testing for other functions where the agonists may differ in their responses [203]. In order to better understand biased agonism and guide drug development, several models have been proposed to quantify agonist bias [204–206].

A number of chemokine receptors have been observed to display biased agonism. For example, the chemokines CCL19 and CCL21 both activate CCR7 to induce G protein activation and calcium mobilization but only CCL19 gives rise to desensitization of CCR7, which is mediated by β-arrestin recruitment [207]. In a systematic study of G protein versus β-arrestin bias for three CC and three CXC chemokine receptors, Rajagopal et al. [208] found significant levels of signaling bias for CCR1, CCR10, and CXCR3. Similarly, Corbisier et al. [209] found significant levels of signaling bias for CCR2, CCR5, and CCR7 in comparisons of G protein activation using several Gα subtypes as well as β-arrestin 2, cAMP, and Ca^{2+} signaling. These recent studies suggest that biased signaling responses to chemokine ligands may be a rather general phenomenon contributing to the different downstream cellular outcomes of chemokine receptor activation.

8. Natural and Pharmacological Inhibitors

8.1. Viral Chemokines and Receptors

Large DNA viruses such as herpesviruses and poxviruses employ numerous strategies to evade the host immune response. One such strategy is molecular mimicry of chemokines and chemokine receptors to modulate the chemokine signaling network, as described in previous reviews [210–212].

Viral chemokines can function as both agonists and antagonists of human chemokine receptors and thereby can promote or inhibit the recruitment of various leukocyte types to infected cells. For instance, viral macrophage inflammatory protein II (vMIP-II or vCCL2), a CC chemokine encoded by Kaposi's sarcoma-associated herpesvirus (KSHV), is unique in that it is a broad spectrum high affinity ligand of many chemokine receptors from all four subfamilies. vMIP-II is an antagonist of CCR1, CCR2, CCR5, CCR10, CXCR4, CX3CR1, and XCR1 but is an agonist of CCR3 and CCR8, which enables this protein to upregulate the Th2-associated immune response, which is associated with delayed viral clearance [213]. The 3D structure of vMIP-II in complex with human CXCR4 has been determined [14].

Viruses can express receptors that interact directly with human chemokines or that regulate the functions of endogenous chemokine receptors. Several viral chemokine receptors are constitutively active, signaling independently of chemokine ligands and coupling promiscuously to several G proteins. For example, ORF74 is a human CXCR2 homologue encoded by KSHV that is constitutively active, but whose activity can be modulated by endogenous chemokines. Human CXCL1, CXCL2/GROβ/MGSA-β, and CXCL3/GROγ/MGSA-γ act as agonists of ORF74, while human CXCL6/GCP-2, CXCL10, CXCL12, CCL1, and CCL15/HCC-2 as well as vMIP-II act as inverse agonists to control the proliferative signaling potential of ORF74 in virus-infected cells [214,215]. By contrast, BILF1 is a constitutively active orphan receptor that can form heterodimeric complexes with human chemokine receptors and thereby impair chemokine receptor signaling at the G protein level, by scavenging a shared pool of G proteins [216]. Finally, US28 is a CX3CR1 homologue that binds chemokines from both the CC and CX3C sub-families. The crystal structure of US28 bound to a human chemokine (CX3CL1) has been determined [13].

8.2. Chemokine-Binding Proteins from Pathogens and Parasites

Large DNA viruses, the parasitic worm *Schistosoma mansoni* [217], and the tick species *Rhipicephalus sanguineus* [218,219] all encode soluble chemokine-binding proteins that disrupt the chemokine signaling network and subsequent activation and recruitment of leukocytes. They do so by hindering the interaction of chemokines with their cognate chemokine receptors and/or GAGs. Most chemokine-binding proteins do not share structural or sequence similarity with chemokine receptors, yet they are sometimes described as soluble chemokine decoy receptors. Many chemokine-binding proteins promiscuously bind many chemokines from multiple sub-families; however, several show specificity for one sub-family. Several detailed reviews of chemokine-binding proteins have been published [220–222].

Viral chemokine-binding proteins vary in selectivity for chemokine ligands, but the majority are able to bind chemokines from more than one sub-family. The poxvirus encoded 35-kDa protein is relatively selective in that it binds with high affinity to nearly all CC chemokines and with only low affinity to CXCL8 and CXCL1 [223]. The structure of this 35-kDa protein showed a globular protein with a β-sandwich domain [224,225]. This fold was found to be conserved in several other viral chemokine-binding proteins, including A41 [226], the SECRET (smallpox virus-encoded chemokine receptor) domain of CrmD [227], and the herpesvirus encoded M3 protein [228]. However, A41 and the CrmD SECRET domain interact with a reduced set of both CC and CXC chemokines, while the M3 protein binds promiscuously to chemokines from all sub-families, despite its structural similarity to the 35 k-Da protein. In contrast, the UL21.5 glycoprotein, encoded by human cytomegalovirus has been reported to bind specifically to CCL5, although only a limited number of chemokines were tested [229].

Parasites such as worms and ticks are also known to produce chemokine-binding proteins, presumably allowing them to evade detection and parasitize their mammalian hosts for longer periods. The 36 kDa chemokine-binding protein of *S. mansoni*, smCKBP, is expressed and secreted by *S. mansoni* eggs and binds to a selection of CC and CXC chemokines [217]; the structure of this protein is yet to be determined. The tick species *R. sangunieus* produces three chemokine-binding proteins, named evasins [218,219]. Evasins-1 and -4 bind exclusively to CC chemokines while evasin-3 binds only CXC chemokines. Evasins-1 and -4 differ in selectivity, with evasin-1 binding to three CC chemokines with high affinity and evasin-4 binding to approximately 20 CC chemokines. The structure of evasin-1 has been determined, revealing a novel fold different from that of viral chemokine-binding proteins [230].

8.3. Pharmacological Approaches towards Inhibition of Chemokines and Receptors

Considering the importance of the chemokine signaling network in numerous inflammatory and autoimmune diseases, considerable effort has been expended developing both small molecules and biologics (antibodies) that modulate the activity of chemokine receptors or chemokines themselves. Reviews of chemokine receptor antagonists have been published previously [231,232]. Here, we provide a brief overview of the main approaches.

A large number of small molecule chemokine receptor antagonists have been developed. Typically these bind to residues in the transmembrane helices of the receptors, stabilizing the inactive conformation of the receptor and/or preventing binding and activation by chemokines. Two such antagonists have reached the market. The CCR5 antagonist Maraviroc (developed by Pfizer) is used as an antiviral agent in HIV infection to block viral entry into macrophages [233], whereas the CXCR4 inhibitor Plerixafor (AMD3100; developed by AnorMED and marketed by Genzyme) blocks homing of hematopoietic stem cells to the bone marrow, thereby mobilizing these cells to the bloodstream, allowing them to be collected for later transplantation [60].

Small molecule agonists of chemokine receptors have also been discovered. In spite of their size, these agonists are generally able to fully activate chemokine receptors, though not always in the same way as chemokine ligands. For example, the functionally selective CCR5 agonist YM-370749 is able to induce internalization of CCR5 from the cell surface but is unable to induce chemotaxis [234]. Thus, it appears that this compound stabilizes a distinct active conformation of the receptor from that stabilized by chemokine ligands.

While less common, small molecules that bind and antagonize chemokines have also been discovered. For instance, the structure of chemokine CXCL12 in complex with an antagonist was determined, showing that this antagonist occupies the site normally bound by the N-terminal regions of the receptor CXCR4 [235].

Whereas small molecules often have the advantage of high oral bioavailability, they may also suffer from fast clearance rates or relatively low specificity, leading to off-target effects. Therefore, a number of biologics (large biomolecule therapeutics) have also been developed. An anti-CXCL8 antibody is marketed in China for the treatment of psoriasis and antibodies targeting CCL2, CCL5, and CXCL10 are in clinical trials [236,237]. The antibody Mogamulizumab (KW-0761), directed against CCR4 [238], is marketed in Japan for adult T-cell leukemia-lymphoma. Recently, Griffiths et al. have described the interesting example of "i-bodies," which are human single domain antibodies (human equivalents of shark V_{NAR}), that antagonize CXCR4 [239]. Finally, an L-stereoisomer oligonucleotide aptamer targeting CCL2 has progressed to a Phase IIa clinical trials in diabetic nephropathy patients [240].

9. Summary and Future Directions

It is widely appreciated that the chemokine-receptor system plays critical roles in immune homeostasis, inflammatory responses, cancer, and several important infectious diseases. The system is inherently complex, consisting of close to fifty chemokines, most of which can activate several receptors, each expressed on a variety of leukocytes and some other cell types. To avoid undesirable inflammation and to ensure appropriate responses to pathogens, this system must be tightly controlled. In this review, we have summarized the major mechanisms that are currently understood to regulate the interactions of chemokines with their receptors.

Although the mechanisms discussed herein together exert substantial biochemical control over the chemokine-receptor network, they also greatly enhance the complexity of the network. For example, post-translational modifications and oligomerization effectively increase the number of chemokines and receptors and vastly expand the number of chemokine-receptor combinations. This presents significant challenges when attempting to inhibit specific targets because inhibitors may not be equally effective against all modified forms of a receptor or chemokine. On the other hand, understanding the mechanisms of regulation also leads to novel opportunities for therapeutic intervention. Thus, in addition to targeting chemokines or receptors directly, it may become possible to influence their activity by indirectly suppressing their expression, altering their localization or blocking downstream signaling pathways. Ongoing studies, such as those reported in this special issue of the *International Journal of Molecular Sciences*, are continuing to reveal novel aspects of chemokine-receptor regulation and to stimulate new approaches to pharmacological control.

Acknowledgments: This work was supported by Australian Research Council Discovery Grant DP120100194 and ANZ Trustees Grant 12-3831 (Martin J. Stone).

Conflicts of Interest: The authors declare no conflict of interest.

Abbreviations

AP2	Adaptin 2
CKBP	Chemokine-binding protein
DC-CK	Dendritic cell-derived CC chemokine
ENA	Epithelial-derived neutrophil-activating
GCP	Granulocyte chemotactic protein
GRO	Growth-regulated protein
IL	Interleukin
IP	Interferon γ-induced protein
IUPHAR	International Union of Basic and Clinical Pharmacology
I-TAC	Interferon-inducible T-cell α chemoattractant
MCP	Monocyte chemoattractant protein
MGSA	Melanoma growth stimulating activity
MIP	Macrophage inflammatory protein
PARC	Pulmonary and activation-regulated chemokine

PF4	Platelet factor 4
RANTES	Regulated on activation, normal T cell expressed and secreted
SDF	Stromal cell-derived factor
SECRET	Smallpox virus-encoded chemokine receptor
SLC	Secondary lymphoid tissue chemokine
SNP	Single nucleotide polymorphism
TARC	Thymus and activation regulated chemokine
TECK	Thymus-expressed chemokine

References

1. Moser, B.; Wolf, M.; Walz, A.; Loetscher, P. Chemokines: Multiple levels of leukocyte migration control. *Trends Immunol.* **2004**, *25*, 75–84. [CrossRef] [PubMed]
2. Baggiolini, M. Chemokines in pathology and medicine. *J. Intern. Med.* **2001**, *250*, 91–104. [CrossRef] [PubMed]
3. Gerard, C.; Rollins, B.J. Chemokines and disease. *Nat. Immunol.* **2001**, *2*, 108–115. [CrossRef] [PubMed]
4. Dimberg, A. Chemokines in angiogenesis. *Curr. Top. Microbiol. Immunol.* **2010**, *341*, 59–80. [PubMed]
5. Speyer, C.L.; Ward, P.A. Role of endothelial chemokines and their receptors during inflammation. *J. Invest. Surg.* **2011**, *24*, 18–27. [CrossRef] [PubMed]
6. Ben-Baruch, A. The multifaceted roles of chemokines in malignancy. *Cancer Metastasis Rev.* **2006**, *25*, 357–371. [CrossRef] [PubMed]
7. Luther, S.A.; Cyster, J.G. Chemokines as regulators of T cell differentiation. *Nat. Immunol.* **2001**, *2*, 102–107. [CrossRef]
8. Choe, H.; Moore, M.J.; Owens, C.M.; Wright, P.L.; Vasilieva, N.; Li, W.; Singh, A.P.; Shakri, R.; Chitnis, C.E.; Farzan, M. Sulphated tyrosines mediate association of chemokines and *Plasmodium vivax* duffy binding protein with the duffy antigen/receptor for chemokines (DARC). *Mol. Microbiol.* **2005**, *55*, 1413–1422. [CrossRef] [PubMed]
9. Alkhatib, G.; Combadiere, C.; Broder, C.C.; Feng, Y.; Kennedy, P.E. CC CKR5: A RANTES, MIP-1a, MIP-1b receptor as a fusion cofactor for macrophage-tropic HIV-1. *Science* **1996**, *272*, 1955–1958. [CrossRef] [PubMed]
10. Proudfoot, A.E. Chemokine receptors: Multifaceted therapeutic targets. *Nat. Rev. Immunol.* **2002**, *2*, 106–115. [CrossRef] [PubMed]
11. Lee, J.; Horuk, R.; Rice, G.C.; Bennett, G.L.; Camerato, T.; Wood, W.I. Characterization of two high affinity human interleukin-8 receptors. *J. Biol. Chem.* **1992**, *267*, 16283–16287. [PubMed]
12. Stone, M.J.; Mayer, K.L. Three dimensional structure of chemokines. In *Chemokines in Allergic Disease*; Rothenberg, M.E., Ed.; Marcel Dekker: New York, NY, USA, 2000; pp. 67–94.
13. Burg, J.S.; Ingram, J.R.; Venkatakrishnan, A.J.; Jude, K.M.; Dukkipati, A.; Feinberg, E.N.; Angelini, A.; Waghray, D.; Dror, R.O.; Ploegh, H.L.; et al. Structural basis for chemokine recognition and activation of a viral G protein–coupled receptor. *Science* **2015**, *347*, 1113–1117. [CrossRef] [PubMed]
14. Qin, L.; Kufareva, I.; Holden, L.G.; Wang, C.; Zheng, Y.; Zhao, C.; Fenalti, G.; Wu, H.; Han, G.W.; Cherezov, V.; et al. Crystal structure of the chemokine receptor CXCR4 in complex with a viral chemokine. *Science* **2015**, *347*, 1117–1122. [CrossRef] [PubMed]
15. Wu, B.; Chien, E.Y.; Mol, C.D.; Fenalti, G.; Liu, W.; Katritch, V.; Abagyan, R.; Brooun, A.; Wells, P.; Bi, F.C.; et al. Structures of the CXCR4 chemokine GPCR with small-molecule and cyclic peptide antagonists. *Science* **2010**, *330*, 1066–1071. [CrossRef] [PubMed]
16. Park, S.H.; Das, B.B.; Casagrande, F.; Tian, Y.; Nothnagel, H.J.; Chu, M.; Kiefer, H.; Maier, K.; de Angelis, A.A.; Marassi, F.M.; et al. Structure of the chemokine receptor CXCR1 in phospholipid bilayers. *Nature* **2012**, *491*, 779–783. [CrossRef] [PubMed]
17. Tan, Q.; Zhu, Y.; Li, J.; Chen, Z.; Han, G.W.; Kufareva, I.; Li, T.; Ma, L.; Fenalti, G.; Zhang, W.; et al. Structure of the CCR5 chemokine receptor-HIV entry inhibitor maraviroc complex. *Science* **2013**, *341*, 1387–1390. [CrossRef] [PubMed]
18. Lubkowski, J.; Bujacz, G.; Boque, L.; Domaille, P.J.; Handel, T.M.; Wlodawer, A. The structure of MCP-1 in two crystal forms provides a rare example of variable quaternary interactions. *Nat. Struct. Biol.* **1997**, *4*, 64–69. [CrossRef] [PubMed]

19. Wescott, M.P.; Kufareva, I.; Paes, C.; Goodman, J.R.; Thaker, Y.; Puffer, B.A.; Berdougo, E.; Rucker, J.B.; Handel, T.M.; Doranz, B.J. Signal transmission through the CXC chemokine receptor 4 (CXCR4) transmembrane helices. *Proc. Natl. Acad. Sci. USA* **2016**, *113*, 9928–9933. [CrossRef] [PubMed]
20. Skelton, N.J.; Quan, C.; Reilly, D.; Lowman, H. Structure of a CXC chemokine-receptor fragment in complex with interleukin-8. *Structure* **1999**, *7*, 157–168. [CrossRef]
21. Veldkamp, C.T.; Seibert, C.; Peterson, F.C.; de la Cruz, N.B.; Haugner, J.C., 3rd; Basnet, H.; Sakmar, T.P.; Volkman, B.F. Structural basis of CXCR4 sulfotyrosine recognition by the chemokine SDF-1/CXCL12. *Sci. Signal.* **2008**, *1*, ra4. [CrossRef] [PubMed]
22. Millard, C.J.; Ludeman, J.P.; Canals, M.; Bridgford, J.L.; Hinds, M.G.; Clayton, D.J.; Christopoulos, A.; Payne, R.J.; Stone, M.J. Structural basis of receptor sulfotyrosine recognition by a CC chemokine: The N-terminal region of CCR3 bound to CCL11/eotaxin-1. *Structure* **2014**, *22*, 1571–1581. [CrossRef] [PubMed]
23. Crump, M.P.; Gong, J.H.; Loetscher, P.; Rajarathnam, K.; Amara, A.; Arenzana-Seisdedos, F.; Virelizier, J.L.; Baggiolini, M.; Sykes, B.D.; Clark-Lewis, I. Solution structure and basis for functional activity of stromal cell-derived factor-1; dissociation of CXCR4 activation from binding and inhibition of HIV-1. *EMBO J.* **1997**, *16*, 6996–7007. [CrossRef] [PubMed]
24. Kleist, A.B.; Getschman, A.E.; Ziarek, J.J.; Nevins, A.M.; Gauthier, P.A.; Chevigne, A.; Szpakowska, M.; Volkman, B.F. New paradigms in chemokine receptor signal transduction: Moving beyond the two-site model. *Biochem. Pharmacol.* **2016**, *114*, 53–68. [CrossRef] [PubMed]
25. Katritch, V.; Cherezov, V.; Stevens, R.C. Diversity and modularity of G protein-coupled receptor structures. *Trends Pharmacol. Sci.* **2012**, *33*, 17–27. [CrossRef] [PubMed]
26. Bajoghli, B.; Aghaallaei, N.; Hess, I.; Rode, I.; Netuschil, N.; Tay, B.H.; Venkatesh, B.; Yu, J.K.; Kaltenbach, S.L.; Holland, N.D.; et al. Evolution of genetic networks underlying the emergence of thymopoiesis in vertebrates. *Cell* **2009**, *138*, 186–197. [CrossRef] [PubMed]
27. Nomiyama, H.; Osada, N.; Yoshie, O. A family tree of vertebrate chemokine receptors for a unified nomenclature. *Dev. Comp. Immunol.* **2011**, *35*, 705–715. [CrossRef] [PubMed]
28. Zlotnik, A.; Yoshie, O. Chemokines: A new classification system and their role in immunity. *Immunity* **2000**, *12*, 121–127. [CrossRef]
29. Zlotnik, A.; Yoshie, O.; Nomiyama, H. The chemokine and chemokine receptor superfamilies and their molecular evolution. *Genome Biol.* **2006**, *7*, 243. [CrossRef] [PubMed]
30. McDermott, D.H.; Yang, Q.; Kathiresan, S.; Cupples, L.A.; Massaro, J.M.; Keaney, J.F., Jr.; Larson, M.G.; Vasan, R.S.; Hirschhorn, J.N.; O'Donnell, C.J.; et al. CCL2 polymorphisms are associated with serum monocyte chemoattractant protein-1 levels and myocardial infarction in the framingham heart study. *Circulation* **2005**, *112*, 1113–1120. [CrossRef] [PubMed]
31. Flex, A.; Gaetani, E.; Papaleo, P.; Straface, G.; Proia, A.S.; Pecorini, G.; Tondi, P.; Pola, P.; Pola, R. Proinflammatory genetic profiles in subjects with history of ischemic stroke. *Stroke* **2004**, *35*, 2270–2275. [CrossRef] [PubMed]
32. Karrer, S.; Bosserhoff, A.K.; Weiderer, P.; Distler, O.; Landthaler, M.; Szeimies, R.M.; Muller-Ladner, U.; Scholmerich, J.; Hellbrand, C. The -2518 promotor polymorphism in the MCP-1 gene is associated with systemic sclerosis. *J. Investig. Dermatol.* **2005**, *124*, 92–98. [CrossRef] [PubMed]
33. Kroner, A.; Maurer, M.; Loserth, S.; Kleinschnitz, C.; Hemmer, B.; Rosche, B.; Toyka, K.V.; Rieckmann, P. Analysis of the monocyte chemoattractant protein 1 -2518 promoter polymorphism in patients with multiple sclerosis. *Tissue Antigens* **2004**, *64*, 70–73. [CrossRef] [PubMed]
34. Gonzalez-Escribano, M.F.; Torres, B.; Aguilar, F.; Rodriguez, R.; Garcia, A.; Valenzuela, A.; Nunez-Roldan, A. MCP-1 promoter polymorphism in Spanish patients with rheumatoid arthritis. *Hum. Immunol.* **2003**, *64*, 741–744. [CrossRef]
35. Porcellini, E.; Ianni, M.; Carbone, I.; Franceschi, M.; Licastro, F. Monocyte chemoattractant protein-1 promoter polymorphism and plasma levels in Alzheimer's disease. *Immun. Ageing* **2013**, *10*, 6. [CrossRef] [PubMed]
36. Gonzalez, E.; Rovin, B.H.; Sen, L.; Cooke, G.; Dhanda, R.; Mummidi, S.; Kulkarni, H.; Bamshad, M.J.; Telles, V.; Anderson, S.A.; et al. HIV-1 infection and aids dementia are influenced by a mutant MCP-1 allele linked to increased monocyte infiltration of tissues and MCP-1 levels. *Proc. Natl. Acad. Sci. USA* **2002**, *99*, 13795–13800. [CrossRef] [PubMed]

37. Hellier, S.; Frodsham, A.J.; Hennig, B.J.; Klenerman, P.; Knapp, S.; Ramaley, P.; Satsangi, J.; Wright, M.; Zhang, L.; Thomas, H.C.; et al. Association of genetic variants of the chemokine receptor CCR5 and its ligands, RANTES and MCP-2, with outcome of HCV infection. *Hepatology* **2003**, *38*, 1468–1476. [CrossRef] [PubMed]

38. Tsunemi, Y.; Komine, M.; Sekiya, T.; Saeki, H.; Nakamura, K.; Hirai, K.; Kakinuma, T.; Kagami, S.; Fujita, H.; Asano, N.; et al. The -431C→T polymorphism of thymus and activation-regulated chemokine increases the promoter activity but is not associated with susceptibility to atopic dermatitis in Japanese patients. *Exp. Dermatol.* **2004**, *13*, 715–719. [CrossRef] [PubMed]

39. Winkler, C.; Modi, W.; Smith, M.W.; Nelson, G.W.; Wu, X.; Carrington, M.; Dean, M.; Honjo, T.; Tashiro, K.; Yabe, D.; et al. Genetic restriction of AIDS pathogenesis by an SDF-1 chemokine gene variant. Alive study, hemophilia growth and development study (HGDS), multicenter AIDS cohort study (MACS), multicenter hemophilia cohort study (MHCS), San Francisco city cohort (SFCC). *Science* **1998**, *279*, 389–393. [CrossRef] [PubMed]

40. Reiche, E.M.; Bonametti, A.M.; Voltarelli, J.C.; Morimoto, H.K.; Watanabe, M.A. Genetic polymorphisms in the chemokine and chemokine receptors: Impact on clinical course and therapy of the human immunodeficiency virus type 1 infection (HIV-1). *Curr. Med. Chem.* **2007**, *14*, 1325–1334. [CrossRef] [PubMed]

41. Ortlepp, J.R.; Krantz, C.; Kimmel, M.; von Korff, A.; Vesper, K.; Schmitz, F.; Mevissen, V.; Janssens, U.; Franke, A.; Hanrath, P.; et al. Additive effects of the chemokine receptor 2, vitamin D receptor, interleukin-6 polymorphisms and cardiovascular risk factors on the prevalence of myocardial infarction in patients below 65 years. *Int. J. Cardiol.* **2005**, *105*, 90–95. [CrossRef] [PubMed]

42. Petrkova, J.; Cermakova, Z.; Drabek, J.; Lukl, J.; Petrek, M. CC chemokine receptor (CCR)2 polymorphism in Czech patients with myocardial infarction. *Immunol. Lett.* **2003**, *88*, 53–55. [CrossRef]

43. Miyagishi, R.; Niino, M.; Fukazawa, T.; Yabe, I.; Kikuchi, S.; Tashiro, K. C-C chemokine receptor 2 gene polymorphism in Japanese patients with multiple sclerosis. *J. Neuroimmunol.* **2003**, *145*, 135–138. [CrossRef] [PubMed]

44. Goulding, C.; McManus, R.; Murphy, A.; MacDonald, G.; Barrett, S.; Crowe, J.; Hegarty, J.; McKiernan, S.; Kelleher, D. The CCR5-D32 mutation: Impact on disease outcome in individuals with hepatitis C infection from a single source. *Gut* **2005**, *54*, 1157–1161. [CrossRef] [PubMed]

45. Navratilova, Z. Polymorphisms in CCL2 & CCL5 chemokines/chemokine receptors genes and their association with diseases. *Biomed. Pap. Med. Fac. Univ. Palacky Olomouc Czechoslov.* **2006**, *150*, 191–204.

46. Smith, M.W.; Dean, M.; Carrington, M.; Winkler, C.; Huttley, G.A.; Lomb, D.A.; Goedert, J.J.; O'Brien, T.R.; Jacobson, L.P.; Kaslow, R.; et al. Contrasting genetic influence of CCR2 and CCR5 variants on HIV-1 infection and disease progression. Hemophilia growth and development study (HGDS), multicenter aids cohort study (MACS), multicenter hemophilia cohort study (MHCS), San Francisco city cohort (SFCC), alive study. *Science* **1997**, *277*, 959–965. [PubMed]

47. Burton, C.T.; Gotch, F.M.; Imami, N. CCR2/64I mutation detection in a HIV-1-positive patient with slow CD4 T-cell decline and delay in disease progression. *Int. J. STD AIDS* **2005**, *16*, 392–394. [CrossRef] [PubMed]

48. Huang, Y.; Paxton, W.A.; Wolinsky, S.M.; Neumann, A.U.; Zhang, L.; He, T.; Kang, S.; Ceradini, D.; Jin, Z.; Yazdanbakhsh, K.; et al. The role of a mutant CCR5 allele in HIV-1 transmission and disease progression. *Nat. Med.* **1996**, *2*, 1240–1243. [CrossRef] [PubMed]

49. Zimmerman, P.A.; Buckler-White, A.; Alkhatib, G.; Spalding, T.; Kubofcik, J.; Combadiere, C.; Weissman, D.; Cohen, O.; Rubbert, A.; Lam, G.; et al. Inherited resistance to HIV-1 conferred by an inactivating mutation in CC chemokine receptor 5: Studies in populations with contrasting clinical phenotypes, defined racial background, and quantified risk. *Mol. Med.* **1997**, *3*, 23–36. [PubMed]

50. Suresh, P.; Wanchu, A. Chemokines and chemokine receptors in HIV infection: Role in pathogenesis and therapeutics. *J. Postgrad. Med.* **2006**, *52*, 210–217. [PubMed]

51. Paxton, W.A.; Kang, S. Chemokine receptor allelic polymorphisms: Relationships to HIV resistance and disease progression. *Semin. Immunol.* **1998**, *10*, 187–194. [CrossRef] [PubMed]

52. Walton, R.T.; Rowland-Jones, S.L. HIV and chemokine binding to red blood cells—DARC matters. *Cell Host Microbe* **2008**, *4*, 3–5. [CrossRef] [PubMed]

53. Charo, I.F.; Myers, S.J.; Herman, A.; Franci, C.; Connolly, A.J.; Coughlin, S.R. Molecular cloning and functional expression of two monocyte chemoattractant protein 1 receptors reveals alternative splicing of the carboxyl-terminal tails. *Proc. Natl. Acad. Sci. USA* **1994**, *91*, 2752–2756. [CrossRef] [PubMed]

54. Bartoli, C.; Civatte, M.; Pellissier, J.F.; Figarella-Branger, D. CCR2A and CCR2B, the two isoforms of the monocyte chemoattractant protein-1 receptor are up-regulated and expressed by different cell subsets in idiopathic inflammatory myopathies. *Acta Neuropathol.* **2001**, *102*, 385–392. [PubMed]

55. Berchiche, Y.A.; Sakmar, T.P. CXC chemokine receptor 3 alternative splice variants selectively activate different signaling pathways. *Mol. Pharmacol.* **2016**, *90*, 483–495. [CrossRef] [PubMed]

56. Zlotnik, A.; Burkhardt, A.M.; Homey, B. Homeostatic chemokine receptors and organ-specific metastasis. *Nat. Rev. Immunol.* **2011**, *11*, 597–606. [CrossRef] [PubMed]

57. Deshmane, S.L.; Kremlev, S.; Amini, S.; Sawaya, B.E. Monocyte chemoattractant protein-1 (MCP-1): An overview. *J. Interferon Cytokine Res.* **2009**, *29*, 313–326. [CrossRef] [PubMed]

58. Nelson, P.J.; Krensky, A.M. Chemokines, chemokine receptors, and allograft rejection. *Immunity* **2001**, *14*, 377–386. [CrossRef]

59. Link, D.C. Neutrophil homeostasis: A new role for stromal cell-derived factor-1. *Immunol. Res.* **2005**, *32*, 169–178. [CrossRef]

60. Uy, G.L.; Rettig, M.P.; Cashen, A.F. Plerixafor, a CXCR4 antagonist for the mobilization of hematopoietic stem cells. *Expert. Opin. Biol. Ther.* **2008**, *8*, 1797–1804. [CrossRef] [PubMed]

61. Vicari, A.P.; Figueroa, D.J.; Hedrick, J.A.; Foster, J.S.; Singh, K.P.; Menon, S.; Copeland, N.G.; Gilbert, D.J.; Jenkins, N.A.; Bacon, K.B.; et al. Teck: A novel CC chemokine specifically expressed by thymic dendritic cells and potentially involved in T cell development. *Immunity* **1997**, *7*, 291–301. [CrossRef]

62. Link, A.; Vogt, T.K.; Favre, S.; Britschgi, M.R.; Acha-Orbea, H.; Hinz, B.; Cyster, J.G.; Luther, S.A. Fibroblastic reticular cells in lymph nodes regulate the homeostasis of naive T cells. *Nat. Immunol.* **2007**, *8*, 1255–1265. [CrossRef] [PubMed]

63. Takada, K.; Jameson, S.C. Naive T cell homeostasis: From awareness of space to a sense of place. *Nat. Rev. Immunol.* **2009**, *9*, 823–832. [CrossRef] [PubMed]

64. Marchese, A. Endocytic trafficking of chemokine receptors. *Curr. Opin. Cell Biol.* **2014**, *27*, 72–77. [CrossRef] [PubMed]

65. Iwamoto, T.; Okamoto, H.; Toyama, Y.; Momohara, S. Molecular aspects of rheumatoid arthritis: Chemokines in the joints of patients. *FEBS J.* **2008**, *275*, 4448–4455. [CrossRef] [PubMed]

66. Niwa, Y.; Akamatsu, H.; Niwa, H.; Sumi, H.; Ozaki, Y.; Abe, A. Correlation of tissue and plasma RANTES levels with disease course in patients with breast or cervical cancer. *Clin. Cancer. Res.* **2001**, *7*, 285–289. [PubMed]

67. Soria, G.; Ben-Baruch, A. The inflammatory chemokines CCL2 and CCL5 in breast cancer. *Cancer Lett.* **2008**, *267*, 271–285. [CrossRef] [PubMed]

68. Ueno, T.; Toi, M.; Saji, H.; Muta, M.; Bando, H.; Kuroi, K.; Koike, M.; Inadera, H.; Matsushima, K. Significance of macrophage chemoattractant protein-1 in macrophage recruitment, angiogenesis, and survival in human breast cancer. *Clin. Cancer. Res.* **2000**, *6*, 3282–3289. [PubMed]

69. Neel, N.F.; Schutyser, E.; Sai, J.; Fan, G.H.; Richmond, A. Chemokine receptor internalization and intracellular trafficking. *Cytokine Growth Factor Rev.* **2005**, *16*, 637–658. [CrossRef] [PubMed]

70. Baugher, P.J.; Richmond, A. The carboxyl-terminal PDZ ligand motif of chemokine receptor CXCR2 modulates post-endocytic sorting and cellular chemotaxis. *J. Biol. Chem.* **2008**, *283*, 30868–30878. [CrossRef] [PubMed]

71. Delhaye, M.; Gravot, A.; Ayinde, D.; Niedergang, F.; Alizon, M.; Brelot, A. Identification of a post-endocytic sorting sequence in CCR5. *Mol. Pharmacol.* **2007**, *72*, 1497–1507. [CrossRef] [PubMed]

72. Busillo, J.M.; Benovic, J.L. Regulation of CXCR4 signaling. *Biochim. Biophys. Acta* **2007**, *1768*, 952–963. [CrossRef] [PubMed]

73. Marchese, A.; Benovic, J.L. Agonist-promoted ubiquitination of the G protein-coupled receptor CXCR4 mediates lysosomal sorting. *J. Biol. Chem.* **2001**, *276*, 45509–45512. [CrossRef] [PubMed]

74. Canals, M.; Scholten, D.J.; de Munnik, S.; Han, M.K.; Smit, M.J.; Leurs, R. Ubiquitination of CXCR7 controls receptor trafficking. *PLoS ONE* **2012**, *7*, e34192. [CrossRef] [PubMed]

75. Schaeuble, K.; Hauser, M.A.; Rippl, A.V.; Bruderer, R.; Otero, C.; Groettrup, M.; Legler, D.F. Ubiquitylation of the chemokine receptor CCR7 enables efficient receptor recycling and cell migration. *J. Cell Sci.* **2012**, *125*, 4463–4474. [CrossRef] [PubMed]

76. Bachelerie, F.; Ben-Baruch, A.; Burkhardt, A.M.; Combadiere, C.; Farber, J.M.; Graham, G.J.; Horuk, R.; Sparre-Ulrich, A.H.; Locati, M.; Luster, A.D.; et al. International union of basic and clinical pharmacology. LXXXIX. Update on the extended family of chemokine receptors and introducing a new nomenclature for atypical chemokine receptors. *Pharmacol. Rev.* **2014**, *66*, 1–79. [CrossRef] [PubMed]

77. Bachelerie, F.; Graham, G.J.; Locati, M.; Mantovani, A.; Murphy, P.M.; Nibbs, R.; Rot, A.; Sozzani, S.; Thelen, M. New nomenclature for atypical chemokine receptors. *Nat. Immunol.* **2014**, *15*, 207–208. [CrossRef] [PubMed]

78. Bonecchi, R.; Savino, B.; Borroni, E.M.; Mantovani, A.; Locati, M. Chemokine decoy receptors: Structure-function and biological properties. *Curr. Top. Microbiol. Immunol.* **2010**, *341*, 15–36. [PubMed]

79. Massara, M.; Bonavita, O.; Mantovani, A.; Locati, M.; Bonecchi, R. Atypical chemokine receptors in cancer: Friends or foes? *J. Leukoc. Biol.* **2016**, *99*, 927–933. [CrossRef] [PubMed]

80. Mantovani, A.; Bonecchi, R.; Locati, M. Tuning inflammation and immunity by chemokine sequestration: Decoys and more. *Nat. Rev. Immunol.* **2006**, *6*, 907–918. [CrossRef] [PubMed]

81. Vacchini, A.; Locati, M.; Borroni, E.M. Overview and potential unifying themes of the atypical chemokine receptor family. *J. Leukoc. Biol.* **2016**, *99*, 883–892. [CrossRef] [PubMed]

82. Fra, A.M.; Locati, M.; Otero, K.; Sironi, M.; Signorelli, P.; Massardi, M.L.; Gobbi, M.; Vecchi, A.; Sozzani, S.; Mantovani, A. Cutting edge: Scavenging of inflammatory CC chemokines by the promiscuous putatively silent chemokine receptor D6. *J. Immunol.* **2003**, *170*, 2279–2282. [CrossRef] [PubMed]

83. Jamieson, T.; Cook, D.N.; Nibbs, R.J.; Rot, A.; Nixon, C.; McLean, P.; Alcami, A.; Lira, S.A.; Wiekowski, M.; Graham, G.J. The chemokine receptor D6 limits the inflammatory response in vivo. *Nat. Immunol.* **2005**, *6*, 403–411. [CrossRef] [PubMed]

84. Wang, X.; Sharp, J.S.; Handel, T.M.; Prestegard, J.H. Chemokine oligomerization in cell signaling and migration. *Prog. Mol. Biol. Transl. Sci.* **2013**, *117*, 531–578. [PubMed]

85. Salanga, C.L.; Handel, T.M. Chemokine oligomerization and interactions with receptors and glycosaminoglycans: The role of structural dynamics in function. *Exp. Cell Res.* **2011**, *317*, 590–601. [CrossRef] [PubMed]

86. Proudfoot, A.E.I.; Handel, T.M.; Johnson, Z.; Lau, E.K.; LiWang, P.; Clark-Lewis, I.; Borlat, F.; Wells, T.N.C.; Kosco-Vilbois, M.H. Glycosaminoglycan binding and oligomerization are essential for the in vivo activity of certain chemokines. *Proc. Natl. Acad. Sci. USA* **2003**, *100*, 1885–1890. [CrossRef] [PubMed]

87. Gangavarapu, P.; Rajagopalan, L.; Kolli, D.; Guerrero-Plata, A.; Garofalo, R.P.; Rajarathnam, K. The monomer-dimer equilibrium and glycosaminoglycan interactions of chemokine CXCL8 regulate tissue-specific neutrophil recruitment. *J. Leukoc. Biol.* **2012**, *91*, 259–265. [CrossRef] [PubMed]

88. Middleton, J.; Patterson, A.M.; Gardner, L.; Schmutz, C.; Ashton, B.A. Leukocyte extravasation: Chemokine transport and presentation by the endothelium. *Blood* **2002**, *100*, 3853–3860. [CrossRef] [PubMed]

89. Moelants, E.A.; Mortier, A.; van Damme, J.; Proost, P. In vivo regulation of chemokine activity by post-translational modification. *Immunol. Cell Biol.* **2013**, *91*, 402–407. [CrossRef] [PubMed]

90. Mortier, A.; van Damme, J.; Proost, P. Regulation of chemokine activity by posttranslational modification. *Pharmacol. Ther.* **2008**, *120*, 197–217. [CrossRef] [PubMed]

91. Starr, A.E.; Dufour, A.; Maier, J.; Overall, C.M. Biochemical analysis of matrix metalloproteinase activation of chemokines CCL15 and CCL23 and increased glycosaminoglycan binding of CCL16. *J. Biol. Chem.* **2012**, *287*, 5848–5860. [CrossRef] [PubMed]

92. Mortier, A.; Berghmans, N.; Ronsse, I.; Grauwen, K.; Stegen, S.; van Damme, J.; Proost, P. Biological activity of CXCL8 forms generated by alternative cleavage of the signal peptide or by aminopeptidase-mediated truncation. *PLoS ONE* **2011**, *6*, e23913. [CrossRef] [PubMed]

93. Moelants, E.A.; Loozen, G.; Mortier, A.; Martens, E.; Opdenakker, G.; Mizgalska, D.; Szmigielski, B.; Potempa, J.; van Damme, J.; Teughels, W.; et al. Citrullination and proteolytic processing of chemokines by porphyromonas gingivalis. *Infect. Immun.* **2014**, *82*, 2511–2519. [CrossRef] [PubMed]

94. Detheux, M.; Standker, L.; Vakili, J.; Munch, J.; Forssmann, U.; Adermann, K.; Pohlmann, S.; Vassart, G.; Kirchhoff, F.; Parmentier, M.; et al. Natural proteolytic processing of hemofiltrate CC chemokine 1 generates a potent CC chemokine receptor (CCR)1 and CCR5 agonist with anti-HIV properties. *J. Exp. Med.* **2000**, *192*, 1501–1508. [CrossRef] [PubMed]

95. Forssmann, U.; Hartung, I.; Balder, R.; Fuchs, B.; Escher, S.E.; Spodsberg, N.; Dulkys, Y.; Walden, M.; Heitland, A.; Braun, A.; et al. *N*-nonanoyl-CC chemokine ligand 14, a potent CC chemokine ligand 14 analogue that prevents the recruitment of eosinophils in allergic airway inflammation. *J. Immunol.* **2004**, *173*, 3456–3466. [CrossRef] [PubMed]

96. Savino, B.; Borroni, E.M.; Torres, N.M.; Proost, P.; Struyf, S.; Mortier, A.; Mantovani, A.; Locati, M.; Bonecchi, R. Recognition versus adaptive up-regulation and degradation of CC chemokines by the chemokine decoy receptor d6 are determined by their N-terminal sequence. *J. Biol. Chem.* **2009**, *284*, 26207–26215. [CrossRef] [PubMed]

97. Eckhard, U.; Huesgen, P.F.; Schilling, O.; Bellac, C.L.; Butler, G.S.; Cox, J.H.; Dufour, A.; Goebeler, V.; Kappelhoff, R.; Keller, U.A.; et al. Active site specificity profiling of the matrix metalloproteinase family: Proteomic identification of 4300 cleavage sites by nine mmps explored with structural and synthetic peptide cleavage analyses. *Matrix Biol.* **2016**, *49*, 37–60. [CrossRef] [PubMed]

98. Wolf, M.; Clark-Lewis, I.; Buri, C.; Langen, H.; Lis, M.; Mazzucchelli, L. Cathepsin D specifically cleaves the chemokines macrophage inflammatory protein-1 a, macrophage inflammatory protein-1 b, and SLC that are expressed in human breast cancer. *Am. J. Pathol.* **2003**, *162*, 1183–1190. [CrossRef]

99. Jiang, Y.; Tabak, L.A.; Valente, A.J.; Graves, D.T. Initial characterization of the carbohydrate structure of MCP-1. *Biochem. Biophys. Res. Commun.* **1991**, *178*, 1400–1404. [CrossRef]

100. Jiang, Y.; Valente, A.J.; Williamson, M.J.; Zhang, L.; Graves, D.T. Post-translational modification of a monocyte-specific chemoattractant synthesized by glioma, osteosarcoma, and vascular smooth muscle cells. *J. Biol. Chem.* **1990**, *265*, 18318–18321. [PubMed]

101. Noso, N.; Bartels, J.; Mallet, A.I.; Mochizuki, M.; Christophers, E.; Schroder, J.M. Delayed production of biologically active *O*-glycosylated forms of human eotaxin by tumor-necrosis-factor-α-stimulated dermal fibroblasts. *Eur. J. Biochem.* **1998**, *253*, 114–122. [CrossRef]

102. Richter, R.; Schulz-Knappe, P.; John, H.; Forssmann, W.G. Posttranslationally processed forms of the human chemokine HCC-1. *Biochemistry* **2000**, *39*, 10799–10805. [CrossRef] [PubMed]

103. Kameyoshi, Y.; Dorschner, A.; Mallet, A.I.; Christophers, E.; Schroder, J.M. Cytokine RANTES released by thrombin-stimulated platelets is a potent attractant for human eosinophils. *J. Exp. Med.* **1992**, *176*, 587–592. [CrossRef] [PubMed]

104. Hermand, P.; Pincet, F.; Carvalho, S.; Ansanay, H.; Trinquet, E.; Daoudi, M.; Combadiere, C.; Deterre, P. Functional adhesiveness of the cx3cl1 chemokine requires its aggregation. Role of the transmembrane domain. *J. Biol. Chem.* **2008**, *283*, 30225–30234. [CrossRef] [PubMed]

105. Liu, Y.D.; Goetze, A.M.; Bass, R.B.; Flynn, G.C. N-terminal glutamate to pyroglutamate conversion in vivo for human IgG2 antibodies. *J. Biol. Chem.* **2011**, *286*, 11211–11217. [CrossRef] [PubMed]

106. Uguccioni, M.; Loetscher, P.; Forssmann, U.; Dewald, B.; Li, H.D.; Lima, S.H.; Li, Y.L.; Kreider, B.; Garotta, G.; Thelen, M.; et al. Monocyte chemotactic protein 4 (MCP-4), a novel structural and functional analogue of MCP-3 and eotaxin. *J. Exp. Med.* **1996**, *183*, 2379–2384. [CrossRef] [PubMed]

107. Vandamme, J.; Proost, P.; Lenaerts, J.P.; Opdenakker, G. Structural and functional identification of 2 human, tumor-derived monocyte chemotactic proteins (MCP-2 and MCP-3) belonging to the chemokine family. *J. Exp. Med.* **1992**, *176*, 59–65. [CrossRef]

108. Yoshimura, T.; Robinson, E.A.; Appella, E.; Matsushima, K.; Showalter, S.D.; Skeel, A.; Leonard, E.J. 3 forms of monocyte-derived neutrophil chemotactic factor (MDNCF) distinguished by different lengths of the amino-terminal sequence. *Mol. Immunol.* **1989**, *26*, 87–93. [PubMed]

109. Cynis, H.; Hoffmann, T.; Friedrich, D.; Kehlen, A.; Gans, K.; Kleinschmidt, M.; Rahfeld, J.U.; Wolf, R.; Wermann, M.; Stephan, A.; et al. The isoenzyme of glutaminyl cyclase is an important regulator of monocyte infiltration under inflammatory conditions. *EMBO Mol. Med.* **2011**, *3*, 545–558. [CrossRef] [PubMed]

110. Gong, J.H.; Clarklewis, I. Antagonists of monocyte chemoattractant protein-1 identified by modification of functionally critical NH_2-terminal residues. *J. Exp. Med.* **1995**, *181*, 631–640. [CrossRef] [PubMed]

111. Hartlage-Rubsamen, M.; Waniek, A.; Meissner, J.; Morawski, M.; Schilling, S.; Jager, C.; Kleinschmidt, M.; Cynis, H.; Kehlen, A.; Arendt, T.; et al. Isoglutaminyl cyclase contributes to CCL2-driven neuroinflammation in Alzheimer's disease. *Acta Neuropathol.* **2015**, *129*, 565–583. [CrossRef] [PubMed]
112. Barker, C.E.; Ali, S.; O'Boyle, G.; Kirby, J.A. Transplantation and inflammation: Implications for the modification of chemokine function. *Immunology* **2014**, *143*, 138–145. [CrossRef] [PubMed]
113. Proost, P.; Loos, T.; Mortier, A.; Schutyser, E.; Gouwy, M.; Noppen, S.; Dillen, C.; Ronsse, I.; Conings, R.; Struyf, S.; et al. Citrullination of CXCL8 by peptidylarginine deiminase alters receptor usage, prevents proteolysis, and dampens tissue inflammation. *J. Exp. Med.* **2008**, *205*, 2085–2097. [CrossRef] [PubMed]
114. Loos, T.; Opdenakker, G.; van Damme, J.; Proost, P. Citrullination of CXCL8 increases this chemokine's ability to mobilize neutrophils into the blood circulation. *Haematologica* **2009**, *94*, 1346–1353. [CrossRef] [PubMed]
115. Mortier, A.; Loos, T.; Gouwy, M.; Ronsse, I.; van Damme, J.; Proost, P. Posttranslational modification of the NH_2-terminal region of CXCL5 by proteases or peptidylarginine deiminases (PAD) differently affects its biological activity. *J. Biol. Chem.* **2010**, *285*, 29750–29759. [CrossRef] [PubMed]
116. Loos, T.; Mortier, A.; Gouwy, M.; Ronsse, I.; Put, W.; Lenaerts, J.P.; van Damme, J.; Proost, P. Citrullination of CXCL10 and CXCL11 by peptidylarginine deiminase: A naturally occurring posttranslational modification of chemokines and new dimension of immunoregulation. *Blood* **2008**, *112*, 2648–2656. [CrossRef] [PubMed]
117. Struyf, S.; Noppen, S.; Loos, T.; Mortier, A.; Gouwy, M.; Verbeke, H.; Huskens, D.; Luangsay, S.; Parmentier, M.; Geboes, K.; et al. Citrullination of CXCL12 differentially reduces CXCR4 and CXCR7 binding with loss of inflammatory and anti-HIV-1 activity via CXCR4. *J. Immunol.* **2009**, *182*, 666–674. [CrossRef] [PubMed]
118. Molon, B.; Ugel, S.; Del Pozzo, F.; Soldani, C.; Zilio, S.; Avella, D.; de Palma, A.; Mauri, P.; Monegal, A.; Rescigno, M.; et al. Chemokine nitration prevents intratumoral infiltration of antigen-specific T cells. *J. Exp. Med.* **2011**, *208*, 1949–1962. [CrossRef] [PubMed]
119. Sato, E.; Simpson, K.L.; Grisham, M.B.; Koyama, S.; Robbins, R.A. Effects of reactive oxygen and nitrogen metabolites on MCP-1-induced monocyte chemotactic activity in vitro. *Am. J. Physiol.* **1999**, *277*, L543–L549. [PubMed]
120. Sato, E.; Simpson, K.L.; Grisham, M.B.; Koyama, S.; Robbins, R.A. Effects of reactive oxygen and nitrogen metabolites on RANTES- and IL-5-induced eosinophil chemotactic activity in vitro. *Am. J. Pathol.* **1999**, *155*, 591–598. [CrossRef]
121. Pi, X.; Wu, Y.; Ferguson, J.E., 3rd; Portbury, A.L.; Patterson, C. SDF-1a stimulates JNK3 activity via enos-dependent nitrosylation of MKP7 to enhance endothelial migration. *Proc. Natl. Acad. Sci. USA* **2009**, *106*, 5675–5680. [CrossRef] [PubMed]
122. Yasuoka, H.; Tsujimoto, M.; Yoshidome, K.; Nakahara, M.; Kodama, R.; Sanke, T.; Nakamura, Y. Cytoplasmic CXCR4 expression in breast cancer: Induction by nitric oxide and correlation with lymph node metastasis and poor prognosis. *BMC Cancer* **2008**, *8*, 340. [CrossRef] [PubMed]
123. Huttenrauch, F.; Pollok-Kopp, B.; Oppermann, M. G protein-coupled receptor kinases promote phosphorylation and β-arrestin-mediated internalization of CCR5 homo- and hetero-oligomers. *J. Biol. Chem.* **2005**, *280*, 37503–37515. [CrossRef] [PubMed]
124. Barker, B.L.; Benovic, J.L. G protein-coupled receptor kinase 5 phosphorylation of HIP regulates internalization of the chemokine receptor CXCR4. *Biochemistry* **2011**, *50*, 6933–6941. [CrossRef] [PubMed]
125. Raghuwanshi, S.K.; Su, Y.; Singh, V.; Haynes, K.; Richmond, A.; Richardson, R.M. The chemokine receptors CXCR1 and CXCR2 couple to distinct G protein-coupled receptor kinases to mediate and regulate leukocyte functions. *J. Immunol.* **2012**, *189*, 2824–2832. [CrossRef] [PubMed]
126. Pu, Q.; Yu, C. Glycosyltransferases, glycosylation and atherosclerosis. *Glycoconj. J.* **2014**, *31*, 605–611. [CrossRef] [PubMed]
127. Grodecka, M.; Czerwinski, M.; Duk, M.; Lisowska, E.; Wasniowska, K. Analysis of recombinant Duffy protein-linked N-glycans using lectins and glycosidases. *Acta Biochim. Pol.* **2010**, *57*, 49–53. [PubMed]
128. Sarmiento, J.; Kypreos, K.E.; Prado, G.N.; Suetomi, K.; Stanzel, C.; Maxwell, C.; Shumate, D.; Tandang-Silvas, M.R.; Rajarathnam, K.; Navarro, J. Adenovirus mediated expression "in vivo" of the chemokine receptor CXCR1. *J. Struct. Funct. Genomics* **2009**, *10*, 17–23. [CrossRef] [PubMed]

129. Czerwinski, M.; Kern, J.; Grodecka, M.; Paprocka, M.; Krop-Watorek, A.; Wasniowska, K. Mutational analysis of the *N*-glycosylation sites of Duffy antigen/receptor for chemokines. *Biochem. Biophys. Res. Commun.* **2007**, *356*, 816–821. [CrossRef] [PubMed]

130. Margulies, B.J.; Gibson, W. The chemokine receptor homologue encoded by US27 of human cytomegalovirus is heavily glycosylated and is present in infected human foreskin fibroblasts and enveloped virus particles. *Virus Res.* **2007**, *123*, 57–71. [CrossRef] [PubMed]

131. Gutierrez, J.; Kremer, L.; Zaballos, A.; Goya, I.; Martinez, A.C.; Marquez, G. Analysis of post-translational CCR8 modifications and their influence on receptor activity. *J. Biol. Chem.* **2004**, *279*, 14726–14733. [CrossRef]

132. Blackburn, P.E.; Simpson, C.V.; Nibbs, R.J.; O'Hara, M.; Booth, R.; Poulos, J.; Isaacs, N.W.; Graham, G.J. Purification and biochemical characterization of the D6 chemokine receptor. *Biochem. J.* **2004**, *379*, 263–272. [CrossRef] [PubMed]

133. Chabot, D.J.; Chen, H.; Dimitrov, D.S.; Broder, C.C. N-linked glycosylation of CXCR4 masks coreceptor function for CCR5-dependent human immunodeficiency virus type 1 isolates. *J. Virol.* **2000**, *74*, 4404–4413. [CrossRef] [PubMed]

134. Bannert, N.; Craig, S.; Farzan, M.; Sogah, D.; Santo, N.V.; Choe, H.; Sodroski, J. Sialylated *O*-glycans and sulfated tyrosines in the NH$_2$-terminal domain of CC chemokine receptor 5 contribute to high affinity binding of chemokines. *J. Exp. Med.* **2001**, *194*, 1661–1673. [CrossRef] [PubMed]

135. Preobrazhensky, A.A.; Dragan, S.; Kawano, T.; Gavrilin, M.A.; Gulina, I.V.; Chakravarty, L.; Kolattukudy, P.E. Monocyte chemotactic protein-1 receptor CCR2B is a glycoprotein that has tyrosine sulfation in a conserved extracellular N-terminal region. *J. Immunol.* **2000**, *165*, 5295–5303. [CrossRef] [PubMed]

136. Hauser, M.A.; Kindinger, I.; Laufer, J.M.; Spate, A.K.; Bucher, D.; Vanes, S.L.; Krueger, W.A.; Wittmann, V.; Legler, D.F. Distinct CCR7 glycosylation pattern shapes receptor signaling and endocytosis to modulate chemotactic responses. *J. Leukoc. Biol.* **2016**, *99*, 993–1007. [CrossRef] [PubMed]

137. Kiermaier, E.; Moussion, C.; Veldkamp, C.T.; Gerardy-Schahn, R.; de Vries, I.; Williams, L.G.; Chaffee, G.R.; Phillips, A.J.; Freiberger, F.; Imre, R.; et al. Polysialylation controls dendritic cell trafficking by regulating chemokine recognition. *Science* **2016**, *351*, 186–190. [CrossRef] [PubMed]

138. Ludwig, A.; Ehlert, J.E.; Flad, H.D.; Brandt, E. Identification of distinct surface-expressed and intracellular CXC-chemokine receptor 2 glycoforms in neutrophils: *N*-glycosylation is essential for maintenance of receptor surface expression. *J. Immunol.* **2000**, *165*, 1044–1052. [CrossRef] [PubMed]

139. Hartl, D.; Latzin, P.; Hordijk, P.; Marcos, V.; Rudolph, C.; Woischnik, M.; Krauss-Etschmann, S.; Koller, B.; Reinhardt, D.; Roscher, A.A.; et al. Cleavage of CXCR1 on neutrophils disables bacterial killing in cystic fibrosis lung disease. *Nat. Med.* **2007**, *13*, 1423–1430. [CrossRef] [PubMed]

140. Stone, M.J.; Chuang, S.; Hou, X.; Shoham, M.; Zhu, J.Z. Tyrosine sulfation: An increasingly recognised post-translational modification of secreted proteins. *New Biotechnol.* **2009**, *25*, 299–317. [CrossRef]

141. Ludeman, J.P.; Stone, M.J. The structural role of receptor tyrosine sulfation in chemokine recognition. *Brit. J. Pharmacol.* **2014**, *171*, 1167–1179. [CrossRef] [PubMed]

142. Farzan, M.; Mirzabekov, T.; Kolchinsky, P.; Wyatt, R.; Cayabyab, M.; Gerard, N.P.; Gerard, C.; Sodroski, J.; Choe, H. Tyrosine sulfation of the amino terminus of CCR5 facilitates HIV-1 entry. *Cell* **1999**, *96*, 667–676. [CrossRef]

143. Farzan, M.; Babcock, G.J.; Vasilieva, N.; Wright, P.L.; Kiprilov, E.; Mirzabekov, T.; Choe, H. The role of post-translational modifications of the CXCR4 amino terminus in stromal-derived factor 1a association and HIV-1 entry. *J. Biol. Chem.* **2002**, *277*, 29484–29489. [CrossRef] [PubMed]

144. Stone, M.J.; Payne, R.J. Homogeneous sulfopeptides and sulfoproteins: Synthetic approaches and applications to characterize the effects of tyrosine sulfation on biochemical function. *Acc. Chem. Res.* **2015**, *48*, 2251–2261. [CrossRef] [PubMed]

145. Simpson, L.S.; Zhu, J.Z.; Widlanski, T.S.; Stone, M.J. Regulation of chemokine recognition by site-specific tyrosine sulfation of receptor peptides. *Chem. Biol.* **2009**, *16*, 153–161. [CrossRef] [PubMed]

146. Zhu, J.Z.; Millard, C.J.; Ludeman, J.P.; Simpson, L.S.; Clayton, D.J.; Payne, R.J.; Widlanski, T.S.; Stone, M.J. Tyrosine sulfation influences the chemokine binding selectivity of peptides derived from chemokine receptor CCR3. *Biochemistry* **2011**, *50*, 1524–1534. [CrossRef] [PubMed]

147. Tan, J.H.Y.; Ludeman, J.P.; Wedderburn, J.; Canals, M.; Hall, P.; Butler, S.J.; Taleski, D.; Christopoulos, A.; Hickey, M.J.; Payne, R.J.; et al. Tyrosine sulfation of chemokine receptor CCR2 enhances interactions with both monomeric and dimeric forms of the chemokine monocyte chemoattractant protein-1 (MCP-1). *J. Biol. Chem.* **2013**, *288*, 10024–10034. [CrossRef] [PubMed]

148. Veldkamp, C.T.; Seibert, C.; Peterson, F.C.; Sakmar, T.P.; Volkman, B.F. Recognition of a CXCR4 sulfotyrosine by the chemokine stromal cell-derived factor-1α (SDF-1α/CXCL12). *J. Mol. Biol.* **2006**, *359*, 1400–1409. [CrossRef] [PubMed]

149. Huma, Z.E.; Ludeman, J.P.; Wilkinson, B.L.; Payne, R.J.; Stone, M.J. NMR characterization of cooperativity: Fast ligand binding coupled to slow protein dimerization. *Chem. Sci.* **2014**, *5*, 2783–2788. [CrossRef]

150. Rajarathnam, K.; Prado, G.N.; Fernando, H.; Clark-Lewis, I.; Navarro, J. Probing receptor binding activity of interleukin-8 dimer using a disulfide trap. *Biochemistry* **2006**, *45*, 7882–7888. [CrossRef] [PubMed]

151. Nasser, M.W.; Raghuwanshi, S.K.; Grant, D.J.; Jala, V.R.; Rajarathnam, K.; Richardson, R.M. Differential activation and regulation of CXCR1 and CXCR2 by CXCL8 monomer and dimer. *J. Immunol.* **2009**, *183*, 3425–3432. [CrossRef] [PubMed]

152. Drury, L.J.; Ziarek, J.J.; Gravel, S.; Veldkamp, C.T.; Takekoshi, T.; Hwang, S.T.; Heveker, N.; Volkman, B.F.; Dwinell, M.B. Monomeric and dimeric CXCL12 inhibit metastasis through distinct CXCR4 interactions and signaling pathways. *Proc. Natl. Acad. Sci. USA* **2011**, *108*, 17655–17660. [CrossRef] [PubMed]

153. Ravindran, A.; Sawant, K.V.; Sarmiento, J.; Navarro, J.; Rajarathnam, K. Chemokine CXCL1 dimer is a potent agonist for the CXCR2 receptor. *J. Biol. Chem.* **2013**, *288*, 12244–12252. [CrossRef] [PubMed]

154. Ravindran, A.; Joseph, P.R.; Rajarathnam, K. Structural basis for differential binding of the interleukin-8 monomer and dimer to the CXCR1 N-domain: Role of coupled interactions and dynamics. *Biochemistry* **2009**, *48*, 8795–8805. [CrossRef] [PubMed]

155. Tan, J.H.Y.; Canals, M.; Ludeman, J.P.; Wedderburn, J.; Boston, C.; Butler, S.J.; Carrick, A.M.; Parody, T.R.; Taleski, D.; Christopoulos, A.; et al. Design and receptor interactions of obligate dimeric mutant of chemokine monocyte chemoattractant protein-1 (MCP-1). *J. Biol. Chem.* **2012**, *287*, 14692–14702. [CrossRef] [PubMed]

156. Jin, H.; Shen, X.; Baggett, B.R.; Kong, X.; LiWang, P.J. The human CC chemokine MIP-1b dimer is not competent to bind to the CCR5 receptor. *J. Biol. Chem.* **2007**, *282*, 27976–27983. [CrossRef] [PubMed]

157. St. Charles, R.; Walz, D.A.; Edwards, B.F. The three-dimensional structure of bovine platelet factor 4 at 3.0-a resolution. *J. Biol. Chem.* **1989**, *264*, 2092–2099.

158. Skelton, N.J.; Aspiras, F.; Ogez, J.; Schall, T.J. Proton NMR assignments and solution conformation of RANTES, a chemokine of the C-C type. *Biochemistry* **1995**, *34*, 5329–5342. [CrossRef] [PubMed]

159. Wang, X.; Watson, C.; Sharp, J.S.; Handel, T.M.; Prestegard, J.H. Oligomeric structure of the chemokine CCL5/RANTES from NMR, MS, and SAXS data. *Structure* **2011**, *19*, 1138–1148. [CrossRef] [PubMed]

160. Zhao, B.; LiWang, P.J. Characterization of the interactions of vMIP-II, and a dimeric variant of vMIP-II, with glycosaminoglycans. *Biochemistry* **2010**, *49*, 7012–7022. [CrossRef] [PubMed]

161. Salanga, C.L.; O'Hayre, M.; Handel, T. Modulation of chemokine receptor activity through dimerization and crosstalk. *Cell. Mol. Life Sci.* **2009**, *66*, 1370–1386. [CrossRef] [PubMed]

162. Yu, Y.; Sweeney, M.D.; Saad, O.M.; Crown, S.E.; Hsu, A.R.; Handel, T.M.; Leary, J.A. Chemokine-glycosaminoglycan binding: Specificity for CCR2 ligand binding to highly sulfated oligosaccharides using FTICR mass spectrometry. *J. Biol. Chem.* **2005**, *280*, 32200–32208. [CrossRef] [PubMed]

163. Nesmelova, I.V.; Sham, Y.; Dudek, A.Z.; van Eijk, L.I.; Wu, G.; Slungaard, A.; Mortari, F.; Griffioen, A.W.; Mayo, K.H. Platelet factor 4 and interleukin-8 CXC chemokine heterodimer formation modulates function at the quaternary structural level. *J. Biol. Chem.* **2005**, *280*, 4948–4958. [CrossRef] [PubMed]

164. Nesmelova, I.V.; Sham, Y.; Gao, J.; Mayo, K.H. CXC and CC chemokines form mixed heterodimers: Association free energies from molecular dynamics simulations and experimental correlations. *J. Biol. Chem.* **2008**, *283*, 24155–24166. [CrossRef] [PubMed]

165. Carlson, J.; Baxter, S.A.; Dreau, D.; Nesmelova, I.V. The heterodimerization of platelet-derived chemokines. *Biochim. Biophys. Acta* **2013**, *1834*, 158–168. [CrossRef] [PubMed]

166. Paavola, C.D.; Hemmerich, S.; Grunberger, D.; Polsky, I.; Bloom, A.; Freedman, R.; Mulkins, M.; Bhakta, S.; McCarley, D.; Wiesent, L.; et al. Monomeric monocyte chemoattractant protein-1 (MCP-1) binds and activates the MCP-1 receptor CCR2B. *J. Biol. Chem.* **1998**, *273*, 33157–33165. [CrossRef] [PubMed]

167. Tuinstra, R.L.; Peterson, F.C.; Kutlesa, S.; Elgin, E.S.; Kron, M.A.; Volkman, B.F. Interconversion between two unrelated protein folds in the lymphotactin native state. *Proc. Natl. Acad. Sci. USA* **2008**, *105*, 5057–5062. [CrossRef] [PubMed]

168. Fox, J.C.; Tyler, R.C.; Guzzo, C.; Tuinstra, R.L.; Peterson, F.C.; Lusso, P.; Volkman, B.F. Engineering metamorphic chemokine lymphotactin/XCL1 into the GAG-binding, HIV-inhibitory dimer conformation. *ACS Chem. Biol.* **2015**, *10*, 2580–2588. [CrossRef] [PubMed]

169. Stephens, B.; Handel, T.M. Chemokine receptor oligomerization and allostery. *Prog. Mol. Biol. Transl. Sci.* **2013**, *115*, 375–420. [PubMed]

170. Kraemer, S.; Alampour-Rajabi, S.; El Bounkari, O.; Bernhagen, J. Hetero-oligomerization of chemokine receptors: Diversity and relevance for function. *Curr. Med. Chem.* **2013**, *20*, 2524–2536. [CrossRef] [PubMed]

171. Munoz, L.M.; Holgado, B.L.; Martinez, A.C.; Rodriguez-Frade, J.M.; Mellado, M. Chemokine receptor oligomerization: A further step toward chemokine function. *Immunol. Lett.* **2012**, *145*, 23–29. [CrossRef] [PubMed]

172. Munoz, L.M.; Lucas, P.; Holgado, B.L.; Barroso, R.; Vega, B.; Rodriguez-Frade, J.M.; Mellado, M. Receptor oligomerization: A pivotal mechanism for regulating chemokine function. *Pharmacol. Ther.* **2011**, *131*, 351–358. [CrossRef] [PubMed]

173. Hernanz-Falcon, P.; Rodriguez-Frade, J.M.; Serrano, A.; Juan, D.; del Sol, A.; Soriano, S.F.; Roncal, F.; Gomez, L.; Valencia, A.; Martinez, A.C.; et al. Identification of amino acid residues crucial for chemokine receptor dimerization. *Nat. Immunol.* **2004**, *5*, 216–223. [CrossRef] [PubMed]

174. Percherancier, Y.; Berchiche, Y.A.; Slight, I.; Volkmer-Engert, R.; Tamamura, H.; Fujii, N.; Bouvier, M.; Heveker, N. Bioluminescence resonance energy transfer reveals ligand-induced conformational changes in CXCR4 homo- and heterodimers. *J. Biol. Chem.* **2005**, *280*, 9895–9903. [CrossRef] [PubMed]

175. El-Asmar, L.; Springael, J.Y.; Ballet, S.; Andrieu, E.U.; Vassart, G.; Parmentier, M. Evidence for negative binding cooperativity within CCR5-CCR2B heterodimers. *Mol. Pharmacol.* **2005**, *67*, 460–469. [CrossRef] [PubMed]

176. Mellado, M.; Rodriguez-Frade, J.M.; Vila-Coro, A.J.; Fernandez, S.; Martin de Ana, A.; Jones, D.R.; Toran, J.L.; Martinez, A.C. Chemokine receptor homo- or heterodimerization activates distinct signaling pathways. *EMBO J.* **2001**, *20*, 2497–2507. [CrossRef] [PubMed]

177. Chakera, A.; Seeber, R.M.; John, A.E.; Eidne, K.A.; Greaves, D.R. The duffy antigen/receptor for chemokines exists in an oligomeric form in living cells and functionally antagonizes CCR5 signaling through hetero-oligomerization. *Mol. Pharmacol.* **2008**, *73*, 1362–1370. [CrossRef] [PubMed]

178. Mustafa, S.; See, H.B.; Seeber, R.M.; Armstrong, S.P.; White, C.W.; Ventura, S.; Ayoub, M.A.; Pfleger, K.D. Identification and profiling of novel α1a-adrenoceptor-CXC chemokine receptor 2 heteromer. *J. Biol. Chem.* **2012**, *287*, 12952–12965. [CrossRef] [PubMed]

179. Suzuki, S.; Chuang, L.F.; Yau, P.; Doi, R.H.; Chuang, R.Y. Interactions of opioid and chemokine receptors: Oligomerization of m, k, and d with CCR5 on immune cells. *Exp. Cell Res.* **2002**, *280*, 192–200. [CrossRef] [PubMed]

180. Pello, O.M.; Martinez-Munoz, L.; Parrillas, V.; Serrano, A.; Rodriguez-Frade, J.M.; Toro, M.J.; Lucas, P.; Monterrubio, M.; Martinez, A.C.; Mellado, M. Ligand stabilization of CXCR4/d-opioid receptor heterodimers reveals a mechanism for immune response regulation. *Eur. J. Immunol.* **2008**, *38*, 537–549. [CrossRef] [PubMed]

181. Parenty, G.; Appelbe, S.; Milligan, G. CXCR2 chemokine receptor antagonism enhances DOP opioid receptor function via allosteric regulation of the CXCR2-DOP receptor heterodimer. *Biochem. J.* **2008**, *412*, 245–256. [CrossRef] [PubMed]

182. Chen, C.; Li, J.; Bot, G.; Szabo, I.; Rogers, T.J.; Liu-Chen, L.Y. Heterodimerization and cross-desensitization between the m-opioid receptor and the chemokine CCR5 receptor. *Eur. J. Pharmacol.* **2004**, *483*, 175–186. [CrossRef] [PubMed]

183. Lefkowitz, R.J. Historical review: A brief history and personal retrospective of seven-transmembrane receptors. *Trends Pharmacol. Sci.* **2004**, *25*, 413–422. [CrossRef] [PubMed]

184. Hamm, H.E. The many faces of G protein signaling. *J. Biol. Chem.* **1998**, *273*, 669–672. [CrossRef] [PubMed]

185. Logothetis, D.E.; Kurachi, Y.; Galper, J.; Neer, E.J.; Clapham, D.E. The b g subunits of GTP-binding proteins activate the muscarinic K+ channel in heart. *Nature* **1987**, *325*, 321–326. [CrossRef] [PubMed]

186. Violin, J.D.; Lefkowitz, R.J. b-arrestin-biased ligands at seven-transmembrane receptors. *Trends Pharmacol. Sci.* **2007**, *28*, 416–422. [CrossRef] [PubMed]
187. DeWire, S.M.; Ahn, S.; Lefkowitz, R.J.; Shenoy, S.K. b-arrestins and cell signaling. *Annu. Rev. Physiol.* **2007**, *69*, 483–510. [CrossRef] [PubMed]
188. Lefkowitz, R.J.; Shenoy, S.K. Transduction of receptor signals by b-arrestins. *Science* **2005**, *308*, 512–517. [CrossRef] [PubMed]
189. Shenoy, S.K.; Drake, M.T.; Nelson, C.D.; Houtz, D.A.; Xiao, K.; Madabushi, S.; Reiter, E.; Premont, R.T.; Lichtarge, O.; Lefkowitz, R.J. b-arrestin-dependent, G protein-independent ERK1/2 activation by the b2 adrenergic receptor. *J. Biol. Chem.* **2006**, *281*, 1261–1273. [CrossRef] [PubMed]
190. Zheng, H.; Chu, J.; Qiu, Y.; Loh, H.H.; Law, P.Y. Agonist-selective signaling is determined by the receptor location within the membrane domains. *Proc. Natl. Acad. Sci. USA* **2008**, *105*, 9421–9426. [CrossRef] [PubMed]
191. Stewart, A.; Fisher, R.A. Introduction: G protein-coupled receptors and RGS proteins. *Prog. Mol. Biol. Transl. Sci.* **2015**, *133*, 1–11. [PubMed]
192. Berman, D.M.; Wilkie, T.M.; Gilman, A.G. GAIP and RGS4 are GTPase-activating proteins for the Gi subfamily of G protein a subunits. *Cell* **1996**, *86*, 445–452. [CrossRef]
193. Ross, E.M.; Wilkie, T.M. GTPase-activating proteins for heterotrimeric G proteins: Regulators of G protein signaling (RGS) and RGS-like proteins. *Annu. Rev. Biochem.* **2000**, *69*, 795–827. [CrossRef] [PubMed]
194. Chini, B.; Parenti, M. G-protein coupled receptors in lipid rafts and caveolae: How, when and why do they go there? *J. Mol. Endocrinol.* **2004**, *32*, 325–338. [CrossRef] [PubMed]
195. Escriba, P.V.; Wedegaertner, P.B.; Goni, F.M.; Vogler, O. Lipid-protein interactions in GPCR-associated signaling. *Biochim. Biophys. Acta* **2007**, *1768*, 836–852. [CrossRef] [PubMed]
196. Ogilvie, P.; Bardi, G.; Clark-Lewis, I.; Baggiolini, M.; Uguccioni, M. Eotaxin is a natural antagonist for CCR2 and an agonist for CCR5. *Blood* **2001**, *97*, 1920–1924. [CrossRef] [PubMed]
197. Martinelli, R.; Sabroe, I.; LaRosa, G.; Williams, T.J.; Pease, J.E. The CC chemokine eotaxin (CCL11) is a partial agonist of CC chemokine receptor 2B. *J. Biol. Chem.* **2001**, *276*, 42957–42964. [CrossRef] [PubMed]
198. Parody, T.R.; Stone, M.J. High level expression, activation, and antagonism of CC chemokine receptors CCR2 and CCR3 in Chinese hamster ovary cells. *Cytokine* **2004**, *27*, 38–46. [CrossRef] [PubMed]
199. Prazeres, D.M.; Martins, S.A. G protein-coupled receptors: An overview of signaling mechanisms and screening assays. *Methods Mol. Biol.* **2015**, *1272*, 3–19. [PubMed]
200. Berchiche, Y.A.; Gravel, S.; Pelletier, M.E.; St-Onge, G.; Heveker, N. Different effects of the different natural CC chemokine receptor 2B ligands on b-arrestin recruitment, G_{ai} signaling, and receptor internalization. *Mol. Pharmacol.* **2011**, *79*, 488–498. [CrossRef] [PubMed]
201. Urban, J.D.; Clarke, W.P.; von Zastrow, M.; Nichols, D.E.; Kobilka, B.; Weinstein, H.; Javitch, J.A.; Roth, B.L.; Christopoulos, A.; Sexton, P.M.; et al. Functional selectivity and classical concepts of quantitative pharmacology. *J Pharmacol Exp Ther* **2007**, *320*, 1–13. [CrossRef] [PubMed]
202. Shonberg, J.; Lopez, L.; Scammells, P.J.; Christopoulos, A.; Capuano, B.; Lane, J.R. Biased agonism at G protein-coupled receptors: The promise and the challenges—A medicinal chemistry perspective. *Med. Res. Rev.* **2014**, *34*, 1286–1330. [CrossRef] [PubMed]
203. Rajagopal, S.; Rajagopal, K.; Lefkowitz, R.J. Teaching old receptors new tricks: Biasing seven-transmembrane receptors. *Nat. Rev. Drug Discov.* **2010**, *9*, 373–386. [CrossRef] [PubMed]
204. Kenakin, T.; Watson, C.; Muniz-Medina, V.; Christopoulos, A.; Novick, S. A simple method for quantifying functional selectivity and agonist bias. *ACS Chem. Neurosci.* **2012**, *3*, 193–203. [CrossRef] [PubMed]
205. Rajagopal, S.; Ahn, S.; Rominger, D.H.; Gowen-MacDonald, W.; Lam, C.M.; Dewire, S.M.; Violin, J.D.; Lefkowitz, R.J. Quantifying ligand bias at seven-transmembrane receptors. *Mol. Pharmacol.* **2011**, *80*, 367–377. [CrossRef] [PubMed]
206. Kenakin, T.; Christopoulos, A. Measurements of ligand bias and functional affinity. *Nat. Rev. Drug Discov.* **2013**, *12*, 483. [CrossRef] [PubMed]
207. Kohout, T.A.; Nicholas, S.L.; Perry, S.J.; Reinhart, G.; Junger, S.; Struthers, R.S. Differential desensitization, receptor phosphorylation, b-arrestin recruitment, and ERK1/2 activation by the two endogenous ligands for the CC chemokine receptor 7. *J. Biol. Chem.* **2004**, *279*, 23214–23222. [CrossRef] [PubMed]

208. Rajagopal, S.; Bassoni, D.L.; Campbell, J.J.; Gerard, N.P.; Gerard, C.; Wehrman, T.S. Biased agonism as a mechanism for differential signaling by chemokine receptors. *J. Biol. Chem.* **2013**, *288*, 35039–35048. [CrossRef] [PubMed]

209. Corbisier, J.; Gales, C.; Huszagh, A.; Parmentier, M.; Springael, J.Y. Biased signaling at chemokine receptors. *J. Biol. Chem.* **2015**, *290*, 9542–9554. [CrossRef] [PubMed]

210. Montaner, S.; Kufareva, I.; Abagyan, R.; Gutkind, S.J. Molecular mechanisms deployed by virally encoded G protein–coupled receptors in human diseases. *Annu. Rev. Pharmacol. Toxicol.* **2013**, *53*, 331–354. [CrossRef] [PubMed]

211. Dagna, L.; Lusso, P. Virus-encoded chemokines, chemokine receptors and chemokine-binding proteins: New paradigms for future therapy. *Futur. Virol.* **2007**, *2*, 353–368. [CrossRef]

212. Vischer, H.F.; Siderius, M.; Leurs, R.; Smit, M.J. Herpesvirus-encoded GPCRs: Neglected players in inflammatory and proliferative diseases? *Nat. Rev. Drug Discov.* **2014**, *13*, 123–139. [CrossRef] [PubMed]

213. Sozzani, S.; Luini, W.; Bianchi, G.; Allavena, P.; Wells, T.N.C.; Napolitano, M.; Bernardini, G.; Vecchi, A.; D'Ambrosio, D.; Mazzeo, D.; et al. The viral chemokine macrophage inflammatory protein-II is a selective Th2 chemoattractant. *Blood* **1998**, *92*, 4036–4039. [PubMed]

214. Gershengorn, M.C.; Geras-Raaka, E.; Varma, A.; Clark-Lewis, I. Chemokines activate Kaposi's sarcoma-associated herpesvirus G protein-coupled receptor in mammalian cells in culture. *J. Clin. Investig.* **1998**, *102*, 1469–1472. [CrossRef] [PubMed]

215. Kledal, T.N.; Rosenkilde, M.M.; Coulin, F.; Simmons, G.; Johnsen, A.H.; Alouani, S.; Power, C.A.; Luttichau, H.R.; Gerstoft, J.; Clapham, P.R.; et al. A broad-spectrum chemokine antagonist encoded by Kaposi's sarcoma-associated herpesvirus. *Science* **1997**, *277*, 1656–1659. [CrossRef] [PubMed]

216. Nijmeijer, S.; Leurs, R.; Smit, M.J.; Vischer, H.F. The Epstein-Barr virus-encoded G protein-coupled receptor BILF1 hetero-oligomerizes with human CXCR4, scavenges G_ai proteins, and constitutively impairs CXCR4 functioning. *J. Biol. Chem.* **2010**, *285*, 29632–29641. [CrossRef] [PubMed]

217. Smith, P.K.; Fallon, R.E.; Mangan, N.E.; Walsh, C.M.; Saraiva, M.; Sayers, J.R.; McKenzie, A.N.J.; Alcami, A.; Fallon, P.G. *Schistosoma mansoni* secretes a chemokine binding protein with anti-inflammatory activity. *J. Exp. Med.* **2005**, *202*, 1319–1325. [CrossRef] [PubMed]

218. Deruaz, M.; Frauenschuh, A.; Alessandri, A.L.; Dias, J.M.; Coelho, F.M.; Russo, R.C.; Ferreira, B.R.; Graham, G.J.; Shaw, J.P.; Wells, T.N.; et al. Ticks produce highly selective chemokine binding proteins with anti-inflammatory activity. *J. Exp. Med.* **2008**, *205*, 2019–2031. [CrossRef] [PubMed]

219. Frauenschuh, A.; Power, C.A.; Deruaz, M.; Ferreira, B.R.; Silva, J.S.; Teixeira, M.M.; Dias, J.M.; Martin, T.; Wells, T.N.; Proudfoot, A.E. Molecular cloning and characterization of a highly selective chemokine-binding protein from the tick *Rhipicephalus sanguineus*. *J. Biol. Chem.* **2007**, *282*, 27250–27258. [CrossRef] [PubMed]

220. Seet, B.T.; McFadden, G. Viral chemokine-binding proteins. *J. Leukoc. Biol.* **2002**, *72*, 24–34. [PubMed]

221. Heidarieh, H.; Hernaez, B.; Alcami, A. Immune modulation by virus-encoded secreted chemokine binding proteins. *Virus Res.* **2015**, *209*, 67–75. [CrossRef] [PubMed]

222. Proudfoot, A.E.; Bonvin, P.; Power, C.A. Targeting chemokines: Pathogens can, why can't we? *Cytokine* **2015**, *74*, 259–267. [CrossRef] [PubMed]

223. Burns, J.M.; Dairaghi, D.J.; Deitz, M.; Tsang, M.; Schall, T.J. Comprehensive mapping of poxvirus vCCI chemokine-binding protein: Expanded range of ligand interactions and unusual dissociation kinetics. *J. Biol. Chem.* **2002**, *277*, 2785–2789. [CrossRef] [PubMed]

224. Carfí, A.; Smith, C.A.; Smolak, P.J.; McGrew, J.; Wiley, D.C. Structure of a soluble secreted chemokine inhibitor vCCI (p35) from cowpox virus. *Proc. Natl. Acad. Sci. USA* **1999**, *96*, 12379–12383. [CrossRef] [PubMed]

225. Zhang, L.; DeRider, M.; McCornack, M.A.; Jao, S.; Isern, N.; Ness, T.; Moyer, R.; LiWang, P.J. Solution structure of the complex between poxvirus-encoded CC chemokine inhibitor vCCI and human MIP-1b. *Proc. Natl. Acad. Sci. USA* **2006**, *103*, 13985–13990. [CrossRef] [PubMed]

226. Bahar, M.W.; Kenyon, J.C.; Putz, M.M.; Abrescia, N.G.; Pease, J.E.; Wise, E.L.; Stuart, D.I.; Smith, G.L.; Grimes, J.M. Structure and function of A41, a vaccinia virus chemokine binding protein. *PLoS Path.* **2008**, *4*, e5. [CrossRef] [PubMed]

227. Xue, X.; Lu, Q.; Wei, H.; Wang, D.; Chen, D.; He, G.; Huang, L.; Wang, H.; Wang, X. Structural basis of chemokine sequestration by CrmD, a poxvirus-encoded tumor necrosis factor receptor. *PLoS Path.* **2011**, *7*. [CrossRef] [PubMed]

228. Alexander, J.M.; Nelson, C.A.; van Berkel, V.; Lau, E.K.; Studts, J.M.; Brett, T.J.; Speck, S.H.; Handel, T.M.; Virgin, H.W.; Fremont, D.H. Structural basis of chemokine sequestration by a herpesvirus decoy receptor. *Cell* **2002**, *111*, 343–356. [CrossRef]

229. Wang, D.; Bresnahan, W.; Shenk, T. Human cytomegalovirus encodes a highly specific RANTES decoy receptor. *Proc. Natl. Acad. Sci. USA* **2004**, *101*, 16642–16647. [CrossRef] [PubMed]

230. Dias, J.M.; Losberger, C.; Deruaz, M.; Power, C.A.; Proudfoot, A.E.; Shaw, J.P. Structural basis of chemokine sequestration by a tick chemokine binding protein: The crystal structure of the complex between evasin-1 and CCL3. *PLoS ONE* **2009**, *4*, e8514. [CrossRef] [PubMed]

231. Pease, J.; Horuk, R. Chemokine receptor antagonists. *J. Med. Chem.* **2012**, *55*, 9363–9392. [CrossRef] [PubMed]

232. Scholten, D.J.; Canals, M.; Maussang, D.; Roumen, L.; Smit, M.J.; Wijtmans, M.; de Graaf, C.; Vischer, H.F.; Leurs, R. Pharmacological modulation of chemokine receptor function. *Br. J. Pharmacol.* **2012**, *165*, 1617–1643. [CrossRef] [PubMed]

233. Dorr, P.; Westby, M.; Dobbs, S.; Griffin, P.; Irvine, B.; Macartney, M.; Mori, J.; Rickett, G.; Smith-Burchnell, C.; Napier, C.; et al. Maraviroc (UK-427,857), a potent, orally bioavailable, and selective small-molecule inhibitor of chemokine receptor CCR5 with broad-spectrum anti-human immunodeficiency virus type 1 activity. *Antimicrob. Agents Chemother.* **2005**, *49*, 4721–4732. [CrossRef] [PubMed]

234. Saita, Y.; Kodama, E.; Orita, M.; Kondo, M.; Miyazaki, T.; Sudo, K.; Kajiwara, K.; Matsuoka, M.; Shimizu, Y. Structural basis for the interaction of CCR5 with a small molecule, functionally selective CCR5 agonist. *J. Immunol.* **2006**, *177*, 3116–3122. [CrossRef] [PubMed]

235. Smith, E.W.; Liu, Y.; Getschman, A.E.; Peterson, F.C.; Ziarek, J.J.; Li, R.; Volkman, B.F.; Chen, Y. Structural analysis of a novel small molecule ligand bound to the CXCL12 chemokine. *J. Med. Chem.* **2014**, *57*, 9693–9699. [CrossRef] [PubMed]

236. Mao-Yu, Z.; Jin-Jian, L.; Wang, L.; Zi-Chao, G.; Hu, H.; Carolina Oi Lam, U.; Yi-Tao, W. Development of monoclonal antibodies in China: Overview and prospects. *BioMed Res. Int.* **2015**, *2015*, 168935. [CrossRef]

237. Klarenbeek, A.; Maussang, D.; Blanchetot, C.; Saunders, M.; van der Woning, S.; Smit, M.; de Haard, H.; Hofman, E. Targeting chemokines and chemokine receptors with antibodies. *Drug Discov. Today Technol.* **2012**, *9*, e237–e244. [CrossRef] [PubMed]

238. Duvic, M.; Evans, M.; Wang, C. Mogamulizumab for the treatment of cutaneous T-cell lymphoma: Recent advances and clinical potential. *Therap. Adv. Hematol.* **2016**, *7*, 171–174. [CrossRef] [PubMed]

239. Griffiths, K.; Dolezal, O.; Cao, B.; Nilsson, S.K.; See, H.B.; Pfleger, K.D.G.; Roche, M.; Gorry, P.R.; Pow, A.; Viduka, K.; et al. I-bodies, human single domain antibodies that antagonize chemokine receptor CXCR4. *J. Biol. Chem.* **2016**, *291*, 12641–12657. [CrossRef] [PubMed]

240. Oberthür, D.; Achenbach, J.; Gabdulkhakov, A.; Buchner, K.; Maasch, C.; Falke, S.; Rehders, D.; Klussmann, S.; Betzel, C. Crystal structure of a mirror-image L-RNA aptamer (Spiegelmer) in complex with the natural L-protein target CCL2. *Nat. Commun.* **2015**, *6*, 6923. [CrossRef] [PubMed]

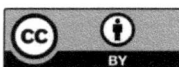

International Journal of
Molecular Sciences

MDPI

Review

Chemokines from a Structural Perspective

Michelle C. Miller and Kevin H. Mayo *

Department of Biochemistry, Molecular Biology & Biophysics, University of Minnesota,
Minneapolis, MN 55455, USA; mill0935@umn.edu
* Correspondence: mayox001@umn.edu; Tel.: +1-612-625-9968, Fax: +1-612-624-5121

Received: 21 August 2017; Accepted: 26 September 2017; Published: 2 October 2017

Abstract: Chemokines are a family of small, highly conserved cytokines that mediate various biological processes, including chemotaxis, hematopoiesis, and angiogenesis, and that function by interacting with cell surface G-Protein Coupled Receptors (GPCRs). Because of their significant involvement in various biological functions and pathologies, chemokines and their receptors have been the focus of therapeutic discovery for clinical intervention. There are several sub-families of chemokines (e.g., CXC, CC, C, and CX3C) defined by the positions of sequentially conserved cysteine residues. Even though all chemokines also have a highly conserved, three-stranded β-sheet/α-helix tertiary structural fold, their quarternary structures vary significantly with their sub-family. Moreover, their conserved tertiary structures allow for subunit swapping within and between sub-family members, thus promoting the concept of a "chemokine interactome". This review is focused on structural aspects of CXC and CC chemokines, their functional synergy and ability to form heterodimers within the chemokine interactome, and some recent developments in structure-based chemokine-targeted drug discovery.

Keywords: chemokine; structure; NMR; heterodimers; interactome

1. Chemokine Structures

Chemokines are a family of small, highly conserved proteins (8 to 12 kDa) involved in many biological processes, including chemotaxis [1], leukocyte degranulation [2], hematopoiesis [3], and angiogenesis [4,5]. Chemokines are usually categorized into sub-families based on the sequential positioning of the first two of four highly conserved cysteine residues: CXC, CC, and CX3C [6]. The C chemokine sub-family is the exception, with only one N-terminal cysteine residue. In the largest subfamilies, CC and CXC, the first two cysteines are adjacent (CC motif) or separated by one amino acid residue (CXC motif). C type chemokines lack the first and third of these cysteines, and CX3C chemokines have three amino acids between the first two cysteine residues. Even though sequence identity between chemokines varies from about 20% to 90%, their sequences overall are highly conserved. Nevertheless, all chemokines adopt essentially the same fold as illustrated in Figure 1 with the superposition of seven chemokines (monomer units): CXCL4, CXCL8, CXCL12, CXCL13, CCL5, CCL14, and CCL20. These structures all consist of a flexible N-terminus and N-terminal loop, followed by a three-stranded antiparallel β-sheet on to which is folded a C-terminal α-helix [7], exemplified early on by CXCL4 [8], CXCL7 [9], CXCL8 [10], and CCL2 [11]. Only atoms within the three-stranded β-sheet have been superimposed (Figure 1A), and RMSD values for backbone atoms of these β-strands range between ~1.3 and ~1.7 Å, with loops being more variable due in part to increased flexibility and differences in amino acid type and number of residues. Note that when the β strands are superimposed, the C-terminal helices are folded onto the β-sheet at somewhat different angles (Figure 1B). The highly conserved cysteine residues (four in CXC and CC chemokines) pair up to form disulfide bridges that are crucial to maintaining structural integrity, which is a prerequisite for chemokine binding to their respective GPCRs [12].

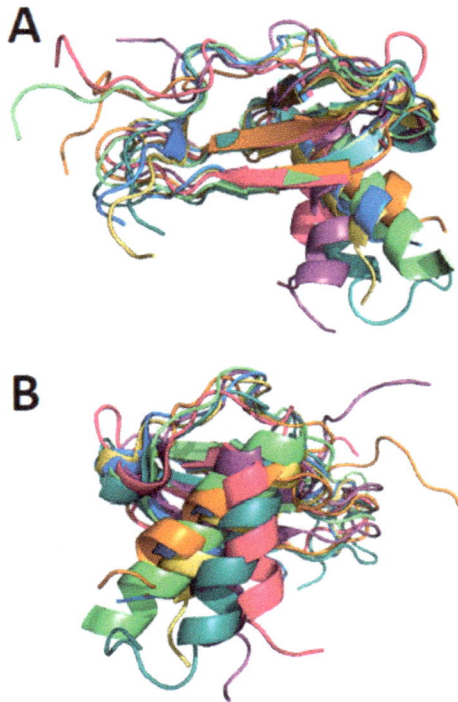

Figure 1. Superposition of seven monomer subunits from reported structures of CXC and CC chemokine homodimers is shown: CXCL4 M2 variant (Protein Data Bank, PDB: 1PFM), CXCL8 (PDB: 1IL8), CXCL12 (PDB: 3HP3), CXCL13 (PDB: 4ZAI), CCL5 (PDB: 5COY), CCL14 (PDB: 2Q8R), and CCL20 (PDB: 1HA6). (**A**) Only atoms within the three-stranded β-sheet are superimposed with RMSD values ranging between ~1.3 and ~1.7 Å; (**B**) Superimposed structures shown in panel A are rotated by about 180° to illustrate how C-terminal helices are folded onto the β-sheet at somewhat different angles.

Chemokine monomers usually associate to form oligomers, primarily dimers, but some are also known to form tetramers [13,14] and higher-order species, e.g., [15,16]. Despite their highly conserved monomer structures, chemokines form different types of oligomer structures depending on the sub-family to which they belong [7]. Within each chemokine sub-family, dimer structures are essentially the same. Figure 2A,B illustrates the dimer structures for CXC chemokine CXCL8 (Interleukin-8 [10]) and CC chemokine CCL5 (RANTES [17]). The more globular CXC-type dimer is formed by interactions between β1 strands from each monomer subunit that extends the three stranded anti-parallel β-sheet from each monomer into a six-stranded β-sheet, on top of which are folded the two C-terminal α-helices, running antiparallel (Figure 2A). On the other hand, CC-type chemokines form elongated end-to end type dimers through contacts between short N-terminal β-strands (labeled βN) with the two C-terminal helices running almost perpendicular to each other on opposite sides of the molecule (Figure 2B). Nevertheless, some CC-type dimer structures like CCL5 have been reported to differ in the relative orientation of some secondary structure elements (e.g., C-terminal α-helices), which may be related to differences in structural dynamics and/or crystal lattice effects [15].

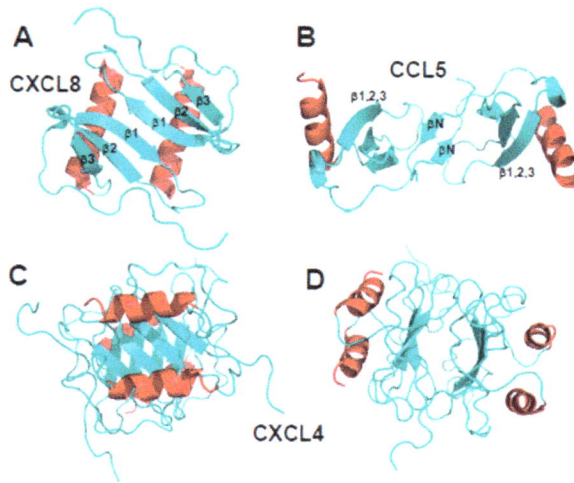

Figure 2. Structures of CXC chemokine CXCL8 (Interleukin-8, PDB access code 1IL8, [10]) (panel **A**) and CC chemokine CCL5 (RANTES, PDB access code 5COY, [17]) (panel **B**) are shown. Two orientations of the CXCL4 M2 tetramer structure (platelet factor-4, PF4; PDB access code 1PFM, [18]) are shown in panels (**C,D**). C-terminal helices are colored red, and the remaining sequences are colored cyan.

An example of a chemokine tetramer formation is shown in Figure 2C,D with the structure of CXCL4 M2 variant (platelet factor-4, [18]). In this example, two CXC-type dimers associate to form a β-sandwich, with the β-sheet of one dimer lying on top of the β-sheet of the other dimer (Figure 2C). The β-sandwich is rotated by ~90° in Figure 2D to better illustrate the contacts between β-sheets and show the center of the CXCL4 tetramer structure. Tetramers have also been observed for other chemokines, e.g., CXCL7 [19]. Moreover, the tetramer structures of different chemokines can vary considerably. For example, two distinct tetramers were reported for CXCL10 [20], one having both CC- and CXC-type dimer topologies and displaying an entirely new conformation. Furthermore, comparison of CXCL4 tetramers [21] and CCL2 tetramers [22] show that they both display CC- and CXC-type dimer motifs.

In other instances, higher order oligomer chemokine structures have not been observed, e.g., CXCL8 or CXCL1 (Growth-related protein-α, Gro-α) (e.g., [23]), but this may be due to the presence of only very low oligomer populations and limitations of experimental techniques used to investigate them. Some CC-type chemokines are not known to form tetramers, yet they do associate to form higher-order oligomers, like CCL5 [15] and CCL27 [16]. Figure 3A illustrates a proposed oligomer structure of CCL5 deduced from analysis of NMR, MS, and SAXS data [15]. This model shows the CCL5 oligomers consisting of chemokine CC-type dimers assemble in a linear fashion. Figure 3B shows the modeled oligomer structure of CCL3 [17], which shows how a CC-type dimer can associate in a somewhat different fashion into a higher order oligomer. Aside from standard CXC- and CC-type inter-subunit interactions seen in the CCL3 oligomer structure (Figure 3B, [17], energetically favorable interactions are also observed between the post-β3 loop of one subunit (Thr43-Arg44-Lys45 and Arg47) and the helix (Glu66) and β1 strand (Glu26-Try27) of the opposing subunit, respectively, suggesting that other types of heterodimers may associate in situ. Nevertheless, whereas these studies underscore the importance of the chemokine CC-type dimer as a building block for larger chemokine oligomers, the idea of a single, well-described dimer structure defining the topology of larger oligomers may be too simplistic.

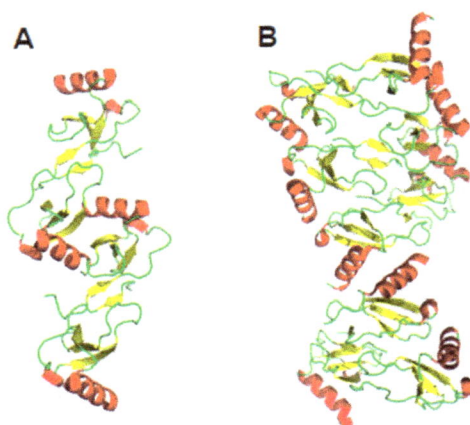

Figure 3. Higher-order oligomer structures of CCL5. (**A**) Proposed oligomer structure of CCL5 deduced from analysis of NMR, MS, and SAXS data (PDB access code: 2L9H, [15]; (**B**) Modeled oligomer structure of CCL3 (PDB access code: 5L2U, [17]) is shown to illustrate how a CC-type dimer could associate in a somewhat different fashion into a higher order oligomer. C-terminal helices are colored red; β-strands are colored yellow, and aperiodic sequences/loops are colored green.

Chemokine monomers, dimers, and higher-order oligomers exist in a complex equilibrium where distinct oligomer structures co-exist and interconvert within a dynamic distribution [15,21,24–28]. For example, distinct co-existing structures have been reported for the monomers and dimers of the chemokines XCL1 and CCL27 [16]. Early on, this was well exemplified by NMR studies on CXCL4 [13,29], low affinity CXCL4 [30], and CXCL7 (platelet basic protein, [19]) and its N-terminal degradation products CTAP-III (connective tissue-activating peptide III) and NAP-2 (neutrophil-activating peptide-2) [31]. In general, the weighting of oligomer populations is dictated by the amino acid composition and conformation of inter-subunit interfaces [32]. This in turn determines the thermodynamic stability of the complexes, with some chemokines forming stronger oligomers and others much weaker ones or remaining as monomers/dimers. This equilibrium distribution can be perturbed by changing solution conditions (e.g., lower pH, buffer type, ionic strength, presence of ligands like heparin) as reported e.g., with CXCL4 [13,29,33], CXCL7 [34], CXCL12 [35,36], and CCL11 [37]. Relatedly, oligomer subunit exchange is the primary reason why not all chemokines can be crystallized or why their structures cannot be solved using NMR spectroscopy.

2. Chemokine Heterodimers

Because chemokine monomer structures are highly conserved, chemokine quaternary structures are determined primarily by the amino acid residues present at the particular inter-subunit interface [32]. Therefore, monomers of different chemokines may be swapped if the arrangement and composition of residues at a given monomer–monomer interface in a heterodimer make for an energetically favorable state relative to that in either homodimer. Indeed, Guan et al. [38] demonstrated that CC chemokines CCL3/4 and CCL2/8 (macrophage inflammatory protein 1α (MIP-1α) and 1β (MIP-1β), respectively) form heterodimers in vitro, as well as being secreted as heterodimers from activated human monocytes and peripheral blood lymphocytes, suggesting that this CC chemokine-based heterodimer may impact on intracellular signaling via binding to, and activation of, its receptor CCR5 [38]. It has also been shown that at least three members of the CXC chemokine sub-family, CXCL4, its N-terminal chimera PF4-M2 [18], and CXCL8, readily exchange subunits to form heterodimers that exhibit similar equilibrium dimerization constants (K_d) as observed for homodimers [39,40]. CXC and CC chemokine heterodimers (i.e., CXCL4 and CCL5) were also shown to form in cells in culture, as well as in vivo [41,42].

Nesmelova et al. [32] explored the energetic basis for heterodimerization of CXC and CC chemokines by using molecular mechanics and the Poisson–Boltzmann surface area (MM-PBSA) approach to calculate binding free energies and to predict which pairs of CXC and CC chemokines would likely form in solution. This study indicated that heterodimers within and between members of CXC and CC sub-families can occur. Calculations were done to assess also which type of heterodimer might form, i.e., CXC-type vs. CC-type heterodimers. In this regard, it was reported that CXCL4 could make thermodynamically favorable interactions with CXCL1, CXCL7, and CXCL8, as well as CXCL1/L8, CXCL7/L8 and CXCL1/L7, with all pairs forming only CXC-type dimers. CC chemokine CCL2 could also favorably pair up with CCL5 and CCL8, with CXC-type heterodimers being favored with the CCL2/CCL8 pair. Several CXC/CC mixed chemokine pairs were also examined, with CCL2/CXCL4 and CCL2/CXCL8 favoring CXC-type heterodimer formation, and CCL5/CXCL4 greatly favoring the CC-type dimer, and CXCL8/CCL5 forming either equally well. Modeled structures of the CCXL4/CCL5 heterodimer are shown in Figure 4A,B for both CXC- and CC-type dimers, with the CC-type heterodimer being highly energetically favored over the CXC-type heterodimer. Some of these, like the CXCL4/CCL5 heterodimer, have been experimentally validated in vitro and/or in vivo [42].

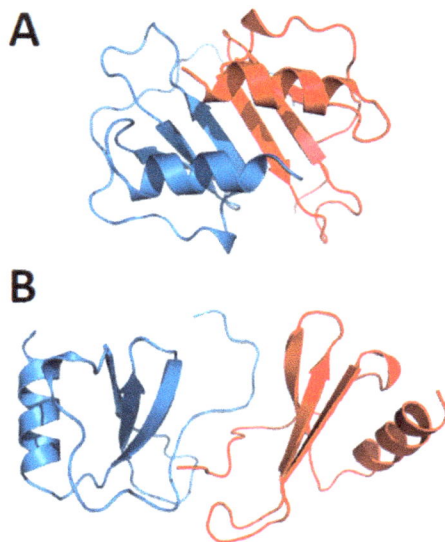

Figure 4. Modeled structures of CXCL4/CCL5 heterodimers. These structures are based on NMR chemical shift and intensity changes from HSQC experiments on CXCL4 and CCL5. NMR data were used to direct manual docking and energy minimization using Molecular Dynamics (MD) simulations, as discussed in von Hundelshausen et al. [42]. MD simulations and energy minimization were done with CCL5 and CXCL4 monomer subunits initially docked as a CXC-type dimer (**A**) or a CC-type dimer (**B**), with the CC-type heterodimer being energetically favored. CXCL4 monomer subunits are shown in red, and CCL5 monomer subunits are shown in blue. These structures were produced by Dr. Kanin Wichapong, Maastricht University, The Netherlands.

Chemokines bind strongly and specifically to glycosaminoglycans (GAGs) [27,43–46] that are comprised of sulfated LacNAc disaccharide repeat units and can vary in chain length and sulfation pattern. For example, CCL5 homo-dimers interact with GAGs in a specific manner [47–49], with

GAG binding affinity depending on both the type of GAG and its sulfation pattern [49]. This has also been reported for CCL2 [50] and CCL11 [43]. In general, highly negatively charged GAGs interact electrostatically with positively charged amino acid residues in chemokines. Contrary to some CXCL4/GAG binding models, which center around the cluster of lysines within the chemokine C-terminal α-helix, Mayo et al. [51] used NMR and site-directed mutagenesis to demonstrate that the loop containing Arg20, Arg22, His23 and Thr25, as well as Lys46 and Arg49, play a greater role in GAG/heparin binding. Moreover, even though electrostatic interactions are understood to play a key role in GAG binding to chemokines, other forces also contribute to their binding specificity (e.g., CXCL4, [51] and XCL1, [52]).

Chemokine homo-oligomers have also been known for some time for their ability to bind relatively strongly to GAGs [48], and conversely, binding to GAGs can induce chemokine homo-oligomer formation, as exemplified by CCL5 homo-oligomer formation [27,53,54]. GAG binding can also have a significant effect on chemokine structure [27,50], structural dynamics [47], homo-oligomerization [55], and chemokine receptor dimerization, e.g., CCR2 [56]. For example, Rek et al. [27] reported that CCL5 undergoes a structural transition upon GAG binding, and Verkaar et al. [57] found that GAG binding affects chemokine cooperativity. Furthermore, Mikhailov et al. [23] demonstrated early on that heparin dodecasaccharide binding to CXCL4 induces higher-order oligomer formation that is dependent upon the chemokine:GAG molar ratio.

Chemokine hetero-oligomers are also stabilized by binding to GAGs [24]. Crown et al. [56] characterized the effects of GAG binding on heterodimerization of CCR2 ligands CCL2 (MCP-1), CCL8 (MCP-2), CCL7 (MCP-3), CCL13 (MCP-4), and CCL11 (eotaxin). These authors reported that CCL2 and CCL8 form strong and specific CC-type heterodimers, whereas CCL2/CCL13, CCL2/CCL11, and CCL8/CCL13 heterodimers are only moderately stable, and CCL7 did not form heterodimers with any other CCR2 chemokine ligand. Moreover, heterodimer formation was enhanced by chemokine binding to GAGs (heparin pentasaccharide, Arixtra). In their study, Arixtra promoted formation of CCL8/CCL11 and CCL2/CCL11 heterodimers, which otherwise either did not form or formed only weakly.

3. Functional Impact of Chemokine Structure

Chemokines play a significant role in biology and are involved in many pathologic disorders, including cancer, HIV/AIDS, and atherosclerosis [58–60]. About fifty chemokines are involved in various aspects of cell interactions and communication with the immune system. In general, chemokines trigger their functional activities by binding to cell surface G-protein coupled receptors (GPCRs) [61–64]. For example, CXCL12 binds to and activates the CXCR4 receptor; CXCL7 (platlet basic protein and its *N*-terminal degradation product NAP-2) signals through both CXCR1 and CXCR2 receptors, and CXCL9, CXCL10 and CXCL11 work through CXCR3 receptor [65].

The best way to understand how chemokines function on their respective receptors is through a structural knowledge of the chemokine ligand/receptor complex [66]. However, the determination of high-resolution structures of chemokine ligand/receptor complexes is highly challenging, and no such structures are presently available. Nevertheless, structural biology plays a major role in delineating how chemokines interact with their GPCR receptors, which in turn relates to how chemokines trigger cell signaling, information that is crucial to designing chemokine antagonists. Given the size of GPCRs and the general difficulties of working with them in vitro, little is known about which residues within any GPCR direct chemokine ligand binding. However, existing evidence indicates that the N termini of some GPCRs are involved in binding chemokine ligands [67–71].

Most studies have focused on defining those residues within the chemokine ligands themselves that are primarily responsible for binding to and activating GPCRs. In particular, the tripeptide ELR sequence (Glu-Leu-Arg) within the dynamic N-terminus of some CXC chemokines was determined to be crucial for interactions with GPCRs. In terms of function, CXC chemokines with the ELR motif (ELR1: CXCL1, 2, 3, 5, 6, 7, 8) generally promote angiogenesis and those lacking the ELR motif

(ELR2: CXCL4, 9, 10) have angiostatic properties [5,72]. Residues within the N-loop between the two N-terminal cysteines, as well as in the helix, can also be involved in GPCR binding [14,73]. Even though the Arg-Phe-Phe-Arg-Glu-Ser-His sequence within this region of CXCL12 is important for receptor binding affinity [74], this is not always the case, and a number of residues throughout the surface of other chemokines have been found to be crucial for receptor binding. In CXCL10 and CCL2, the loops between β-strands are also important for high-affinity receptor binding [71,75]. Binding interactions can also vary depending on the chemokine and which GPCR is involved in their interplay.

Recently, Handel et al. and Volkman et al. have taken the lead in studies aimed at defining structurally crucial interactions between chemokine ligands and their respective GPCRs. Hemmerich et al. [71] showed early on, using primarily mutagenesis studies, that the complex between CCR2 and CCL2 was mediated in part by a few basic amino acid residues in CCL2 and acidic residues (particularly a DYDY tyrosine sulfation motif) in CCR2. Their model suggests that the DYDY motif might bind to a basic residue pocket on CCL2. Such electrostatic interactions from acidic and basic side chains that were also found to be important within the CXCR4:vCCL2 complex [76,77]. vCCL2 (viral macrophage inflammatory protein-II) is expressed by human herpes virus-8 and can bind to multiple chemokine receptors, including CCR5 and CXCR4, thus vCCL2 is quite interesting due to its ability to inhibit HIV infection.

Other studies have reported on chemokine ligand interactions with CXCR4 and CCR2. Ziarek et al. [78] merged information on the NMR-derived structure of a constitutively monomeric CXCL12 variant bound to the amino terminus of CXCR4 with a crystal structure of the trans-membrane domain of CXCR4. Their work showed that the CXCL12:CXCR4 interface allowed previously unknown interactions to be identified, which raised questions about the classical "two-site model" for chemokine-receptor recognition. Moreover, the study demonstrated that the CXCR4 contacts with monomeric CXCL12 were different from those made by dimeric CXCL12, which only stimulates GPCR-dependent signaling.

Using a different approach, Kufareva et al. [79] employed disulfide trapping to identify how chemokines bind their receptors in order to guide molecular modeling. Early attempts in disulfide crosslinking between CXCR4 and CXCL12 were guided by the NMR structure of a CXCL12 dimer in complex with a 38-residue peptide isolated from the N-terminus of CXCR4 (CRS1) [80]. This work with CXCL12 and CXCR4 was recently continued with a combination of computational modeling, functional assays, and biophysical approaches to assess the stoichiometry and geometry of the interaction in this chemokine ligand/receptor pair [81]. In fact, their cysteine trapping experiments allowed residue proximities to be derived enabling construction and validation of a 1:1 receptor:chemokine model consistent with the two-site model of receptor activation and accumulating evidence supporting monomers as the minimal functional unit of binding to GPCRs [81].

Nevertheless, the simple two-site model in chemokine receptor signal transduction may be inadequate to explain chemokine function in all instances, and new paradigms are required [82]. For example, chemokine monomers and homodimers can interact with and activate their cell surface receptors somewhat differently, as exemplified with CXCL12 where its oligomer state directs the inhibition of metastasis through distinct CXCR4 interactions and signaling pathways [83]. Moreover, chemokine activities can be quite varied. For example, while CXCL9 and CXCL10 both have potent antitumor activities through attraction of cytotoxic T lymphocytes and inhibition of angiogenesis, CXCL11 is more potent in terms of its antitumor activity [84]. The modulation of chemokine responses in terms of synergy and cooperativity has been nicely reviewed by Proudfoot et al. [85].

Understanding chemokine structure-function relationships has been complicated by reports that chemokine heterodimers and/or hetero-oligomers can also form and are associated with some cellular responses [25,32,38–42,86–88]. This has been demonstrated e.g., with the formation of the CXCL8/CXCL4 heterodimer, which enhances both CXCL4-induced endothelial cell proliferation, and CXCL8-induced migration of Baf3 cells [40]. The presence of angiogenic CXCL8 in solution with the angiostatic chemokine CXCL4 increases the anti-proliferative activity of CXCL4 against endothelial cells [40]. In addition, the co-presence of CXCL4 and CXCL8, in turn, attenuates the CXCL8-mediated rise in intracellular calcium in the amyloid progenitor cell line and enhances CXCL8-induced migration of bone-marrow-derived pro-B-cells (Baf/3) [39,40]. Moreover, heterodimerization between members of the CXC and CC sub-families has also been reported with CXCL4 and CCL5 [41,42,86], as well as with CCL21 (secondary lymphoid tissue chemokine) and CXCL13 (B cell attracting chemokine-1) [25]. The functional result is that hetero-dimerization dramatically modulates biological activities of these chemokines in vitro and in vivo. In this regard, chemokine heterodimerization can modulate the overall signaling response of GPCRs, thereby providing a general mechanism for regulating chemokine function. The recent synthesis and in vitro/in vivo testing of a covalently-linked CXCL4/CCL5 heterodimer has validated the functional relevance of chemokine heterodimers in GPCR-mediated signal transduction [42,89].

GAGs are essential to chemokine function in vivo [54], and their structures and localization are altered after injury and during inflammation [90,91]. While the exact role of GAGs is quite diverse, it appears that chondroitin sulfate can induce a specific CCL5/CXCL4 hetero-oligomer structure that promotes atherosclerosis [41,86]. The exact molecular structure of this "active" CCL5/CXCL4 heterooligomer is unknown. The possibility of functionally relevant, structurally distinct oligomer conformations as a result of GAG/chemokine interactions has previously been postulated [47,92]. For some chemokines, homo-oligomerization is coupled to GAG binding, e.g., CCL5 and CCL3 [93]. Mikhailov et al. [23] demonstrated early on that GAG (heparin dodecasaccharide) binding to CXCL4 induces higher-order oligomer formation, dependent upon the chemokine:GAG molar ratio, which can lead to the development of thrombocytopenia. Although the role of higher-order chemokine oligomers has been widely recognized to play a role in cell signal transduction, their mechanism of action is poorly understood.

Even though there is evidence that chemokine heterodimers and/or hetero-oligomers impact biological activity, this does not exclude the occurrence of individual chemokines working in concert on their respective GPCRs to elicit synergistic effects. In fact, Gouwy et al. [94–96] have shown that blocking one of the two chemokine receptors negates synergistic interactions, suggesting that synergy requires each chemokine to bind to its respective cell receptor leading to intra-cellular signaling. Gouwy et al. [94] reported that CXCR4 and CCR5 ligands cooperate in monocyte and lymphocyte migration and in the inhibition of dual-tropic (R5/X4) HIV-1 infection. Gouwy et al. [96] demonstrated that chemokines and other GPCR ligands synergize in receptor-mediated migration of monocyte-derived immature and mature dendritic cells. These authors also observed synergy between chemokines and chemotactic non-chemokine GPCR agonists, including fMLP, C5a and SAA. In view of these results, it is likely that there are several ways to obtain synergy between these chemo-attractants [97].

4. Chemokine Antagonists

Given the important roles that chemokines and their cell surface GPCR receptors play in biology and pathological disorders, a number of chemokines and their GPCR partners have become targets for therapeutic drug development [98–100]. Moreover, because chemokines are major players in inflammation, pathological disorders that involve chemokines in tissue inflammation, primarily via leukocyte recruitment and activation, have been central to these efforts [101]. Various strategies have been used to intervene with chemokine systems for therapeutic purposes [102]. Knowledge of chemokine oligomer structures [103] and how chemokines interact with their receptors (see above) has been crucial to the development of chemokine antagonists. Here, we provide a limited presentation of some of these, and discuss how targeting chemokine hetero-oligomers may be another fruitful approach going forward.

One of the major strategies in this field has been the direct inhibition of GPCRs. Small molecule inhibitors targeting chemokine receptors CCR3 and CCR4 have been reported to attenuate lung inflammation in animal models [104–106]. A modest effect targeting CXCL8 with a mAb has been reported in a Phase II clinical trial against chronic obstructive pulmonary disease (COPD) [107].

However, this approach targeted the free CXCL8 ligand and not the ligand-receptor bound state, which is likely to be the actual "bioactive" state, thus possibly explaining the limited success using this mAb. In the rheumatoid arthritis arena, two inhibitors have shown promise: one is a CCR2/CCL2 inhibitor INCB3344 [108] and the other is a monomeric variant P8A-CCL2 antagonist [109]. However, both agents had mixed results. In fact, anti-CCR2 depleting antibody MC-21 actually exacerbated the disease [110], and three phase II clinical trials using an anti-MCP-1 antibody, an anti-CCR2 antibody, and a CCR2 inhibitor [111] all failed.

Overall, the development of highly effective chemokine antagonists has been slow. Part of the problem is that most chemokine/receptor interactions are not very selective [60,112], and thus there has been limited success in the clinic. Nevertheless, recent success with the anti-HIV drug Maraviroc has underscored the therapeutic value of interfering with chemokines in receptor binding and cell signaling [113]. There are some other exceptions that have shown potential. For example, the orally active, small molecule inhibitor CCX282-B, which targets CCR9, has shown efficacy in a colitis model in animals [114], as well as promising results in clinical trials against colitis. CCR5 and CXCR3 are central to alloimmune responses and thus are potential targets for post-transplant immunosuppression, and another small molecule antagonist of CCR5 (TAK-779) has been shown to prolong allograft survival in transplant models by attenuating recruitment of $CD4^+$, $CD8^+$ and $CD11^+$ cells and to attenuate development of chronic vasculopathy, fibrosis, and cellular infiltration [115].

Using a quite different approach, others have demonstrated that DNA viruses can control the immune response to infection by expressing chemokine ligand [116,117] and receptor [118] homologs, as well as small chemokine-binding compounds [119]. Phage display has been used to identify the pharmacophore of CC chemokine-binding proteins Evasin-1 and -4 with the goal of developing novel drugs to target this system [120]. Another interesting approach is to "lock" a chemokine ligand into its homodimer structure, as exemplified by CXCL12 [121]. Due to enhanced serum stability, this dimeric CXCL12 variant was shown to inhibit pulmonary metastasis of CXCR4-expressing melanoma cells. CXCL12 is a popular target for drug development, as exemplified with a structure-based drug design approach leading to the development of an interesting CXCL12 antagonist [122,123]. Relatedly, Ziarek et al. [124] employed a fragment-based strategy to optimize small molecule CXCL12 inhibitors that antagonize the CXCL12/CXCR4 interaction. More recently, analysis of the CCR2 structure has led to the identification of orthosteric and allosteric antagonists of this receptor [125].

Another approach has exploited GAG–chemokine binding [126]. Evidence indicates that functional and tissue-specific selectivity are introduced into the chemokine system via the formation of chemokine oligomers that are modulated by GAG binding [54,57]. Nellen et al. [127] reported that interference with CCL5 oligomerization and GAG binding improves liver injury. Heparin oligosaccharides have been used to inhibit CXCL12-mediated cardio-protection by binding to the chemokine dimerization interface to promote oligomerization and compete with binding to the N-terminus of its receptor CXCR4 [128]. Another polysaccharide-related approach is use of a 30 kDa secreted protein, TSG-6, a member of the hyaluronan-binding protein family (hyaladherins) that contains a hyaluronan-binding LINK domain. TSG-6 inhibits neutrophil migration via direct interaction with CXCL8 [129].

Even though early reports of chemokine heterodimers [32,38–40] were somewhat controversial in terms of their biological relevance, this concept has been validated experimentally and does present a novel paradigm for designing chemokine antagonists [40–42]. Koenen et al. [41] reported on the use of CCL5-derived peptides, e.g., CKEY, that function as chemokine heterodimer agonists. The term "chemokine interactome" was recently introduced to promote the chemokine heterodimer concept and present further empirical evidence as to which CXC and CC chemokines interact physically with each other [42]. This large sampling of chemokines demonstrated that not all of them have the potential to form hetero-oligomers, which imparts selectivity to interactions between mixed chemokines. Moreover, the GAG chondroitin sulfate appears to induce a specific CCL5/CXCL4 heterodimer that enhances atherosclerotic development [41,86]. Evidence suggests that this "active" form of CCL5:CXCL4 is a promising target for therapeutic intervention selective to sites of atherosclerotic lesions [41]. Based on these studies, other chemokine-derived peptides were designed and shown to be effective chemokine antagonists [42]. However, it was the design and synthesis of a covalently-linked CXCL4/CCL5 heterodimer [89] that has provided the most compelling evidence in vitro and in vivo it validated the biological relevance of chemokine heterodimers [42]. These studies may contribute to the development and promise of novel chemokine antagonists for use in the clinic.

Note: Given the breadth of the chemokine field and the numerous labs involved in it, we apologize for the inadvertent omission of many excellent works.

Conflicts of Interest: The authors declare no conflict of interest.

References

1. Baggiolini, M. Chemokines and leukocyte traffic. *Nature* **1998**, *392*, 565–568. [CrossRef] [PubMed]
2. Mackay, C.R. Chemokines:Immunology's high impact factors. *Nat. Immunol.* **2001**, *2*, 95–101. [CrossRef] [PubMed]
3. Youn, B.S.; Mantel, C.; Broxmeyer, H.E. Chemokines, chemokine receptors and hematopoiesis. *Immunol. Rev.* **2000**, *177*, 150–174. [CrossRef] [PubMed]
4. Koch, A.E.; Polverini, P.J.; Kunkel, S.L.; Harlow, L.A.; DiPietro, L.A.; Elner, V.M.; Elner, S.G.; Strieter, R.M. Interleukin-8 as a macrophage-derived mediator of angiogenesis. *Science* **1992**, *258*, 1798–1801. [CrossRef]
5. Belperio, J.A.; Keane, M.P.; Arenberg, D.A.; Addison, C.L.; Ehlert, J.E.; Burdick, M.D.; Strieter, R.M. CXC Chemokines in Angiogenesis. *J. Leukoc. Biol.* **2000**, *68*, 1–8. [PubMed]
6. Zlotnik, A.; Yoshie, O. Chemokines: A new classification system and their role in immunity. *Immunity* **2000**, *12*, 121–127. [CrossRef]
7. Clore, G.M.; Gronenborn, A.M. Three-dimensional structures of alpha and beta chemokines. *FASEB J.* **1995**, *9*, 57–62. [PubMed]
8. St. Charles, R.; Walz, D.A.; Edwards, B.F. Crystal structure of bovine platelet factor-4. *J. Biol. Chem.* **1989**, *264*, 2092–2099.
9. Mayo, K.H.; Yang, Y.; Daly, T.J.; Barry, J.K.; La Rosa, G.J. Secondary Structure of Neutrophil Activating Peptide-2 Determined by ^{1}H-NMR Spectroscopy. *Biochem. J.* **1994**, *303*, 371–376. [CrossRef]
10. Clore, G.M.; Appella, E.; Yamada, M.; Matsushima, K.; Gronenborn, A.M. Three dimensional structure of interleukin 8 in solution. *Biochemistry* **1990**, *29*, 1689–1696. [CrossRef] [PubMed]
11. Handel, T.M.; Domaille, P.J. Heteronuclear (^{1}H, ^{13}C, ^{15}N) NMR assignments and solution structure of the monocyte chemoattractant protein-1 (MCP-1) dimer. *Biochemistry* **1996**, *35*, 6569–6584. [CrossRef] [PubMed]
12. Thomas, M.A.; Buelow, B.J.; Nevins, A.M.; Jones, S.E.; Peterson, F.C.; Gundry, R.L.; Grayson, M.H.; Volkman, B.F. Structure-function analysis of CCL28 in the development of post-viral asthma. *J. Biol. Chem.* **2015**, *290*, 4528–4536. [CrossRef] [PubMed]
13. Mayo, K.H.; Chen, M.-J. Human Platelet Factor 4 Monomer- Dimer-Tetramer Equilibria Investigated by NMR Spectroscopy. *Biochemistry* **1989**, *28*, 9469–9478. [CrossRef] [PubMed]
14. Clark-Lewis, I.; Kim, K.S.; Rajarathnam, K.; Gong, J.H.; Dewald, B.; Moser, B.; Baggiolini, M.; Sykes, B.D. Structure-activity relationships of chemokines. *J. Leukoc. Biol.* **1995**, *57*, 703–711. [PubMed]
15. Wang, X.; Watson, C.; Sharp, J.S.; Handel, T.M.; Prestegard, J.H. Oligomeric structure of the chemokine CCL5/RANTES from NMR, MS, and SAXS data. *Structure* **2011**, *19*, 1138–1148. [CrossRef] [PubMed]
16. Jansma, A.L.; Kirkpatrick, J.P.; Hsu, A.R.; Handel, T.M.; Nietlispach, D. NMR analysis of the structure, dynamics, and unique oligomerization properties of the chemokine CCL27. *J. Biol. Chem.* **2010**, *285*, 14424–14437. [CrossRef] [PubMed]
17. Liang, W.G.; Triandafillou, C.G.; Huang, T.Y.; Zulueta, M.M.; Banerjee, S.; Dinner, A.R.; Hung, S.C.; Tang, W.J. Crystal structure of CC chemokine 5 (CCL5). *Proc. Natl. Acad. Sci. USA* **2016**, *113*, 5000–5005. [CrossRef] [PubMed]
18. Mayo, K.H.; Roongta, V.; Barker, S.; Milius, R.; Ilyina, E.; Quinlan, C.; La Rosa, G.; Daly, T. NMR Solution Structure of the 32 kD Tetrameric Platelet Factor-4 ELR-Motif N-terminal Chimer: A Symmetric Tetramer. *Biochemistry* **1995**, *34*, 11399–11409. [CrossRef] [PubMed]

19. Yang, Y.; Mayo, K.H.; Daly, T.; Barry, J.K.; La Rosa, G.J. Subunit Association and Structural Analysis of Platelet Basic Protein and Related Proteins Investigated by ^{1}H-NMR Spectroscopy and Circular Dichroism. *J. Biol. Chem.* **1994**, *269*, 20110–20118. [PubMed]

20. Swaminathan, G.J.; Holloway, D.E.; Colvin, R.A.; Campanella, G.K.; Papageorgiou, A.C.; Luster, A.D.; Acharya, K.R. Crystal Structures of Oligomeric Forms of the IP-10/CXCL10 Chemokine. *Structure* **2003**, *11*, 521–532. [CrossRef]

21. Zhang, X.; Chen, L.; Bancroft, D.P.; Lai, C.K.; Maione, T.E. Crystal structure of recombinant human platelet factor 4. *Biochemistry* **1994**, *33*, 8361–8366. [CrossRef] [PubMed]

22. Lubkowski, J.; Bujacz, G.; Boqué, L.; Domaille, P.J.; Handel, T.M.; Wlodawer, A. The structure of MCP-1 in two crystal forms provides a rare example of variable quaternary interactions. *Nat. Struct. Biol.* **1997**, *4*, 64–69. [CrossRef] [PubMed]

23. Mikhailov, D.V.; Young, H.; Linhardt, R.J.; Mayo, K.H. Heparin Dodecasaccharide Binding to Platelet Factor-4 and Growth-related Protein-α: Induction of a Partially Folded State and Implications for Heparin-Induced Thrombocytopenia. *J. Biol. Chem.* **1999**, *274*, 25317–25329. [CrossRef] [PubMed]

24. Jansma, A.; Handel, T.M.; Hamel, D.J. Chapter 2. Homo- and hetero-oligomerization of chemokines. *Methods Enzymol.* **2009**, *461*, 31–50. [PubMed]

25. Paoletti, S.; Petkovic, V.; Sebastiani, S.; Danelon, M.G.; Uguccioni, M.; Gerber, B.O. A rich chemokine environment strongly enhances leukocyte migration and activities. *Blood* **2005**, *105*, 3405–3412. [CrossRef] [PubMed]

26. Campanella, G.S.; Grimm, J.; Manice, L.A.; Colvin, R.A.; Medoff, B.D.; Wojtkiewicz, G.R.; Weissleder, R.; Luster, A.D. Oligomerization of CXCL10 Is Necessary for Endothelial Cell Presentation and In Vivo Activity. *J. Immunol.* **2006**, *177*, 6991–6998. [CrossRef] [PubMed]

27. Rek, A.; Brandner, B.; Geretti, E.; Kungl, A.J. A biophysical insight into the RANTES–glycosamino- glycan interaction. *Biochim. Biophys. Acta* **2009**, *1794*, 577–582. [CrossRef] [PubMed]

28. Ren, M.; Guo, Q.; Guo, L.; Lenz, M.; Qian, F.; Koenen, R.R.; Xu, H.; Schilling, A.B.; Weber, C.; Ye, R.D.; et al. Polymerization of MIP-1 chemokine (CCL3 and CCL4) and clearance of MIP1 by insulin-degrading enzyme. *EMBO J.* **2010**, *29*, 3952–3966. [CrossRef] [PubMed]

29. Chen, M.J.; Mayo, K.H. Human Platelet Factor 4 Subunit Association-Dissociation Thermodynamics and Kinetics. *Biochemistry* **1991**, *30*, 6402–6411. [CrossRef] [PubMed]

30. Mayo, K.H. Low Affinity Platelet Factor 4 1H-NMR Derived Aggregate Equilibria Indicate Physiological Preference for Monomers over Dimers and Tetramers. *Biochemistry* **1991**, *30*, 925–934. [CrossRef] [PubMed]

31. Young, H.; Roongta, V.; Daly, T.J.; Mayo, K.H. NMR Structure and Dynamics of Monomeric Neutrophil Activating Peptide-2. *Biochem. J.* **1999**, *338*, 591–598. [CrossRef] [PubMed]

32. Nesmelova, I.V.; Sham, Y.; Gao, J.; Mayo, K.H. CXC-chemokines associate with CC-chemokines to form mixed heterodimers: Rantes and PF4 monomers associate as CC-type heterodimers. *J. Biol. Chem.* **2008**, *283*, 24155–24166. [CrossRef] [PubMed]

33. Yang, Y.; Mayo, K.H. Alcohol-Induced Protein Folding Transitions in Platelet Factor- 4: The O-State. *Biochemistry* **1993**, *32*, 8661–8671. [CrossRef] [PubMed]

34. Yang, Y.; Barker, S.; Chen, M.-J.; Mayo, K.H. Effect of Low Molecular Weight Aliphatic Alcohols and Related Compounds on Platelet Factor-4 Subunit Association. *J. Biol. Chem.* **1993**, *268*, 9223–9229. [PubMed]

35. Veldkamp, C.T.; Ziarek, J.J.; Su, J.; Basnet, H.; Lennertz, R.; Weiner, J.J.; Peterson, F.C.; Baker, J.E.; Volkman, B.F. Monomeric structure of the cardio-protective chemokine SDF-1/CXCL12. *Protein Sci.* **2009**, *18*, 1359–1369. [CrossRef] [PubMed]

36. Veldkamp, C.T.; Peterson, F.C.; Pelzek, A.J.; Volkman, B.F. The monomer-dimer equilibrium of stromal cell-derived factor-1 (CXCL12) is altered by pH, phosphate, sulfate, and heparin. *Protein Sci.* **2005**, *14*, 1071–1081. [CrossRef] [PubMed]

37. Crump, M.P.; Rajarathnam, K.; Kim, K.-S.; Clark-Lewis, I.; Sykes, B.D. Solution Structure of Eotaxin, a Chemokine That Selectively Recruits Eosinophils in Allergic Inflammation. *J. Biol. Chem.* **1998**, *273*, 22471–22479. [CrossRef] [PubMed]

38. Guan, E.; Wang, J.; Norcross, M.A. Identification of Human Macrophage Inflammatory Proteins 1alpha and 1beta as a Native Secreted Heterodimer. *J. Biol. Chem.* **2001**, *276*, 12404–12409. [CrossRef] [PubMed]

39. Dudek, A.Z.; Nesmelova, I.; Mayo, K.H.; Verfaillie, C.M.; Pitchford, E.; Slungaard, A. Platelet Factor 4 Promotes Adhesion of Hematopoietic Progenitor Cells and Binds IL-8: Novel Mechanisms for Modulation of Hematopoiesis. *Blood* **2003**, *101*, 4687–4694. [CrossRef] [PubMed]

40. Nesmelova, I.; Sham, Y.; Dudek, A.Z.; van Eijk, L.I.; Wu, G.; Slungaard, A.; Mortari, F.; Griffioen, A.W.; Mayo, K.H. Platelet Factor 4 and Interleukin-8 CXC Chemokine Heterodimer Formation Modulates Function at the Quaternary Structural Level. *J. Biol. Chem.* **2005**, *280*, 4948–4958. [CrossRef] [PubMed]

41. Koenen, R.; von Hundelhausen, P.; Nesmelova, I.V.; Zernecke, A.; Liehn, E.A.; Sarabi, A.; Kramp, B.K.; Piccinini, A.; Paludan, S.R.; Kowalska, M.A.; et al. Disrupting functional interactions between platelet chemokines inhibits atherosclerosis in hyperlipidemic mice. *Nat. Med.* **2009**, *15*, 97–103. [CrossRef] [PubMed]

42. Von Hundelshausen, P.; Agten, S.; Eckardt, V.; Schmitt, M.; Blanchet, X.; Neideck, C.; Ippel, H.; Bidzhekov, K.; Wichapong, K.; Faussner, A.; et al. Chemokine interactome mapping enables tailored intervention in acute and chronic inflammation. *Sci. Transl. Med.* **2017**, *9*, 384. [CrossRef] [PubMed]

43. Ellyard, J.I.; Simson, L.; Bezos, A.; Johnston, K.; Freeman, C.; Parish, C.R. Eotaxin Selectively Binds Heparin. An interaction that protects eotaxin from proteolysis and potentiates chemotactic activity in vivo. *J. Biol. Chem.* **2007**, *282*, 15238–15247. [CrossRef] [PubMed]

44. Proudfoot, A.E. The BBXB Motif of RANTES Is the Principal Site for Heparin Binding and Controls Receptor Selectivity. *J. Biol. Chem.* **2001**, *276*, 10620–10626. [CrossRef] [PubMed]

45. Sheng, G.J.; Oh, Y.I.; Chang, S.-K.; Hsieh-Wilson, L.C. Tunable Heparan Sulfate Mimetics for Modulating Chemokine Activity. *J. Am. Chem. Soc.* **2013**, *135*, 10898–10901. [CrossRef] [PubMed]

46. Cai, Z.; Yarovoi, S.V.; Zhu, Z.; Rauova, L.; Hayes, V.; Lebedeva, T.; Liu, Q.; Poncz, M.; Arepally, G.; Cines, D.B.; et al. Crystal structure of platelet factor 4 complexed with fondaparinux. *Nat. Commun.* **2015**, *6*, 8277. [CrossRef] [PubMed]

47. Salanga, C.L.; Handel, T.M. Chemokine oligomerization and interactions with receptors and glycosaminoglycans: The role of structural dynamics in function. *Exp. Cell Res.* **2011**, *317*, 590–601. [CrossRef] [PubMed]

48. Proudfoot, A.E. Chemokines and Glycosaminoglycans. *Front. Immunol.* **2015**, *6*, 246. [CrossRef] [PubMed]

49. Shaw, J.P.; Johnson, Z.; Borlat, F.; Zwahlen, C.; Kungl, A.; Roulin, K.; Harrenga, A.; Wells, T.N.; Proudfoot, A.E. The X-Ray Structure of RANTES Heparin-Derived Disaccharides Allows the Rational Design of Chemokine Inhibitors. *Structure* **2004**, *12*, 2081–2093. [CrossRef] [PubMed]

50. Seo, Y.; Andaya, A.; Bleiholder, C.; Leary, J.A. Differentiation of CC vs. CXC Chemokine Dimers with GAG Octasaccharide Binding Partners: An Ion Mobility Mass Spectrometry Approach. *J. Am. Chem. Soc.* **2013**, *135*, 4325–4332. [CrossRef] [PubMed]

51. Mayo, K.H.; Ilyina, E.; Roongta, V.; Dundas, M.; Joseph, J.; Lai, C.K.; Maione, T.; Daly, T. Heparin Binding to Platelet Factor-4. An NMR and Site-Directed Mutagenesis Study: Arginine Residues Crucial for Binding. *Biochem. J.* **1995**, *312*, 357–365. [CrossRef] [PubMed]

52. Fox, J.C.; Tyler, R.C.; Peterson, F.C.; Dyer, D.P.; Zhang, F.; Linhardt, R.J.; Handel, T.M.; Volkman, B.F. Examination of Glycosaminoglycan Binding Sites on the XCL1 Dimer. *Biochemistry* **2016**, *55*, 1214–1225. [CrossRef] [PubMed]

53. Hoogewerf, A.J.; Kuschert, G.S.; Proudfoot, A.E.; Borlat, F.; Clark-Lewis, I.; Power, C.A.; Wells, T.N. Glycosaminoglycans mediate cell surface oligomerization of chemokines. *Biochemistry* **1997**, *36*, 13570–13578. [CrossRef] [PubMed]

54. Proudfoot, A.E.; Handel, T.M.; Johnson, Z.; Lau, E.K.; LiWang, P.; Clark-Lewis, I.; Borlat, F.; Wells, T.N.; Kosco-Vilbois, M.H. Glycosaminoglycan binding and oligomerization are essential for the in vivo activity of certain chemokines. *Proc. Natl. Acad. Sci. USA* **2003**, *100*, 1885–1890. [CrossRef] [PubMed]

55. Dyer, D.P.; Salanga, C.L.; Volkman, B.F.; Kawamura, T.; Handel, T.M. The dependence of chemokine-glycosaminoglycan interactions on chemokine oligomerization. *Glycobiology* **2016**, *26*, 312–326. [CrossRef] [PubMed]

56. Crown, S.E.; Yu, Y.; Sweeney, M.D.; Leary, J.A.; Handel, T.M. Heterodimerization of CCR2 chemokines and regulation by glycosaminoglycan binding. *J. Biol. Chem.* **2006**, *281*, 25438–25446. [CrossRef] [PubMed]

57. Verkaar, F.; van Offenbeek, J.; van der Lee, M.M.C.; van Lith, L.H.C.J.; Watts, A.O.; Rops, A.L.W.M.M.; Aguilar, D.C.; Ziarek, J.J.; van der Vlag, J.; Handel, T.M.; et al. Chemokine cooperativity is caused by competitive glycosaminoglycan binding. *J. Immunol.* **2014**, *192*, 3908–3914. [CrossRef] [PubMed]

58. Koenen, R.R.; Weber, C. Therapeutic targeting of chemokine interactions in atherosclerosis. *Nat. Rev. Drug Discov.* **2010**, *9*, 141–153. [CrossRef] [PubMed]
59. Raman, D.; Sobolik-Delmaire, T.; Richmond, A. Chemokines in health and disease. *Exp. Cell Res.* **2011**, *317*, 575–589. [CrossRef] [PubMed]
60. Viola, A.; Luster, A.D. Chemokines and Their Receptors: Drug Targets in Immunity and Inflammation. *Annu. Rev. Pharmacol. Toxicol.* **2008**, *48*, 171–197. [CrossRef] [PubMed]
61. Allen, S.J.; Crown, S.E.; Handel, T.M. Chemokine: Receptor structure, interactions, and antagonism. *Annu. Rev. Immunol.* **2007**, *25*, 787–820. [CrossRef] [PubMed]
62. Park, S.H.; Das, B.B.; Casagrande, F.; Tian, Y.; Nothnagel, H.J.; Chu, M.; Kiefer, H.; Maier, K.; De Angelis, A.A.; Marassi, F.M.; Opella, S.J. Structure of the chemokine receptor CXCR1 in phospholipid bilayers. *Nature* **2012**, *491*, 779–781. [CrossRef] [PubMed]
63. Thelen, M.; Stein, J.V. How chemokines invite leukocytes to dance. *Nat. Immunol.* **2008**, *9*, 953–959. [CrossRef] [PubMed]
64. Wu, B.; Chien, E.Y.; Mol, C.D.; Fenalti, G.; Liu, W.; Katritch, V.; Abagyan, R.; Brooun, A.; Wells, P.; Bi, F.C.; et al. Structures of the CXCR4 Chemokine GPCR with Small-Molecule and Cyclic Peptide Antagonists. *Science* **2010**, *330*, 1066–1071. [CrossRef] [PubMed]
65. Van Raemdonck, K.; Van den Steen, P.E.; Liekens, S.; Van Damme, J.; Struyf, S. CXCR3 ligands in disease and therapy. *Cytokine Growth Factor Rev.* **2015**, *26*, 311–327. [CrossRef] [PubMed]
66. Rajagopalan, L.; Rajarathnam, K. Structural Basis of Chemokine Receptor Function—A Model for Binding Affinity and Ligand Selectivity. *Biosci. Rep.* **2006**, *26*, 325–339. [CrossRef] [PubMed]
67. Katancik, J.A.; Sharma, A.; Radel, S.J.; De Nardin, E. Mapping of the extracellular binding regions of the human interleukin-8 type B receptor. *Biochem. Biophys. Res. Commun.* **1997**, *232*, 663–668. [CrossRef] [PubMed]
68. Skelton, N.J.; Quan, C.; Reilly, D.; Lowman, H. Structure of a CXC chemokine-receptor fragment in complex with interleukin-8. *Struct. Fold. Des.* **1999**, *7*, 157–168. [CrossRef]
69. Handel, T.M.; Lau, E.K. Chemokine structure and receptor interactions. *Ernst Scher Res. Found. Workshop* **2004**, *2004*, 101–124.
70. Casarosa, P.; Waldhoer, M.; LiWang, P.J.; Vischer, H.F.; Kledal, T.; Timmerman, H.; Schwartz, T.W.; Smit, M.J.; Leurs, R. CC and CX3C chemokines differentially interact with the N terminus of the human cytomegalovirus-encoded US28 receptor. *J. Biol. Chem.* **2005**, *280*, 3275–3285. [CrossRef] [PubMed]
71. Hemmerich, S.; Paavola, C.; Bloom, A.; Bhakta, S.; Freedman, R.; Grunberger, D.; Krstenansky, J.; Lee, S.; McCarley, D.; Mulkins, M.; et al. Identification of residues in the mono cytechemotacticprotein-1 that contact the MCP-1 receptor, CCR2. *Biochemistry* **1999**, *38*, 13013–13025. [CrossRef] [PubMed]
72. Strieter, R.M.; Polverini, P.J.; Kunkel, S.L.; Arenberg, D.A.; Burdick, M.D.; Kasper, J.; Dzuiba, J.; Van Damme, J.; Walz, A.; Marriott, D.; et al. The functional role of the ELR motif in CXC chemokine-mediated angiogenesis. *J. Biol. Chem.* **1995**, *270*, 27348–27357. [CrossRef] [PubMed]
73. Blanpain, C.; Doranz, B.J.; Bondue, A.; Govaerts, C.; De Leener, A.; Vassart, G.; Doms, R.W.; Proudfoot, A.; Parmentier, M. The core domain of chemokines bind CCR5 extracellular domains while their amino terminus interacts with the transmembrane helix bundle. *J. Biol. Chem.* **2003**, *278*, 5179–5187. [CrossRef] [PubMed]
74. Crump, M.P.; Gong, J.H.; Loetscher, P.; Rajarathnam, K.; Amara, A.; Arenzana-Seisdedos, F.; Virelizier, J.L.; Baggiolini, M.; Sykes, B.D.; Clark-Lewis, I. Solution structure and basis for functional activity of stromal cell-derived factor-1; dissociation of CXCR4 activation from binding and inhibition of HIV-1. *EMBO J.* **1997**, *16*, 6996–7007. [CrossRef] [PubMed]
75. Campanella, G.S.; Lee, E.M.; Sun, J.; Luster, A.D. CXCR3 and heparin binding sites of the chemokine IP-10 (CXCL10). *J. Biol. Chem.* **2003**, *278*, 17066–17074. [CrossRef] [PubMed]
76. Qin, L.; Kufareva, I.; Holden, L.G.; Wang, C.; Zheng, Y.; Zhao, C.; Fenalti, G.; Wu, H.; Han, G.W.; Cherezov, V.; et al. Crystal structure of the chemokine receptor CXCR4 in complex with a viral chemokine. *Science* **2015**, *357*, 1117–1122. [CrossRef] [PubMed]
77. Handel, T.M. The structure of a CXCR4-chemokine complex. *Front. Immunol.* **2015**, *6*, 282. [CrossRef] [PubMed]
78. Ziarek, J.J.; Kleist, A.B.; London, N.; Raveh, B.; Montpas, N.; Bonneterre, J.; St-Onge, G.; DiCosmo-Ponticello, C.J.; Koplinski, C.A.; Roy, I.; et al. Structural basis for chemokine recognition by a G protein-coupled receptor and implications for receptor activation. *Sci. Signal.* **2017**, *10*, 471. [CrossRef] [PubMed]

79. Kufareva, I.; Gustavsson, M.; Holden, L.G.; Qin, L.; Zheng, Y.; Handel, T.M. Disulfide trapping for modeling and structure determination of receptor:chemokine complexes. *Methods Enzymol.* **2016**, *570*, 389–420. [PubMed]

80. Veldkamp, C.T.; Seibert, C.; Peterson, F.C.; De la Cruz, N.B.; Haugner, J.C.; Basnet, H.; Sakmar, T.P.; Volkman, B.F. Structural basis of CXCR4 sulfotyrosine recognition by the chemokine SDF-1/CXCL12. *Sci. Signal.* **2008**, *1*, ra4. [CrossRef] [PubMed]

81. Kufareva, I.; Stephens, B.S.; Holden, L.G.; Qin, L.; Zhao, C.; Kawamura, T.; Abagyan, R.; Handel, T.M. Stoichiometry and geometry of the CXC chemokine receptor 4 complex with CXC ligand 12: Molecular modeling and experimental validation. *Proc. Natl. Acad. Sci. USA* **2014**, *111*, 5363–5372. [CrossRef] [PubMed]

82. Kleist, A.B.; Getschman, A.E.; Ziarek, J.J.; Nevins, A.M.; Gauthier, P.A.; Chevigné, A.; Szpakowska, M.; Volkman, B.F. New paradigms in chemokine receptor signal transduction: Moving beyond the two-site model. *Biochem. Pharmacol.* **2016**, *114*, 53–68. [CrossRef] [PubMed]

83. Drury, L.J.; Ziarek, J.J.; Gravel, S.; Veldkamp, C.T.; Takekoshi, T.; Hwang, S.T.; Heveker, N.; Volkman, B.F.; Dwinell, M.B. Monomeric and dimeric CXCL12 inhibit metastasis through distinct CXCR4 interactions and signaling pathways. *Proc. Natl. Acad. Sci. USA* **2011**, *108*, 17655–17660. [CrossRef] [PubMed]

84. Hensbergen, P.J.; Wijnands, P.G.J.; Schreurs, M.W.J.; Scheper, R.J.; Willemze, R.; Tensen, C.P. The CXCR3 Targeting Chemokine CXCL11 Has Potent Antitumor Activity In Vivo Involving Attraction of CD8+ T Lymphocytes But Not Inhibition of Angiogenesis. *J. Immunother.* **2005**, *28*, 343–351. [CrossRef] [PubMed]

85. Proudfoot, A.E.; Uguccioni, M. Modulation of Chemokine Responses: Synergy and Cooperativity. *Front. Immunol.* **2016**, *7*, 183. [CrossRef] [PubMed]

86. Von Hundelshausen, P.; Koenen, R.R.; Sack, M.; Mause, S.F.; Adriaens, W.; Proudfoot, A.E.; Hackeng, T.M.; Weber, C. Heterophilic interactions of platelet factor 4 and RANTES promote monocyte arrest on endothelium. *Blood* **2005**, *105*, 924–930. [CrossRef] [PubMed]

87. Gouwy, M. Synergy between proinflammatory ligands of G protein-coupled receptors in neutrophil activation and migration. *J. Leukoc. Biol.* **2004**, *76*, 185–194. [CrossRef] [PubMed]

88. Gouwy, M.; Struyf, S.; Noppen, S.; Schutyser, E.; Springael, J.Y.; Parmentier, M.; Proost, P.; Van Damme, J. Synergy between Co-produced CC and CXC Chemokines in Monocyte Chemotaxis through Receptor-Mediated Events. *Mol. Pharmacol.* **2008**, *74*, 485–495. [CrossRef] [PubMed]

89. Agten, S.M.; Koenen, R.; Ippel, H.; Eckert, V.; von Hundelshausen, P.; Mayo, K.H.; Weber, C.; Hackeng, T.M. Probing Functional Heteromeric Chemokine Protein-Protein Interactions through Conformation-assisted Oxime-Linkage. *Angew. Chem.* **2016**, *55*, 14963–14966. [CrossRef] [PubMed]

90. Stevens, R.L.; Colombo, M.; Gonzales, J.J.; Hollander, W.; Schmid, K. The glycosaminoglycans of the human artery and their changes in atherosclerosis. *J. Clin. Investig.* **1976**, *58*, 470. [CrossRef] [PubMed]

91. Taylor, K.R.; Gallo, R.L. Glycosaminoglycans and their proteoglycans: Host-associated molecular patterns for initiation and modulation of inflammation. *FASEB J.* **2006**, *20*, 9–22. [CrossRef] [PubMed]

92. Handel, T.M.; Johnson, Z.; Crown, S.E.; Lau, E.K.; Proudfoot, A.E. Regulation of protein function by glycosaminoglycans—As exemplified by chemokines. *Annu. Rev. Biochem.* **2005**, *74*, 385–410. [CrossRef] [PubMed]

93. Wang, X.; Sharp, J.S.; Handel, T.M.; Prestegard, J.H. Chemokine oligomerization in cell signaling and migration. *Prog. Mol. Biol. Transl. Sci.* **2013**, *117*, 531–578. [PubMed]

94. Gouwy, M.; Struyf, S.; Berghmans, N.; Vanormelingen, C.; Schols, D.; Van Damme, J. CXCR4 and CCR5 ligands cooperate in monocyte and lymphocyte migration and in inhibition of dual-tropic (R5/X4) HIV-1 infection. *Eur. J. Immunol.* **2011**, *41*, 963–973. [CrossRef] [PubMed]

95. Gouwy, M.; Schiraldi, M.; Struyf, S.; Van Damme, J.; Uguccioni, M. Possible mechanisms involved in chemokine synergy fine tuning the inflammatory response. *Immunol. Lett.* **2012**, *145*, 10–14. [CrossRef] [PubMed]

96. Gouwy, M.; Struyf, S.; Leutenez, L.; Pörtner, N.; Sozzani, S.; Van Damme, J. Chemokines and other GPCR ligands synergize in receptor-mediated migration of monocyte-derived immature and mature dendritic cells. *Immunobiology* **2014**, *219*, 218–229. [CrossRef] [PubMed]

97. Mortier, A.; Van Damme, J.; Proost, P. Overview of the mechanisms regulating chemokine activity and availability. *Immunol. Lett.* **2012**, *145*, 2–9. [CrossRef] [PubMed]

98. Garin, A.; Proudfoot, A.E. Chemokines as targets for therapy. *Exp. Cell Res.* **2011**, *317*, 602–612. [CrossRef] [PubMed]

99. Allegretti, M.; Cesta, M.C.; Garin, A.; Proudfoot, A.E. Current status of chemokine receptor inhibitors in development. *Immunol. Lett.* **2012**, *145*, 68–78. [CrossRef] [PubMed]
100. Proudfoot, A.E.; Bonvin, P.; Power, C.A. Targeting chemokines: Pathogens can, why can't we? *Cytokine* **2015**, *74*, 259–267. [CrossRef] [PubMed]
101. Proudfoot, A.E.; Power, C.A.; Schwarz, M.K. Anti-chemokine small molecular drugs: A promising future? *Expert Opin. Investig. Drugs* **2010**, *19*, 345–355. [CrossRef] [PubMed]
102. O'Hayre, M.; Salanga, C.L.; Handel, T.M.; Hamel, D.J. Emerging concepts and approaches for chemokine-receptor drug discovery. *Expert Opin. Drug Discov.* **2010**, *5*, 1109–1122. [CrossRef] [PubMed]
103. Kufareva, I.; Salanga, C.L.; Handel, T.M. Chemokine and chemokine receptor structure and interactions: Implications for therapeutic strategies. *Immunol. Cell Biol.* **2015**, *93*, 372–383. [CrossRef] [PubMed]
104. Sato, T.; Komai, M.; Iwase, M.; Kobayashi, K.; Tahara, H.; Ohshima, E.; Arai, H.; Miki, I. Inihbitory effect of the new orally active CCR4 antagonist K327 on CCR4+CD4+ T cell migration into the lung of mice with ovalbumin-induced lung allergic inflammation. *Pharmacology* **2009**, *84*, 171–182. [CrossRef] [PubMed]
105. Perros, F.; Hoogsteden, H.C.; Coyle, A.J.; Lambrecht, B.N.; Hammad, H. Blockade of CCR4 in a humanized model of asthma reveals a critical role for DC-derived CCL17 and CCL22 in attracting Th2 cells and inducing airway inflammation. *Allergy* **2009**, *64*, 995–1002. [CrossRef] [PubMed]
106. Komai, M.; Tanaka, H.; Nagao, K.; Ishizaki, M.; Kajiwara, D.; Miura, T.; Ohashi, H.; Haba, T.; Kawakami, K.; Sawa, E.; et al. A novel CC-chemokine receptor 3 antagonist, Ki19003, inhibits airway eosinophilia and subepithelial/peribronchial fibrosis induced by repeated antigen challenge in mice. *J. Pharmacol. Sci.* **2010**, *112*, 203–213. [CrossRef] [PubMed]
107. Mahler, D.A.; Huang, S.; Tabrizi, M.; Bell, G.M. Efficacy and safety of a monoclonal antibody recognizing interleukin-8 in COPD: A pilot study. *Chest* **2004**, *126*, 926–934. [CrossRef] [PubMed]
108. Brodmerkel, C.M.; Huber, R.; Covington, M.; Diamond, S.; Hall, L.; Collins, R.; Leffet, L.; Gallagher, K.; Feldman, P.; Collier, P.; et al. Discovery and pharmacological characterization of a novel rodent-active CCR2 antagonist, INCB3344. *J. Immunol.* **2005**, *175*, 5370–5378. [CrossRef] [PubMed]
109. Shahrara, S.; Proudfoot, A.E.; Park, C.C.; Volin, M.V.; Haines, G.K.; Woods, J.M.; Handel, T.M.; Pope, R.M. Inhibition of monocyte chemoattractant protein-1 ameliorates rat adjuvant-induced arthritis. *J. Immunol.* **2008**, *180*, 3447–3456. [CrossRef] [PubMed]
110. Brühl, H.; Cihak, J.; Schneider, M.A.; Plachý, J.; Rupp, T.; Wenzel, I.; Shakarami, M.; Milz, S.; Ellwart, J.W.; Stangassinger, M.; et al. Dual role of CCR2 during initiation and progression of collagen-induced arthritis: Evidence for regulatory activity of CCR2+ T cells. *J. Immunol.* **2004**, *172*, 890–898. [CrossRef] [PubMed]
111. Struthers, M.; Pasternak, A. CCR2 antagonists. *Curr. Top. Med. Chem.* **2010**, *10*, 1278–1298. [CrossRef] [PubMed]
112. Horuk, R. Chemokine receptor antagonists: Overcoming developmental hurdles. *Nat. Rev. Drug Discov.* **2008**, *8*, 23–33. [CrossRef] [PubMed]
113. Tan, Q.; Zhu, Y.; Li, J.; Chen, Z.; Han, G.W.; Kufareva, I.; Li, T.; Ma, L.; Fenalti, G.; Li, J.; et al. Structure of the CCR5 Chemokine Receptor-HIV Entry Inhibitor Maraviroc Complex. *Science* **2013**, *341*, 1387–1390. [CrossRef] [PubMed]
114. Walters, M.J.; Wang, Y.; Lai, N.; Baumgart, T.; Zhao, B.N.; Dairaghi, D.J.; Bekker, P.; Ertl, L.S.; Penfold, M.E.; Jaen, J.C.; et al. Characterization of CCX282-B, an orally bioavailable antagonist of the CCR9 chemokine receptor, for treatment of inflammatory bowel disease. *J. Pharm. Exp. Ther.* **2010**, *335*, 61–69. [CrossRef] [PubMed]
115. Akashi, S.; Sho, M.; Kashizuka, H.; Hamada, K.; Ikeda, N.; Kuzumoto, Y.; Tsurui, Y.; Nomi, T.; Mizuno, T.; Kanehiro, H.; et al. A Novel Small-Molecule Compound Targeting CCR5 and CXCR3 Prevents Acute and Chronic Allograft Rejection. *Transplantation* **2005**, *80*, 378–384. [CrossRef] [PubMed]
116. Lüttichau, H.R. The herpesvirus 8 encoded chemokines vCCL2 (vMIP-II) and vCCL3 (vMIP-III) target the human but not the murine lymphotactin receptor. *Virol. J.* **2008**, *5*, 50. [CrossRef] [PubMed]
117. Luz, J.G.; Yu, M.; Su, Y.; Wu, Z.; Zhou, Z.; Sun, R.; Wilson, I.A. Crystal Structure of Viral Macrophage Inflammatory Protein I Encoded by Kaposi's Sarcoma-associated Herpesvirus at 1.7Å. *J. Mol. Biol.* **2005**, *352*, 1019–1028. [CrossRef] [PubMed]
118. Arvanitakis, L.; Geras-Raaka, E.; Varma, A.; Gershengorn, M.C.; Cesarman, E. Human herpesvirus KSHV encodes a constitutively active G-proteincoupled receptor linked to cell proliferation. *Nature* **1997**, *385*, 347–350. [CrossRef] [PubMed]

119. Lalani, A.S.; Masters, J.; Graham, K.; Liu, L.; Lucas, A.; McFadden, G. Role of the Myxoma Virus Soluble CC-Chemokine Inhibitor Glycoprotein, M-T1, during Myxoma Virus Pathogenesis. *Virology* **1999**, *255*, 233–245. [CrossRef] [PubMed]

120. Bonvin, P.; Dunn, S.M.; Rousseau, F.; Dyer, D.P.; Shaw, J.; Power, C.A.; Handel, T.M.; Proudfoot, A.E. Identification of the pharmacophore of the CC chemokine-binding proteins Evasin-1 and -4 using phage display. *J. Biol. Chem.* **2014**, *289*, 31846–31855. [CrossRef] [PubMed]

121. Takekoshi, T.; Ziarek, J.J.; Volkman, B.F.; Hwang, S.T. A locked, dimeric CXCL12 variant effectively inhibits pulmonary metastasis of CXCR4-expressing melanoma cells due to enhanced serum stability. *Mol. Cancer Ther.* **2012**, *11*, 2516–2525. [CrossRef] [PubMed]

122. Veldkamp, C.T.; Ziarek, J.J.; Peterson, F.C.; Chen, Y.; Volkman, B.F. Targeting SDF-1/CXCL12 with a ligand that prevents activation of CXCR4 through structure-based drug design. *J. Am. Chem. Soc.* **2010**, *132*, 7242–7243. [CrossRef] [PubMed]

123. Smith, E.W.; Liu, Y.; Getschman, A.E.; Peterson, F.C.; Ziarek, J.J.; Li, R.; Volkman, B.F.; Chen, Y. Structural analysis of a novel small molecule ligand bound to the CXCL12 chemokine. *J. Med. Chem.* **2014**, *57*, 9693–9699. [CrossRef] [PubMed]

124. Ziarek, J.J.; Liu, Y.; Smith, E.; Zhang, G.; Peterson, F.C.; Chen, J.; Yu, Y.; Chen, Y.; Volkman, B.F.; Li, R. Fragment-based optimization of small molecule CXCL12 inhibitors for antagonizing the CXCL12/CXCR4 interaction. *Curr. Top. Med. Chem.* **2012**, *12*, 2727–2740. [CrossRef] [PubMed]

125. Zheng, Y.; Qin, L.; Zacarías, N.V.; de Vries, H.; Han, G.W.; Gustavsson, M.; Dabros, M.; Zhao, C.; Cherney, R.J.; Carter, P.; et al. Structure of CC chemokine receptor 2 with orthosteric and allosteric antagonists. *Nature* **2016**, *540*, 458–461. [CrossRef] [PubMed]

126. Johnson, Z.; Proudfoot, A.E.; Handel, T.M. Interaction of chemokines and glycosaminoglycans: A new twist in the regulation of chemokine function with opportunities for therapeutic intervention. *Cytokine Growth Factor Rev.* **2005**, *16*, 625–636. [CrossRef] [PubMed]

127. Nellen, A.; Heinrichs, D.; Berres, M.L.; Sahin, H.; Schmitz, P.; Proudfoot, A.E.; Trautwein, C.; Wasmuth, H.E. Interference with oligomerization and glycosaminoglycan binding of the chemokine CCL5 improves experimental liver injury. *PLoS ONE* **2012**, *7*, e36614. [CrossRef] [PubMed]

128. Ziarek, J.J.; Veldkamp, C.T.; ZhaDyerg, F.; Murray, N.J.; Kartz, G.A.; Liang, X.; Su, J.; Baker, J.E.; Linhardt, R.J.; Volkman, B.F. Heparin oligosaccharides inhibit chemokine (CXC motif) ligand 12 (CXCL12) cardio-protection by binding orthogonal to the dimerization interface, promoting oligomerization, and competing with the chemokine (CXC motif) receptor 4 (CXCR4) N terminus. *J. Biol. Chem.* **2013**, *288*, 737–746. [CrossRef] [PubMed]

129. Dyer, D.P.; Thomson, J.M.; Hermant, A.; Jowitt, T.A.; Handel, T.M.; Proudfoot, A.E.; Day, A.J.; Milner, C.M. TSG-6 inhibits neutrophil migration via direct interaction with the chemokine CXCL8. *J. Immunol.* **2014**, *192*, 2177–2185. [CrossRef] [PubMed]

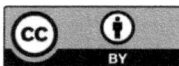

International Journal of
Molecular Sciences

MDPI

Review

Regulation of Chemokine Function: The Roles of GAG-Binding and Post-Translational Nitration

Sarah Thompson [1,†], **Beatriz Martínez-Burgo** [1,†], **Krishna Mohan Sepuru** [2],
Krishna Rajarathnam [2], **John A. Kirby** [1], **Neil S. Sheerin** [1] and **Simi Ali** [1,*]

[1] Applied Immunobiology and Transplantation Group, Institute of Cellular Medicine, Medical School, University of Newcastle upon Tyne, Newcastle upon Tyne NE2 4HH, UK; s.thompson3@ncl.ac.uk (S.T.); b.martinez.burgo@ncl.ac.uk (B.M.-B.); john.kirby@ncl.ac.uk (J.A.K.); neil.sheerin@ncl.ac.uk (N.S.S.)
[2] Department of Biochemistry and Molecular Biology, The University of Texas Medical Branch, 301 University Boulevard, Galveston, TX 77555, USA; kmsepuru@utmb.edu (K.M.S.); krrajara@utmb.edu (K.R.)
* Correspondence: simi.ali@ncl.ac.uk; Tel.: +44-(0)191-208-7158
† These authors contributed equally to this work.

Received: 14 June 2017; Accepted: 30 July 2017; Published: 3 August 2017

Abstract: The primary function of chemokines is to direct the migration of leukocytes to the site of injury during inflammation. The effects of chemokines are modulated by several means, including binding to G-protein coupled receptors (GPCRs), binding to glycosaminoglycans (GAGs), and through post-translational modifications (PTMs). GAGs, present on cell surfaces, bind chemokines released in response to injury. Chemokines bind leukocytes via their GPCRs, which directs migration and contributes to local inflammation. Studies have shown that GAGs or GAG-binding peptides can be used to interfere with chemokine binding and reduce leukocyte recruitment. Post-translational modifications of chemokines, such as nitration, which occurs due to the production of reactive species during oxidative stress, can also alter their biological activity. This review describes the regulation of chemokine function by GAG-binding ability and by post-translational nitration. These are both aspects of chemokine biology that could be targeted if the therapeutic potential of chemokines, like CXCL8, to modulate inflammation is to be realised.

Keywords: chemokine-GAG interaction; synthetic peptide chemistry; PTM; chemokine nitration

1. Introduction

Chemokines are small cytokines (8–17 kDa) with chemoattractant properties that are involved in processes ranging from homeostasis to development and tissue repair. They also play essential roles in pathological conditions such as tumorigenesis, cancer metastasis and inflammatory or autoimmune disorders where they mediate the migration of leukocytes to the site of injury [1–4]. Chemokine biology also plays a role in generating immune tolerance [5]. Chemokines are classified into four subfamilies; C, CC, CXC and CX3C in relation to the location/spacing of cysteine residues within the N-terminal region.

The migration of immune cells is mediated through the formation of dynamic chemokine gradients, which are achieved by the binding of chemokines on glycosaminoglycans (GAGs) present on the surface of endothelial cells and in the extracellular matrix [6]. This creates an equilibrium of free and bound monomer and dimer in the proximity of the injury, resulting in haptotactic and chemotactic gradients. This allows directed movement of leukocytes from circulation to the site of injury via chemokine signalling through the G-protein coupled receptors (GPCR) [7,8]. One of many possible GAG-chemokine-receptor interaction scenarios is shown diagrammatically in Figure 1 below.

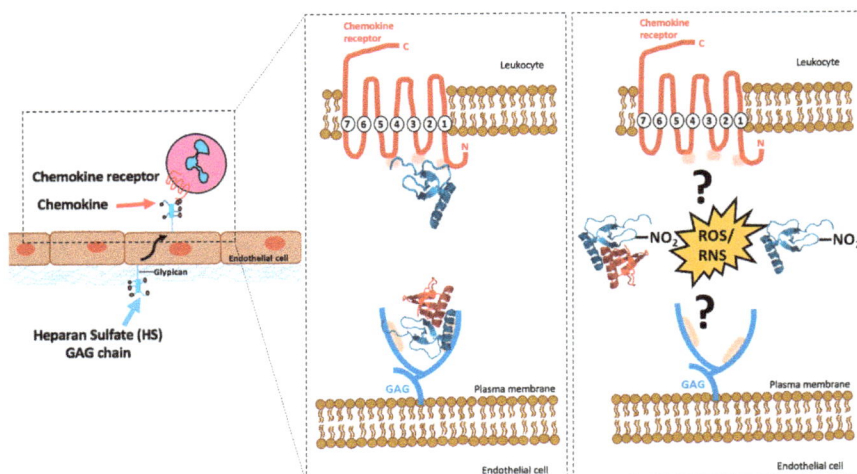

Figure 1. Chemokine interactions with G-protein coupled receptors (GPCRs) and glycosaminoglycans (GAGs). Chemokines bind to GAGs present on the surface of endothelial cells in a dynamic manner, creating a localised chemokine gradient and facilitating the recruitment of leukocytes. Leukocyte recruitment is a multistep process in which leukocytes tether to, roll along, and adhere to the endothelium before transmigrating out of the blood vessels. On the right, magnified image indicating specific chemokine regions involved in GPCR/GAG binding (shaded in orange), and potential consequences of stress (i.e., production of reactive oxygen species/reactive nitrogen species (ROS/RNS respectively)) on regulation of chemokine function. CXCL8 is used as an example chemokine, with the monomer shown in blue and the dimer depicted with one monomer in blue and the other in red.

Regulation of chemokine function is essential in order to prevent excessive inflammation and allow healing after injury. This regulation can occur at many levels and can involve different aspects of chemokine biology, including epigenetic modifications which can affect chemokine production [9], the concentration and oligomeric state of the chemokine (monomer/dimer), the steepness of the chemokine gradient [10,11], the ability of the chemokine to interact with GPCRs and GAGs [7,12], and receptor signalling bias [13,14]. Post-translational modifications (PTMs) such as nitration, glycosylation, phosphorylation, and citrullination also play a critical regulatory role on chemokine function.

In this review, we will describe how chemokine function can be regulated by GAG-binding and post-translational nitration, primarily focusing on CXCL8 as a model CXC chemokine.

2. Chemokine and Chemokine Receptor Interactions

Chemokine receptors all share a similar structure; an extracellular N-terminal domain, seven transmembrane-spanning segments, three extracellular loops, three cytoplasmic loops and a C-terminal segment [15]. Binding of chemokine ligands to their receptors initiates a signalling cascade involving the influx of calcium, which ultimately leads to chemotaxis [7].

Targeting the interaction between chemokines and their receptors is one potential method to regulate the recruitment of leukocytes and modulate inflammation. However, this is limited by the high level of promiscuity displayed by chemokines and their receptors [16]. While some receptor-ligand interactions are specific e.g., CX3CL1-CX3CR1 or CCL20-CCR6 [15], chemokines can often bind multiple receptors, and receptors may in turn be activated by many chemokines, making it difficult to achieve a selective and specific effect when targeting these interactions [17,18]. For example, whereas CXCR1 binds CXCL8 with high affinity and CXCL6 with lower affinity, CXCR2 binds CXCL1/2/3/5/6/7/8 with high affinity [15,19,20]. In addition, there are atypical receptors

Int. J. Mol. Sci. **2017**, *18*, 1692

(ACKR) such as ACKR1/D6 or ACKR2/DARC, that bind chemokines but do not induce G-protein signalling [21]. They act as chemokine scavengers and are thought to be involved in the regulation of the immune response. For instance, DARC present on erythrocytes is known to induce clearance of circulating CXCL8, affecting the chemokine's ability to stimulate neutrophil recruitment [22], hence having a significant role limiting the inflammatory response.

3. Chemokines and GAG Interactions

GAGs such as heparan sulphate (HS), are long linear polysaccharides consisting of a repeating disaccharide unit [23] frequently covalently attached to a core protein forming proteoglycans. The main classes of proteoglycans are defined according to their distribution, homologies, and function. Common examples of HS proteoglycans are glypican, syndecan and perlecan. GAGs display varying patterns of sulphation, which in addition to carboxyl groups, confer a negative charge which is a critical determinant of chemokine binding [24]. GAGs are located primarily on the surface of endothelial cells, as macromolecular complexes with matrix proteins in the extracellular matrix (ECM), and are also secreted/shed during active inflammation [25]. They can be divided into four groups: heparin/heparan sulphate, chondroitin sulphate/dermatan sulphate, keratan sulphate, and hyaluronic acid (a non-sulphated GAG, non-covalently attached to proteins) shown in Figure 2.

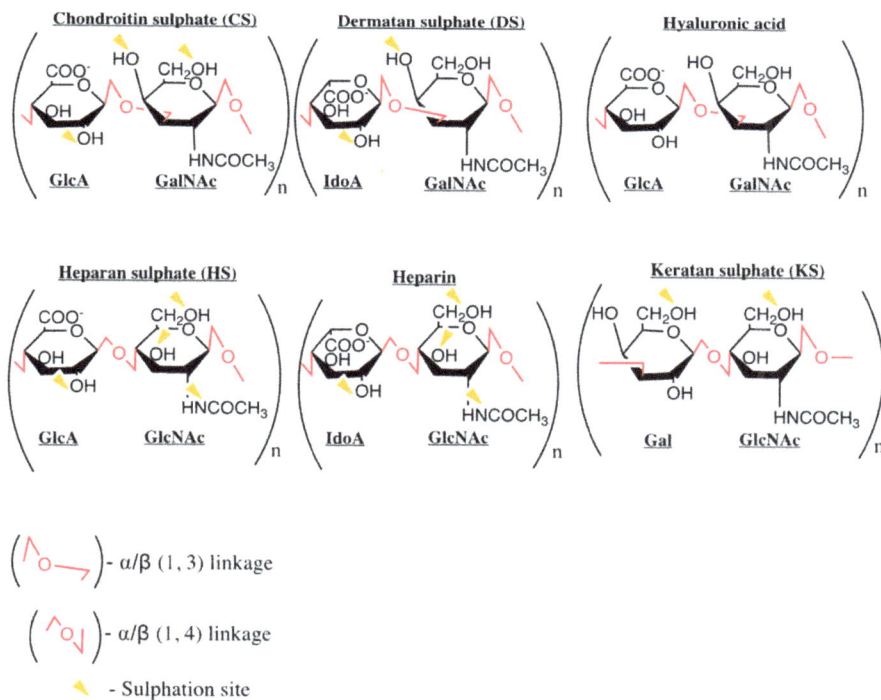

Figure 2. Structure and composition of GAGs. Linkages are shown in red, and sites of sulphation indicated by yellow triangles. The backbone is made up of repeating disaccharide blocks composed of uronic acid (glucuronic acid (GlcA) or iduronic acid (IdoA)), or galactose (Gal) and an amino sugar (*N*-acetyl-galactosamine (GalNAc) or *N*-acetyl-glucosamine (GlcNAc)).

Although chemokines are promiscuous to a degree in terms of receptor binding, data on GAG binding is beginning to show that chemokines interact with GAGs differently, and must be studied individually [26–28]. GAGs have the potential to modulate chemokine heterodimer formation and function, receptor binding and enhance stability [29–31]. GAG binding has been identified as essential for regulating chemotaxis in vivo [12], and could, therefore, be an aspect of chemokine biology to be targeted to modulate function. However, the system is intricate and complex, with the diversity of GAGs (which vary greatly in length, composition and sulphation pattern as shown in Figure 2), the oligomerisation state of the chemokine and the tissue microenvironment all affecting the chemokine-GAG interactions, and increasing the challenge of targeting this aspect of chemokine biology [32,33]. The presence/composition of other molecules beside GAGs also influences binding, for example, studies have shown that sialic acid and mannose-containing glycans are responsible (in addition to GAGs) for the binding of CCL5 to both CCR5+ and CCR5− cells [34]. Furthermore, data are beginning to show that chemokine residues that are involved in receptor interactions are also involved in GAG binding, suggesting GAG-bound chemokines may be unable to bind their receptors [27,29,35,36]. The affinity of the chemokine for different GAGs also changes depending upon whether the chemokine is in the monomer/dimer state, with dimers generally being the higher affinity GAG ligands [37–39]. The ratio of bound to free chemokine is therefore fine-tuned to modulate cellular recruitment.

The highly sulphated and acidic GAGs bind to basic residues within chemokines through electrostatic and H-bonding interactions. This usually involves residues such as arginine, lysine or histidine, which typically form the BBXB or (B)BXX(X/B)BXXB(B) peptide signature, where B is a basic amino acid residue and X a non-conserved amino acid, present in virtually all chemokines. Earlier studies revealed BBXB or (B)BXX(X/B)BXXB(B) as common heparin binding sequences for several chemokines, however, with the characterisation of more GAG-binding regions, it is suggested that GAG-binding motifs can be defined as sequential distant residues that form an optimal binding surface due to spatial orientation in the folded state [40]. This binding regulates the steepness and duration of chemokine gradients, which in turn regulates leukocyte adhesion and infiltration [41,42]. GAG binding has been identified as essential for the induction of chemotaxis, as chemokine mutants that bind receptor but not GAGs have impaired ability to recruit immune cells in vivo [12]. GAG binding could, therefore, be an aspect of chemokine biology to be targeted to modulate function.

Common GAGs: Heparan Sulphate and Heparin

Heparan Sulphate (HS) is an anionic GAG component of the glycocalyx, and the most abundant GAG on the surface of endothelial cells [43]. HS is initially synthesised as a repeating disaccharide composed of the monomeric units N-acetyl-glucosamine (GlcNAc) and glucuronic acid. These units may or may not then be modified by a series of biosynthetic reactions within the Golgi. These give rise to N-, 6-O, or (albeit rarely) 3-O-sulphation of the glucosamine (GlcNS), as well as epimerisation and subsequent 2-O-sulphation of the glucuronic acid. The family of enzymes responsible for these modifications includes N-deacetylase/N-sulphotranferases (NDSTs 1/2/3/4), 2-O-sulphotransferases (HS2ST), 6-O-sulphotransferases (HS6ST), and 3-O-sulphotransferases (HS3ST) [44,45]. Mature HS can also be modified on the cell surface glycocalyx by specific sulphatases (SULF1 and SULF2). Additionally, heparanase, an endo-glycosidase, can cleave the HS polymer releasing smaller fragments from the HS proteoglycan complex.

HS serves homeostatic functions, including maintenance of the endothelial barrier permeability and the activation of antithrombin III. During disease or stress, HS can present inflammatory molecules such as chemokines to leukocytes, facilitating selectin-mediated rolling along the endothelial surface, potentially leading to increased integrin adhesion, intravascular arrest and diapedesis [46] (Figure 1).

In the short term, inflammation such as ischaemia-reperfusion injury can induce the shedding of some HS proteoglycans from the endothelial cell surface, which can then bind and sequester chemokines in the blood and reduce leukocyte migration [47–49]. Upon regeneration of the glycocalyx, upregulation of the expression of NDST enzymes increases the extent of N-sulphation, which in turn enhances the potential of the endothelium to bind and present pro-inflammatory chemokines [50].

This highlights the flexibility and varied regulation of endothelial GAGs and their ability to modulate chemokine binding and subsequent leukocyte migration.

Heparin, a soluble GAG produced by mast cells [51], has essentially the same backbone structure as HS but a different (more uniform) sulphation pattern [52]. Due to heparin's uniform sulphation pattern, and the commercial availability of size-fractionated oligosaccharides of many different sizes, heparin is commonly used for structure—function and chemokine-GAG interaction studies.

4. Post-Translational Modification of Chemokines

The regulation of chemokines through post-translational modification can affect both receptor and GAG binding, and impact upon chemokine function and biological activity [53]. Many forms of modification can occur, such as cleavages by matrix metalloproteinases and other enzymes, as well as modifications of individual residues by citrullination or nitration [54–57].

The heterogeneous nature of post-translational modifications emphasises the need for better understanding, with some modifications enhancing or abrogating function, and others preventing detection using conventional methods [58,59]. This review article will focus on nitration, which occurs naturally during any situation that involves oxidative stress, such as myocardial infarction or organ transplantation.

5. Nitration of Chemokines

The reactive nitrogen species (RNS) peroxynitrite ($ONOO^-$) is formed from the reaction between nitric oxide (NO) with the superoxide anion (O_2^-) [60,61]. $ONOO^-$ has a very short half-life of around 10 ms at physiological pH, and can affect molecules within a 20 μm range of its production [62]. Effects of $ONOO^-$ include protein nitration, lipid peroxidation, DNA strand breakage and the inhibition of cell signalling and metabolism [63].

NO is produced by nitric oxide synthase enzymes present in many cell types and in all tissues [64–66]. O_2^- is produced by a range of enzymes present in many cell types, including nicotinamide adenine dinucleotide phosphate (NADPH) oxidase within the mitochondria [67–69]. Production of both NO [70] and O_2^- [71,72] increases during inflammation and strategies to reduce production are protective in pre-clincial models of injury [73–75] and in human disease [76].

$ONOO^-$ nitrates tyrosine residues to form 3-nitrotyrosine (3-NT), and also modifies tryptophan, cysteine, methionine, lysine and histidine, examples of which are shown in Figure 3 [77,78]. $ONOO^-$ has been implicated in the pathology of many diseases [79], including myocardial reperfusion injury [80], cardiac allograft rejection [81], Fabry disease [82] and kidney diseases including acute tubular necrosis and diabetic nephropathy [83]. An increase in 3-NT was also detected in plasma and synovial fluid in osteoarthritis patients [84], in plasma from patients with interstitial lung disease [85] and type II diabetes mellitus [86].

One way that nitration could be affecting disease progression is through its effect on chemokines and leukocyte recruitment. Chemokine nitration usually results in a decrease in function [59] but for some proteins nitration can enhance function [87].

5.1. Effects of Nitration: Detection of Chemokines

Studies have shown that nitration may alter the ability of antibodies to detect proteins, presumably due to epitope modification by the addition of the NO_2 groups. This has been shown for nitrated CCL2 and CXCL12 [54,88]. This may limit the biological relevance of measuring chemokine concentrations as disease biomarkers if only unmodified chemokine is detected. The amount of unmodified chemokine may be a less informative indicator of disease activity than the ratio of modified to unmodified chemokine.

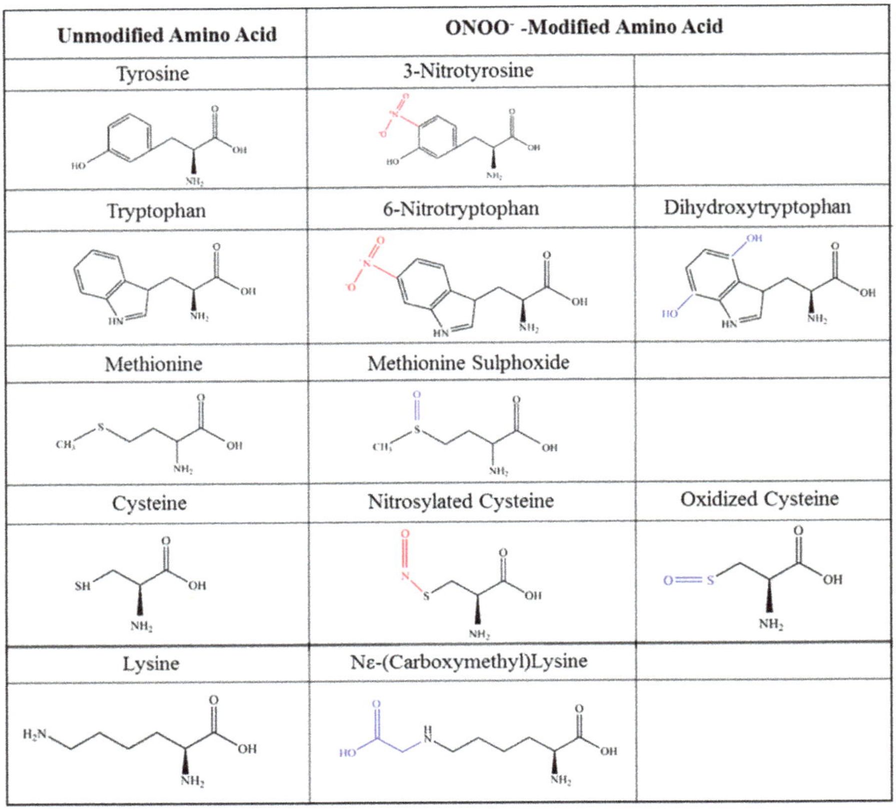

Unmodified Amino Acid	ONOO⁻-Modified Amino Acid	
Tyrosine	3-Nitrotyrosine	
Tryptophan	6-Nitrotryptophan	Dihydroxytryptophan
Methionine	Methionine Sulphoxide	
Cysteine	Nitrosylated Cysteine	Oxidized Cysteine
Lysine	Nε-(Carboxymethyl)Lysine	

Figure 3. Some examples of amino acid modifications by peroxynitrite (ONOO⁻). Modifications involving oxidation are shown in blue, and modifications involving nitration are shown in red.

5.2. Effects of Nitration: Chemotaxis

Nitration affects the chemotactic function of several chemokines but the biological significance of this is not fully understood. Incubation of chemokine with ONOO⁻ inhibits monocyte chemotaxis in response to CCL2 and eosinophil chemotaxis in response to CCL5 [89]. Another study found that CCL2 nitrated by intratumoural RNS was unable to induce CD8+ T cell recruitment to the tumour, but could still induce some recruitment of myeloid cells at high concentrations [88]. Nitration of tyrosine 7 in CXCL12 rendered the chemokine unable to induce lymphocyte chemotaxis both in vitro and in vivo [90]. Nitration could therefore be a negative regulator of inflammation; reducing the chemotactic functions of chemokines and thereby reducing leukocyte infiltration.

5.3. Effects of Nitration: Receptor Binding

The effect that nitration has on the ability of a chemokine to bind/signal through its receptor(s) is complex. Nitrated CCL2 was shown to have a reduced affinity for its receptor CCR2, which may explain its failure to induce chemotaxis of CD8+ T cells (as these cells express low levels of the CCR2 receptor), but retained ability to induce migration of myeloid cells (which express very high levels of CCR2) [88]. Nitration of CXCL12 does not affect its ability to bind the CXCR4 receptor, but does impair its ability to signal through this receptor [90]. In cases where nitration reduces receptor activation capacity, this could influence the receptor signaling bias mentioned previously, and increase the specificity of signaling in situations where many chemokines can bind to the same receptor.

To date, all research on nitration in chemokine biology appears to focus upon nitration of the chemokines themselves. The effect that nitration of the chemokine receptors may have is unknown. The Y188A CXCR1 mutant displayed a decreased affinity for CXCL8 compared with the wild type receptor, indicating the importance of this tyrosine residue in receptor-ligand interactions. As tyrosine is a potential target for nitration by $ONOO^-$, nitration of CXCR1 as well as CXCL8 could affect receptor-ligand interactions [91].

5.4. Effects of Nitration: GAG Binding

Whether or not nitration affects GAG-binding depends upon the chemokine in question. For example, nitrated CXCL12 binds GAGs with a similar affinity as wild type CXCL12 [90], but nitrated CCL2 has been shown to have reduced ability to bind both heparin and heparan sulphate when compared to wild type CCL2 [92].

It is worth noting that soluble/immobilized chemokines can initiate different downstream pathways affecting cell migration, as is the case of the CCR7-CCL19/CCL21 axis. This means that in cases where nitration affects GAG binding (i.e., ability of the chemokine to be immobilized), this can in turn affect receptor signaling and therefore regulation of receptor binding, GAG binding and post-translational modifications are all likely to be linked and influence each other [93].

6. GAGs, Nitration and CXCL8 Function

CXCL8 is a potent neutrophil chemoattractant protein released by many cell types in response to a wide range of stimuli including cytokines, microbial products and hypoxia [94,95]. CXCL8 has also been shown to act on other cell types such as lymphocytes and fibroblasts, and is known to promote angiogenesis [96] and leukocyte degranulation. CXCL8 is therefore implicated in both acute and chronic inflammation [97]. Its modulation could influence the pathology of a wide range of diseases and at multiple disease stages [98].

6.1. Targeting CXCL8-GAG Interactions

Studies have shown that while the CXCL8 monomer is the higher affinity receptor ligand, the CXCL8 dimer (which is the higher affinity GAG ligand) is far less competent at CXCR1 receptor activation (although quite active for CXCR2 [99]). This suggests that CXCL8, when GAG-bound, cannot access the receptor [36,100,101]. The C-terminal alpha helix of CXCL8, in addition to some basic residues located within the N-loop, is critical for GAG binding [102,103] due to its positive electrostatic charge. This binding is mediated by basic amino acids (Arg, Lys, His) core residues and by other secondary residues across its sequence (as shown in Figure 4) [41,104]. Targeted substitution of these basic residues for alanine residues reduced in vivo neutrophil recruitment to the peritoneum [8,32], but increased recruitment to the lungs [32,105]. These different recruitment patterns of neutrophils in response to CXCL8 in the mouse peritoneum compared to lung could be attributed to differences in chemokine gradients caused by different GAG structures and compositions between these tissues, and by differences in binding kinetics or diffusion rates, adding further complexity to this topic [32].

A)

N-loop

C-terminal α-helix

	15 18 20 23		42 47 54 60 64 67 68

CXCL8   SAKELRCQCIKTYSKPFHPKFIKELRVIESGPHCANTEIIVKLSDGRELCLDPKENWVQRVVEKFLKRAENS

GAG-binding
Receptor-binding
Both GAG and receptor-binding
BXXXBXXBB motif: motif associated with GAG-binding, where B is basic aa

B)

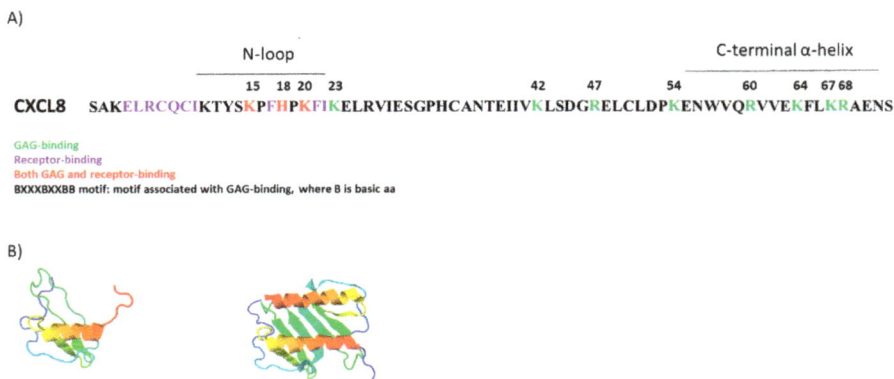

Figure 4. CXCL8 sequence and structure. (**A**) Diagrammatic representation of CXCL8 (72 amino acids long), showing the amino acid sequence. Purple: Receptor-binding residues. Green: GAG-binding residues. Red: residues implicated in both GAG and receptor binding; (**B**) CXCL8 in monomeric form (1KL, PDB) on the left, and dimeric form on the right (1CXCL8, PDB).

6.2. Competitive Displacement of Chemokines

The administration of a GAG, usually heparin, is a method that has been employed in pre-clinical models to modulate inflammation, and is thought to act through disruption of pre-formed chemokine gradients present on cell surface GAGs. Heparin in various forms inhibits leukocyte recruitment to mouse models of arthritis, traumatic brain injury and lipopolysaccharide (LPS) treatment [106–108], although its effectiveness depends upon the dose given and the duration of inflammation [109]. These studies show potential role of GAG mimetics on chemokine-mediated immunomodulation when administered, either local or systemically, however it should be noted that administered heparin is likely to interact with all cytokines due to its highly negative charge, and a more chemokine-specific gradient disruption method could be more beneficial.

Chemokine-GAG interactions also play an essential role in the antiviral immune response. Viruses can evade the chemokine-mediated immune response by expression of viral chemokine binding proteins (vCKBP), which interfere with the GAG binding, GPCR-binding, or both, thus modulating chemokine-mediated migration of leukocytes to the site of infection or tissue damage in vitro and in vivo [110].

6.3. Mutants with Altered GAG Binding

Substitution of basic residues for alanine residues in the GAG binding domain generates a non-GAG binding mutant. These mutant chemokines bind their cognate receptors normally and competitively inhibit binding of their wild type counterparts. Occupation of chemokine receptors by non-GAG binding chemokine variants prevents migration along a gradient and therefore inhibits chemotaxis, as has been shown with CCL5, CCL7 and CXCL12 amongst others [111,112]. Studies have shown that CXCL8 mutants with reduced GAG-binding abilities induced lower recruitment of neutrophils than wild type CXCL8 in the peritoneum but not the lung in vivo [32,105]. This work could be developed in order to create a non-GAG binding CXCL8 mutant with further impaired recruitment capabilities, although clearly biological activity effects in different tissues would need to be fully characterized. Studies conducted on CXCL11, however, showed that a mutant with reduced GAG binding in vitro could still induce cell migration in vivo, highlighting the need for each chemokine to be studied individually [113].

A variant of CXCL8 which has no ability to bind GPCRs but with increased GAG binding affinity inhibits trans-endothelial migration of neutrophils by displacing CXCL8 from the surface of endothelial cells [114]. A similar study by our group showed that a non-GPCR binding, increased-GAG binding CXCL12 variant showed a reduction in cell migration [115]. A CCL2 mutant with increased GAG binding was shown to displace multiple chemokines which could overcome the issues of redundancy [116], however high concentrations of chemokine may be required to occupy binding sites on all GAGs [43,117]. This approach represents another potential method of regulating chemokine function.

6.4. Using Peptides to Block Chemokine-GAG Binding

In addition to whole chemokine mutants, small peptide fragments of chemokines, for example, a CXCL9 C-terminal peptide was successfully able to compete with CXCL8, CXCL11 and CCL2 for binding to heparin, HS or other GAGs [118]. This illustrates the therapeutic potential of peptides to inhibit chemokine function by disrupting the interaction between chemokines and GAGs. In addition, these short chemokine fragments might occur naturally, due to cleavage by proteases such as matrix metalloproteinases (MMPs). Unpublished data from our group suggests that both a synthesised wild type (KENWVQRVVEKFLKRAENS) and mutant E70K CXCL8 peptide (KENWVQRVVEKFLKRAKNS) can successfully inhibit the action of the full length wild type protein, and thereby reduce adhesion of leukocytes to an endothelial cell monolayer under physiological flow conditions.

6.5. Nitration and CXCL8 Function

Neutrophils recruited by CXCL8 produce NO and reactive species generating $ONOO^-$. Therefore nitration of CXCL8 is likely to occur at sites of inflammation. This could be a mechanism by which neutrophils limit further chemo-attraction to prevent tissue injury [119]. Unpublished data from our group suggests that nitration significantly reduces the ability of CXCL8 to induce neutrophil chemotaxis in vitro.

How nitration may affect the function of CXCL8 is as yet undetermined. Y13 is a residue in the N-loop that is known to be important for receptor signaling and a target for $ONOO^-$. Nitration alters the pK_a making tyrosine residues more acidic, increases the mass of the protein by 45 Da per residue nitrated [54], and is also likely to cause some steric hindrance through increasing the surface area of tyrosine's phenolic ring [120]. The nitration of tyrosine also affects its hydrophobicity, although there are conflicting reports in the literature as to whether this makes the residue more hydrophilic [70] or hydrophobic [120]. It is possible that the hydrophobicity of tyrosine is important in the function of CXCL8 in particular, as a Y13L mutant (which maintains hydrophobicity) showed similar if not slightly increased activity when compared to the wild type [121], but Y13E (hydrophilic) and Y13T (neutral) mutants both showed a decrease in receptor affinity [122]. As the core and secondary GAG-binding residues of CXCL8 described previously include histidines and lysines, which are potential targets of $ONOO^-$, it is likely that modification of CXCL8 by $ONOO^-$ could also affect its GAG binding properties [123].

Tyrosine has also been shown to be an important residue within the receptor CXCR1, as a Y188A mutant version showed decreased affinity for CXCL8 in comparison to the wild type receptor [91]. Therefore nitration of the receptors as well as the ligands (particularly tyrosine residues) could affect chemokine-mediated signal transduction and leukocyte chemotaxis. It is possible that the location and function of the aforementioned residues within any given chemokine (and/or receptor) will determine the specific effects of nitration on each one in turn, highlighting the need for further study.

7. Future Research Directions

Factors such as chemokine-GAG binding and post-translational protein modification are increasingly recognised as important determinants of chemokine function in vivo. How these factors affect chemokine function is only starting to emerge and the challenge is now to understand their effects at a whole organ/organism level during both normal tissue homeostasis and in disease. This is not only of biological interest but it may identify new treatment targets.

In this review we have discussed the importance of chemokine-GAG interactions and how this could be modified by soluble GAGs, mutant chemokines or peptide fragments. There is increasing evidence that this can be done in vitro and in pre-clinical disease models. However, we still do not know what the effect of disrupting chemokine gradients in injured tissues would be nor how this could be applied in the clinic. These are all important areas of future research.

The capacity to mount an effective inflammatory response is paramount. However, to maintain tissue integrity, this response has to be regulated. If we understand the natural mechanisms employed to control inflammation we may be able to exploit this to modify disease. One example discussed in this review is the nitration of chemokines, with resultant loss of activity. Currently, the best methods for detecting chemokine nitration involve NMR analysis or Nano-HPLC, however the development of antibodies specific for nitrated chemokines would better facilitate their study; something our group is currently investigating for nitrated CXCL8. This and similar chemokine modifications could be biological 'off switches', limiting unopposed leukocyte accumulation and tissue damage. Studies are beginning to find links between these different regulatory aspects of chemokine biology, and clearly further study is required to discover how post-translational modifications may affect GAG and GPCR binding in order to contribute to a more complete understanding of the biology of chemokine regulation.

Acknowledgments: This work was supported by The British Heart Foundation (FS/15/19/31327) and a Marie Curie Grant from the European Commission (POSAT 606979, FP7-PEOPLE-2013-ITN).

Author Contributions: Sarah Thompson and Beatriz Martinez-Burgo conceived and wrote the manuscript. Simi Ali, Neil S. Sheerin, Krishna Rajarathnam, Krishna Mohan Sepuru and John A. Kirby provided intellectual in-put and helped with the writing of the manuscript.

Conflicts of Interest: The authors declare no conflict of interest.

Abbreviations

ACKR	Atypical chemokine receptor
ECM	Extracellular matrix
GAG	Glycosaminoglycan
Gal	Galactose
GalNAc	*N*-acetyl-galactosamine
GlcA	Glucuronic acid
GlcNAc	*N*-acetyl-glucosamine
GlcNS	Glucosamine
GPCR	G-protein coupled receptor
HS	Heparan sulphate
HS2ST	2-*O*-sulphotransferases
HS6ST	6-*O*-sulphotransferases
HS3ST	3-*O*-sulphotransferases
IdoA	Iduronic acid
LPS	Lipopolysaccharide
MMPs	Matrix metalloproteinases
NADPH	Nicotinamide adenine dinucleotide phosphate
NDSTs+	*N*-deacetylase/*N*-sulphotranferases
NO	Nitric oxide
O_2^-	Superoxide anion
ONOO$^-$	Peroxynitrite
PTM	Post-translational modifications
RNS	Reactive nitrogen species
SULF1/2	Sulphatases
vCKBP	Viral chemokine binding proteins
3-NT	3-Nitrotyrosine

References

1. Lo, D.J.; Weaver, T.A.; Kleiner, D.E.; Mannon, R.B.; Jacobson, L.M.; Becker, B.N.; Swanson, S.J.; Hale, D.A.; Kirk, A.D. Chemokines and their receptors in human renal allotransplantation. *Transplantation* **2011**, *91*, 70–77. [CrossRef] [PubMed]

2. Meloni, F.; Solari, N.; Miserere, S.; Morosini, M.; Cascina, A.; Klersy, C.; Arbustini, E.; Pellegrini, C.; Vigano, M.; Fietta, A.M. Chemokine redundancy in BOS pathogenesis. A possible role also for the CC chemokines: MIP3-β, MIP3-α, MDC and their specific receptors. *Transpl. Immunol.* **2008**, *18*, 275–280. [CrossRef] [PubMed]

3. Collier, J.J.; Sparer, T.E.; Karlstad, M.D.; Burke, S.J. Pancreatic islet inflammation: An emerging role for chemokines. *J. Mol. Endocrinol.* **2017**, *59*, 33–46. [CrossRef] [PubMed]

4. Liao, X.; Pirapakaran, T.; Luo, X.M. Chemokines and chemokine receptors in the development of lupus nephritis. *Mediat. Inflamm.* **2016**, *2016*. [CrossRef] [PubMed]

5. Kulkarni, N.; Pathak, M.; Lal, G. Role of chemokine receptors and intestinal epithelial cells in the mucosal inflammation and tolerance. *J. Leukoc. Biol.* **2017**, *101*, 377–394. [CrossRef] [PubMed]

6. Weber, M.; Hauschild, R.; Schwarz, J.; Moussion, C.; de Vries, I.; Legler, D.F.; Luther, S.A.; Bollenbach, T.; Sixt, M. Interstitial dendritic cell guidance by haptotactic chemokine gradients. *Science* **2013**, *339*, 328–332. [CrossRef] [PubMed]

7. Kufareva, I.; Salanga, C.L.; Handel, T.M. Chemokine and chemokine receptor structure and interactions: Implications for therapeutic strategies. *Immunol. Cell Biol.* **2015**, *93*, 372–383. [CrossRef] [PubMed]

8. Kolaczkowska, E.; Kubes, P. Neutrophil recruitment and function in health and inflammation. *Nat. Rev. Immunol.* **2013**, *13*, 159–175. [CrossRef] [PubMed]

9. Takahashi, A.; de Andres, M.C.; Hashimoto, K.; Itoi, E.; Oreffo, R.O.C. Epigenetic regulation of interleukin-8, an inflammatory chemokine, in osteoarthritis. *Osteoarthr. Cartil.* **2015**, *23*, 1946–1954. [CrossRef] [PubMed]

10. Das, S.T.; Rajagopalan, L.; Guerrero-Plata, A.; Sai, J.; Richmond, A.; Garofalo, R.P.; Rajarathnam, K. Monomeric and dimeric CXCL8 are both essential for in vivo neutrophil recruitment. *PLoS ONE* **2010**, *5*, e11754. [CrossRef] [PubMed]

11. Dyer, D.P.; Salanga, C.L.; Volkman, B.F.; Kawamura, T.; Handel, T.M. The dependence of chemokine-glycosaminoglycan interactions on chemokine oligomerization. *Glycobiology* **2016**, *26*, 312–326. [CrossRef] [PubMed]

12. Proudfoot, A.E.I.; Handel, T.M.; Johnson, Z.; Lau, E.K.; LiWang, P.; Clark-Lewis, I.; Borlat, F.; Wells, T.N.C.; Kosco-Vilbois, M.H. Glycosaminoglycan binding and oligomerization are essential for the in vivo activity of certain chemokines. *Proc. Natl. Acad. Sci. USA* **2003**, *100*, 1885–1890. [CrossRef] [PubMed]

13. Zweemer, A.J.M.; Toraskar, J.; Heitman, L.H.; Ijzerman, A.P. Bias in chemokine receptor signalling. *Trends Immunol.* **2014**, *35*, 243–252. [CrossRef] [PubMed]

14. Zidar, D.A.; Violin, J.D.; Whalen, E.J.; Lefkowitz, R.J. Selective engagement of g protein coupled receptor kinases (GRKS) encodes distinct functions of biased ligands. *Proc. Natl. Acad. Sci. USA* **2009**, *106*, 9649–9654. [CrossRef] [PubMed]

15. Rajagopalan, L.; Rajarathnam, K. Structural basis of chemokine receptor function—A model for binding affinity and ligand selectivity. *Biosci. Rep.* **2006**, *26*, 325–339. [CrossRef] [PubMed]

16. Bromley, S.K.; Mempel, T.R.; Luster, A.D. Orchestrating the orchestrators: Chemokines in control of T cell traffic. *Nat. Immunol.* **2008**, *9*, 970–980. [CrossRef] [PubMed]

17. Kleist, A.B.; Getschman, A.E.; Ziarek, J.J.; Nevins, A.M.; Gauthier, P.-A.; Chevigné, A.; Szpakowska, M.; Volkman, B.F. New paradigms in chemokine receptor signal transduction: Moving beyond the two-site model. *Biochem. Pharmacol.* **2016**, *114*, 53–68. [CrossRef] [PubMed]

18. Kunkel, S.L. Promiscuous chemokine receptors and their redundant ligands play an enigmatic role during HIV-1 infection. *Am. J. Respir. Cell Mol. Biol.* **1999**, *20*, 859–860. [CrossRef] [PubMed]

19. Baggiolini, M.; Dewald, B.; Moser, B. Human chemokines: An update. *Annu. Rev. Immunol.* **1997**, *15*, 675–705. [CrossRef] [PubMed]

20. Gijsbers, K.; van Assche, G.; Joossens, S.; Struyf, S.; Proost, P.; Rutgeerts, P.; Geboes, K.; van Damme, J. CXCR1-binding chemokines in inflammatory bowel diseases: Down-regulated IL-8/CXCL8 production by leukocytes in crohn's disease and selective GCP-2/CXCL6 expression in inflamed intestinal tissue. *Eur. J. Immunol.* **2004**, *34*, 1992–2000. [CrossRef] [PubMed]

21. Bachelerie, F.; Graham, G.J.; Locati, M.; Mantovani, A.; Murphy, P.M.; Nibbs, R.; Rot, A.; Sozzani, S.; Thelen, M. New nomenclature for atypical chemokine receptors. *Nat. Immunol.* **2014**, *15*, 207–208. [CrossRef] [PubMed]

22. Loos, T.; Opdenakker, G.; van Damme, J.; Proost, P. Citrullination of CXCL8 increases this chemokine's ability to mobilize neutrophils into the blood circulation. *Haematologica* **2009**, *94*, 1346–1353. [CrossRef] [PubMed]

23. Fu, B.M.; Tarbell, J.M. Mechano-sensing and transduction by endothelial surface glycocalyx: Composition, structure, and function. *Wiley Interdiscip. Rev. Syst. Biol. Med.* **2013**, *5*, 381–390. [CrossRef] [PubMed]

24. Handel, T.M.; Johnson, Z.; Crown, S.E.; Lau, E.K.; Sweeney, M.; Proudfoot, A.E. Regulation of protein function by glycosaminoglycans-as exemplified by chemokines. *Annu. Rev. Biochem.* **2005**, *74*, 385–410. [CrossRef] [PubMed]

25. Mihov, D.; Spiess, M. Glycosaminoglycans: Sorting determinants in intracellular protein traffic. *Int. J. Biochem. Cell Biol.* **2015**, *68*, 87–91. [CrossRef] [PubMed]

26. Sepuru, K.M.; Rajarathnam, K. CXCL1/MGSA is a novel glycosaminoglycan (GAG)-binding chemokine structural evidence for two distinct non-overlapping binding domains. *J. Biol. Chem.* **2016**, *291*, 4247–4255. [CrossRef] [PubMed]

27. Sepuru, K.M.; Nagarajan, B.; Desai, U.R.; Rajarathnam, K. Molecular basis of chemokine CXCL5-glycosaminoglycan interactions. *J. Biol. Chem.* **2016**, *291*, 20539–20550. [CrossRef] [PubMed]

28. Liang, W.G.; Triandafillou, C.G.; Huang, T.Y.; Zulueta, M.M.L.; Banerjee, S.; Dinner, A.R.; Hung, S.C.; Tang, W.J. Structural basis for oligomerization and glycosaminoglycan binding of CCL5 and CCL3. *Proc. Natl. Acad. Sci. USA* **2016**, *113*, 5000–5005. [CrossRef] [PubMed]

29. Brown, A.J.; Joseph, P.R.B.; Sawant, K.V.; Rajarathnam, K. Chemokine CXCL7 heterodimers: Structural insights, CXCR2 receptor function, and glycosaminoglycan interactions. *Int. J. Mol. Sci.* **2017**, *18*, 748. [CrossRef] [PubMed]

30. Poluri, K.M.; Joseph, P.R.B.; Sawant, K.V.; Rajarathnam, K. Molecular basis of glycosaminoglycan heparin binding to the chemokine CXCL1 dimer. *J. Biol. Chem.* **2013**, *288*, 25143–25153. [CrossRef] [PubMed]

31. Crown, S.E.; Yu, Y.; Sweeney, M.D.; Leary, J.A.; Handel, T.M. Heterodimerization of CCR2 chemokines and regulation by glycosaminoglycan binding. *J. Biol. Chem.* **2006**, *281*, 25438–25446. [CrossRef] [PubMed]

32. Gangavarapu, P.; Rajagopalan, L.; Kolli, D.; Guerrero-Plata, A.; Garofalo, R.P.; Rajarathnam, K. The monomer-dimer equilibrium and glycosaminoglycan interactions of chemokine CXCL8 regulate tissue-specific neutrophil recruitment. *J. Leukoc. Biol.* **2012**, *91*, 259–265. [CrossRef] [PubMed]

33. Proudfoot, A.E. Chemokines and glycosaminoglycans. *Front. Immunol.* **2015**, *6*, 246. [CrossRef] [PubMed]

34. Mbemba, E.; Slimani, H.; Atemezem, A.; Saffar, L.; Gattegno, L. Glycans are involved in rantes binding to CCR5 positive as well as to CCR5 negative cells. *Biochim. Biophys. Acta Biomembr.* **2001**, *1510*, 354–366. [CrossRef]

35. Brown, A.J.; Sepuru, K.M.; Rajarathnam, K. Structural basis of native CXCL7 monomer binding to CXCR2 receptor n-domain and glycosaminoglycan heparin. *Int. J. Mol. Sci.* **2017**, *18*, 508. [CrossRef] [PubMed]

36. Singh, A.; Kett, W.C.; Severin, I.C.; Agyekum, I.; Duan, J.; Amster, I.J.; Proudfoot, A.E.I.; Coombe, D.R.; Woods, R.J. The interaction of heparin tetrasaccharides with chemokine CCL5 is modulated by sulfation pattern and PH. *J. Biol. Chem.* **2015**, *290*, 15421–15436. [CrossRef] [PubMed]

37. Sawant, K.V.; Poluri, K.M.; Dutta, A.K.; Sepuru, K.M.; Troshkina, A.; Garofalo, R.P.; Rajarathnam, K. Chemokine CXCL1 mediated neutrophil recruitment: Role of glycosaminoglycan interactions. *Sci. Rep.* **2016**, *6*. [CrossRef] [PubMed]

38. Ziarek, J.J.; Kleist, A.B.; London, N.; Raveh, B.; Montpas, N.; Bonneterre, J.; St-Onge, G.; DiCosmo-Ponticello, C.J.; Koplinski, C.A.; Roy, I. Structural basis for chemokine recognition by a g protein-coupled receptor and implications for receptor activation. *Sci. Signal.* **2017**, *10*, 5756. [CrossRef] [PubMed]

39. Drury, L.J.; Ziarek, J.J.; Gravel, S.; Veldkamp, C.T.; Takekoshi, T.; Hwang, S.T.; Heveker, N.; Volkman, B.F.; Dwinell, M.B. Monomeric and dimeric CXCL12 inhibit metastasis through distinct CXCR4 interactions and signaling pathways. *Proc. Natl. Acad. Sci. USA* **2011**, *108*, 17655–17660. [CrossRef] [PubMed]

40. Lortat-Jacob, H.; Grosdidier, A.; Imberty, A. Structural diversity of heparan sulfate binding domains in chemokines. *Proc. Natl. Acad. Sci. USA* **2002**, *99*, 1229–1234. [CrossRef] [PubMed]

41. Joseph, P.R.B.; Mosier, P.D.; Desai, U.R.; Rajarathnam, K. Solution NMR characterization of chemokine CXCL8/IL-8 monomer and dimer binding to glycosaminoglycans: Structural plasticity mediates differential binding interactions. *Biochem. J.* **2015**, *472*, 121–133. [CrossRef] [PubMed]

42. Rot, A. Chemokine patterning by glycosaminoglycans and interceptors. *Front. Biosci.* **2009**, *15*, 645–660. [CrossRef]

43. Ali, S.; Hardy, L.A.; Kirby, J.A. Transplant immunobiology: A crucial role for heparan sulfate glycosaminoglycans? *Transplantation* **2003**, *75*, 1773–1782. [CrossRef] [PubMed]

44. Hacker, U.; Nybakken, K.; Perrimon, N. Heparan sulphate proteoglycans: The sweet side of development. *Nat. Rev. Mol. Cell Biol.* **2005**, *6*, 530–541. [CrossRef] [PubMed]

45. Ferreras, L.; Sheerin, N.S.; Kirby, J.A.; Ali, S. Mechanisms of renal graft chronic injury and progression to interstitial fibrosis. *Curr. Transplant. Rep.* **2015**, *2*, 259–268. [CrossRef]

46. Bao, X.; Moseman, E.A.; Saito, H.; Petryanik, B.; Thiriot, A.; Hatakeyama, S.; Ito, Y.; Kawashima, H.; Yamaguchi, Y.; Lowe, J.B.; et al. Endothelial heparan sulfate controls chemokine presentation in recruitment of lymphocytes and dendritic cells to lymph nodes. *Immunity* **2010**, *33*, 817–829. [CrossRef] [PubMed]

47. Parish, C.R. The role of heparan sulphate in inflammation. *Nat. Rev. Immunol.* **2006**, *6*, 633–643. [CrossRef] [PubMed]

48. Marshall, L.J.; Ramdin, L.S.P.; Brooks, T.; Shute, J.K. Plasminogen activator inhibitor-1 supports IL-8-mediated neutrophil transendothelial migration by inhibition of the constitutive shedding of endothelial IL-8/heparan sulfate/syndecan-1 complexes. *J. Immunol.* **2003**, *171*, 2057–2065. [CrossRef] [PubMed]

49. Lipowsky, H.H.; Lescanic, A. Inhibition of inflammation induced shedding of the endothelial glycocalyx with low molecular weight heparin. *Microvasc. Res.* **2017**, *112*, 72–78. [CrossRef] [PubMed]

50. Carter, N.M.; Ali, S.; Kirby, J.A. Endothelial inflammation: The role of differential expression of *N*-deacetylase/*N*-sulphotransferase enzymes in alteration of the immunological properties of heparan sulphate. *J. Cell Sci.* **2003**, *116*, 3591–3600. [CrossRef] [PubMed]

51. Mulloy, B.; Lever, R.; Page, C.P. Mast cell glycosaminoglycans. *Glycoconj. J.* **2016**, *34*, 351–361. [CrossRef] [PubMed]

52. Doster, A.; Schwarzig, U.; Zygmunt, M.; Rom, J.; Schuetz, F.; Fluhr, H. Unfractionated heparin selectively modulates the expression of CXCL8, CCL2 and CCL5 in endometrial carcinoma cells. *Anticancer Res.* **2016**, *36*, 1535–1544. [PubMed]

53. Mortier, A.; Van Damme, J.; Proost, P. Regulation of chemokine activity by posttranslational modification. *Pharmacol. Ther.* **2008**, *120*, 197–217. [CrossRef] [PubMed]

54. Barker, C.E.; Ali, S.; O'Boyle, G.; Kirby, J.A. Transplantation and inflammation: Implications for the modification of chemokine function. *Immunology* **2014**, *143*, 138–145. [CrossRef] [PubMed]

55. Loos, T.; Mortier, A.; Gouwy, M.; Ronsse, I.; Put, W.; Lenaerts, J.P.; Van Damme, J.; Proost, P. Citrullination of CXCL10 and CXCL11 by peptidylarginine deiminase: A naturally occurring posttranslational modification of chemokines and new dimension of immunoregulation. *Blood* **2008**, *112*, 2648–2656. [CrossRef] [PubMed]

56. Proost, P.; Loos, T.; Mortier, A.; Schutyser, E.; Gouwy, M.; Noppen, S.; Dillen, C.; Ronsse, I.; Conings, R.; Struyf, S.; et al. Citrullination of CXCL8 by peptidylarginine deiminase alters receptor usage, prevents proteolysis, and dampens tissue inflammation. *J. Exp. Med.* **2008**, *205*, 2085–2097. [CrossRef] [PubMed]

57. Struyf, S.; Noppen, S.; Loos, T.; Mortier, A.; Gouwy, M.; Verbeke, H.; Huskens, D.; Luangsay, S.; Parmentier, M.; Geboes, K.; et al. Citrullination of CXCL12 differentially reduces CXCR4 and CXCR7 binding with loss of inflammatory and anti-HIV-1 activity via CXCR4. *J. Immunol.* **2009**, *182*, 666–674. [CrossRef] [PubMed]

58. Gole, M.D.; Souza, J.M.; Choi, I.; Hertkorn, C.; Malcolm, S.; Foust, R.F.; Finkel, B.; Lanken, P.N.; Ischiropoulos, H. Plasma proteins modified by tyrosine nitration in acute respiratory distress syndrome. *Am. J. Physiol. Lung Cell. Mol. Physiol.* **2000**, *278*, 961–967.

59. Greenacre, S.A.B.; Ischiropoulos, H. Tyrosine nitration: Localisation, quantification, consequences for protein function and signal transduction. *Free Radic. Res.* **2001**, *34*, 541–581. [CrossRef] [PubMed]

60. Lowenstein, C.J.; Snyder, S.H. Nitric oxide, a novel biologic messenger. *Cell* **1992**, *70*, 705–707. [CrossRef]

61. Lim, C.H.; Dedon, P.C.; Deen, W.M. Kinetic analysis of intracellular concentrations of reactive nitrogen species. *Chem. Res. Toxicol.* **2008**, *21*, 2134–2147. [CrossRef] [PubMed]

62. Szabó, C.; Ischiropoulos, H.; Radi, R. Peroxynitrite: Biochemistry, pathophysiology and development of therapeutics. *Nat. Rev. Drug Discov.* **2007**, *6*, 662–680. [CrossRef] [PubMed]

63. Beckman, J.S. Oxidative damage and tyrosine nitration from peroxynitrite. *Chem. Res. Toxicol.* **1996**, *9*, 836–844. [CrossRef] [PubMed]

64. Vanhoutte, P.M.; Zhao, Y.; Xu, A.; Leung, S.W.S. Thirty years of saying no. *Circ. Res.* **2016**, *119*, 375–396. [CrossRef] [PubMed]

65. Mount, P.F.; Power, D.A. Nitric oxide in the kidney: Functions and regulation of synthesis. *Acta Physiol.* **2005**, *187*, 433–446. [CrossRef] [PubMed]

66. De Oliveira, G.A.; Cheng, R.Y.S.; Ridnour, L.A.; Basudhar, D.; Somasundaram, V.; McVicar, D.W.; Monteiro, H.P.; Wink, D.A. Inducible nitric oxide synthase in the carcinogenesis of gastrointestinal cancers. *Antioxid. Redox Signal.* **2016**, *26*, 1059–1077. [CrossRef] [PubMed]

67. Epstein, F.H.; Weiss, S.J. Tissue destruction by neutrophils. *N. Engl. J. Med.* **1989**, *320*, 365–376. [CrossRef] [PubMed]

68. Inauen, W.; Suzuki, M.; Granger, D.N. Mechanisms of cellular injury: Potential sources of oxygen free radicals in ischemia/reperfusion. *Microcirc. Endothel. Lymphat.* **1988**, *5*, 143–155.

69. Biswas, S.K. Does the interdependence between oxidative stress and inflammation explain the antioxidant paradox? *Oxidative Med. Cell. Longev.* **2016**, *2016*, 1–9. [CrossRef] [PubMed]

70. Turko, I.V.; Murad, F. Protein nitration in cardiovascular diseases. *Pharmacol. Rev.* **2002**, *54*, 619–634. [CrossRef] [PubMed]

71. Thompson-Gorman, S.L.; Zweier, J.L. Evaluation of the role of xanthine oxidase in myocardial reperfusion injury. *J. Biol. Chem.* **1990**, *265*, 6656–6663. [PubMed]

72. Gondouin, B.; Jourde-Chiche, N.; Sallee, M.; Dou, L.; Cerini, C.; Loundou, A.; Morange, S.; Berland, Y.; Burtey, S.; Brunet, P.; et al. Plasma xanthine oxidase activity is predictive of cardiovascular disease in patients with chronic kidney disease, independently of uric acid levels. *Nephron* **2015**, *131*, 167–174. [CrossRef] [PubMed]

73. Choi, E.K.; Jung, H.; Kwak, K.H.; Yi, S.J.; Lim, J.A.; Park, S.H.; Park, J.M.; Kim, S.; Jee, D.L.; Lim, D.G. Inhibition of oxidative stress in renal ischemia-reperfusion injury. *Anesth. Anal.* **2017**, *124*, 204–213. [CrossRef] [PubMed]

74. Shin, J.H.; Chun, K.S.; Na, Y.G.; Song, K.H.; Kim, S.I.; Lim, J.S.; Kim, G.H. Allopurinol protects against ischemia/reperfusion-induced injury in rat urinary bladders. *Oxidative Med. Cell. Longev.* **2015**, *2015*, 1–8. [CrossRef] [PubMed]

75. Saavedra, W.F.; Paolocci, N.; John, M.E.S.; Skaf, M.W.; Stewart, G.C.; Xie, J.S.; Harrison, R.W.; Zeichner, J.; Mudrick, D.; Marbán, E.; et al. Imbalance between xanthine oxidase and nitric oxide synthase signaling pathways underlies mechanoenergetic uncoupling in the failing heart. *Circ. Res.* **2002**, *90*, 297–304. [CrossRef] [PubMed]

76. Cappola, T.P.; Kass, D.A.; Nelson, G.S.; Berger, R.D.; Rosas, G.O.; Kobeissi, Z.A.; Marbán, E.; Hare, J.M. Allopurinol improves myocardial efficiency in patients with idiopathic dilated cardiomyopathy. *Circulation* **2001**, *104*, 2407–2411. [CrossRef] [PubMed]

77. Pacher, P.; Beckman, J.S.; Liaudet, L. Nitric oxide and peroxynitrite in health and disease. *Physiol. Rev.* **2007**, *87*, 315–424. [CrossRef] [PubMed]

78. Nagai, R.; Unno, Y.; Hayashi, M.C.; Masuda, S.; Hayase, F.; Kinae, N.; Horiuchi, S. Peroxynitrite induces formation of $N\varepsilon$-(carboxymethyl) lysine by the cleavage of amadori product and generation of glucosone and glyoxal from glucose. *Diabetes* **2002**, *51*, 2833–2839. [CrossRef] [PubMed]

79. Batthyány, C.; Bartesaghi, S.; Mastrogiovanni, M.; Lima, A.; Demicheli, V.; Radi, R. Tyrosine-nitrated proteins: Proteomic and bioanalytical aspects. *Antioxid. Redox Signal.* **2016**, *26*, 313–328. [CrossRef] [PubMed]

80. Lee, W.H.; Gounarides, J.S.; Roos, E.S.; Wolin, M.S. Influence of peroxynitrite on energy metabolism and cardiac function in a rat ischemia-reperfusion model. *Am. J. Physiol. Heart Circ. Physiol.* **2003**, *285*, 1385–1395. [CrossRef] [PubMed]

81. Sakurai, M.; Fukuyama, N.; Iguchi, A.; Akimoto, H.; Ohmi, M.; Yokoyama, H.; Nakazawa, H.; Tabayashi, K. Quantitative analysis of cardiac 3-L-nitrotyrosine during acute allograft rejection in an experimental heart transplantation1. *Transplantation* **1999**, *68*, 1818–1822. [CrossRef] [PubMed]

82. Chimenti, C.; Scopelliti, F.; Vulpis, E.; Tafani, M.; Villanova, L.; Verardo, R.; de Paulis, R.; Russo, M.A.; Frustaci, A. Increased oxidative stress contributes to cardiomyocyte dysfunction and death in patients with fabry disease cardiomyopathy. *Hum. Pathol.* **2015**, *46*, 1760–1768. [CrossRef] [PubMed]

83. Thuraisingham, R.C.; Nott, C.A.; Dodd, S.M.; Yaqoob, M.M. Increased nitrotyrosine staining in kidneys from patients with diabetic nephropathy. *Kidney Int.* **2000**, *57*, 1968–1972. [CrossRef] [PubMed]

84. Ahmed, U.; Anwar, A.; Savage, R.S.; Thornalley, P.J.; Rabbani, N. Protein oxidation, nitration and glycation biomarkers for early-stage diagnosis of osteoarthritis of the knee and typing and progression of arthritic disease. *Arthritis Res. Ther.* **2016**, *18*, 250. [CrossRef] [PubMed]

85. Pennathur, S.; Vivekanandan-Giri, A.; Locy, M.L.; Kulkarni, T.; Zhi, D.; Zeng, L.; Byun, J.; de Andrade, J.A.; Thannickal, V.J. Oxidative modifications of protein tyrosyl residues are increased in plasma of human subjects with interstitial lung disease. *Am. J. Respir. Crit. Care Med.* **2016**, *193*, 861–868. [CrossRef] [PubMed]

86. Aydın, A.; Orhan, H.; Sayal, A.; Özata, M.; Şahin, G.; Işımer, A. Oxidative stress and nitric oxide related parameters in type II diabetes mellitus: Effects of glycemic control. *Clin. Biochem.* **2001**, *34*, 65–70. [CrossRef]

87. Balafanova, Z.; Bolli, R.; Zhang, J.; Zheng, Y.; Pass, J.M.; Bhatnagar, A.; Tang, X.-L.; Wang, O.; Cardwell, E.; Ping, P. Nitric oxide (NO) induces nitration of protein kinase Cε (PKCE), facilitating PKCE translocation via enhanced PKCE–RACK2 interactions a novel mechanism of no-triggered activation of PKCE. *J. Biol. Chem.* **2002**, *277*, 15021–15027. [CrossRef] [PubMed]

88. Molon, B.; Ugel, S.; Del Pozzo, F.; Soldani, C.; Zilio, S.; Avella, D.; De Palma, A.; Mauri, P.; Monegal, A.; Rescigno, M.; et al. Chemokine nitration prevents intratumoral infiltration of antigen-specific T cells. *J. Exp. Med.* **2011**, *208*, 1949–1962. [CrossRef] [PubMed]

89. Sato, E.; Simpson, K.L.; Grisham, M.B.; Koyama, S.; Robbins, R.A. Effects of reactive oxygen and nitrogen metabolites on rantes and IL-5-induced eosinophil chemotactic activity in vitro. *Am. J. Pathol.* **1999**, *155*, 591–598. [CrossRef]

90. Janssens, R.; Mortier, A.; Boff, D.; Vanheule, V.; Gouwy, M.; Franck, C.; Larsen, O.; Rosenkilde, M.M.; Van Damme, J.; Amaral, F.A.; et al. Natural nitration of CXCL12 reduces its signaling capacity and chemotactic activity in vitro and abrogates intra-articular lymphocyte recruitment in vivo. *Oncotarget* **2016**, *7*, 62439–62459. [CrossRef] [PubMed]

91. Leong, S.R.; Kabakoff, R.C.; Hebert, C.A. Complete mutagenesis of the extracellular domain of interleukin-8 (IL-8) type a receptor identifies charged residues mediating IL-8 binding and signal transduction. *J. Biol. Chem.* **1994**, *269*, 19343–19348. [PubMed]

92. Barker, C.E.; Thompson, S.; O'boyle, G.; Lortat-Jacob, H.; Sheerin, N.S.; Ali, S.; Kirby, J.A. CCL2 nitration is a negative regulator of chemokine-mediated inflammation. *Sci. Rep.* **2017**, *7*, 44384. [CrossRef] [PubMed]

93. Hauser, M.A.; Legler, D.F. Common and biased signaling pathways of the chemokine receptor CCR7 elicited by its ligands CCL19 and CCL21 in leukocytes. *J. Leukoc. Biol.* **2016**, *99*, 869–882. [CrossRef] [PubMed]

94. De Oliveira, S.; Reyes-Aldasoro, C.C.; Candel, S.; Renshaw, S.A.; Mulero, V.; Calado, Â. CXCL8 (IL-8) mediates neutrophil recruitment and behavior in the zebrafish inflammatory response. *J. Immunol.* **2013**, *190*, 4349–4359. [CrossRef] [PubMed]

95. Rot, A. Neutrophil attractant/activation protein-1 (interleukin-8) induces in vitro neutrophil migration by haptotactic mechanism. *Eur. J. Immunol.* **1993**, *23*, 303–306. [CrossRef] [PubMed]

96. Mehrad, B.; Keane, M.P.; Strieter, R.M. Chemokines as mediators of angiogenesis. *Thromb. Haemost.* **2007**, *97*, 755. [CrossRef] [PubMed]

97. Kendrick, A.A.; Holliday, M.J.; Isern, N.G.; Zhang, F.; Camilloni, C.; Huynh, C.; Vendruscolo, M.; Armstrong, G.; Eisenmesser, E.Z. The dynamics of interleukin-8 and its interaction with human CXC receptor I peptide. *Protein Sci.* **2014**, *23*, 464–480. [CrossRef] [PubMed]

98. Ranganathan, P.; Jayakumar, C.; Manicassamy, S.; Ramesh, G. CXCR2 knockout mice are protected against DSS-colitis-induced acute kidney injury and inflammation. *Am. J. Physiol. Ren. Physiol.* **2013**, *305*, 1422–1427. [CrossRef] [PubMed]

99. Nasser, M.W.; Raghuwanshi, S.K.; Grant, D.J.; Jala, V.R.; Rajarathnam, K.; Richardson, R.M. Differential activation and regulation of CXCR1 and CXCR2 by CXCL8 monomer and dimer. *J. Immunol.* **2009**, *183*, 3425–3432. [CrossRef] [PubMed]

100. Fernando, H.; Chin, C.; Rösgen, J.; Rajarathnam, K. Dimer dissociation is essential for interleukin-8 (IL-8) binding to CXCR1 receptor. *J. Biol. Chem.* **2004**, *279*, 36175–36178. [CrossRef] [PubMed]

101. Rajarathnam, K.; Prado, G.N.; Fernando, H.; Clark-Lewis, I.; Navarro, J. Probing receptor binding activity of interleukin-8 dimer using a disulfide trap. *Biochemistry* **2006**, *45*, 7882–7888. [CrossRef] [PubMed]

102. Webb, L.M.C.; Clark-Lewis, I.; Alcami, A. The gammaherpesvirus chemokine binding protein binds to the N terminus of CXCL8. *J. Virol.* **2003**, *77*, 8588–8592. [CrossRef] [PubMed]

103. Falsone, A.; Wabitsch, V.; Geretti, E.; Potzinger, H.; Gerlza, T.; Robinson, J.; Adage, T.; Teixeira, M.M.; Kungl, A.J. Designing CXCL8-based decoy proteins with strong anti-inflammatory activity in vivo. *Biosci. Rep.* **2013**, *33*. [CrossRef] [PubMed]

104. Kuschert, G.S.V.; Hoogewerf, A.J.; Proudfoot, A.E.I.; Chung, C.-W.; Cooke, R.M.; Hubbard, R.E.; Wells, T.N.C.; Sanderson, P.N. Identification of a glycosaminoglycan binding surface on human interleukin-8. *Biochemistry* **1998**, *37*, 11193–11201. [CrossRef] [PubMed]

105. Tanino, Y.; Coombe, D.R.; Gill, S.E.; Kett, W.C.; Kajikawa, O.; Proudfoot, A.E.I.; Wells, T.N.C.; Parks, W.C.; Wight, T.N.; Martin, T.R.; et al. Kinetics of chemokine-glycosaminoglycan interactions control neutrophil migration into the airspaces of the lungs. *J. Immunol.* **2010**, *184*, 2677–2685. [CrossRef] [PubMed]

106. Al Faruque, H.; Kang, J.H.; Hwang, S.R.; Sung, S.; Alam, M.M.; Sa, K.H.; Nam, E.J.; Byun, Y.R.; Kang, Y.M. Stepwise inhibition of T cell recruitment at post-capillary venules by orally active desulfated heparins in inflammatory arthritis. *PLoS ONE* **2017**, *12*. [CrossRef] [PubMed]

107. Nagata, K.; Kumasaka, K.; Browne, K.D.; Li, S.; St-Pierre, J.; Cognetti, J.; Marks, J.; Johnson, V.E.; Smith, D.H.; Pascual, J.L. Unfractionated heparin after TBI reduces in vivo cerebrovascular inflammation, brain edema and accelerates cognitive recovery. *J. Trauma Acute Care Surg.* **2016**, *81*, 1088–1094. [CrossRef] [PubMed]

108. Riffo-Vasquez, Y.; Somani, A.; Man, F.; Amison, R.; Pitchford, S.; Page, C.P. A non-anticoagulant fraction of heparin inhibits leukocyte diapedesis into the lung by an effect on platelets. *Am. J. Respir. Cell Mol. Biol.* **2016**, *55*, 554–563. [CrossRef] [PubMed]

109. Arimateia, D.S.; da Silva Brito, A.; de Azevedo, F.M.; de Andrade, G.P.V.; Chavante, S.F. Heparin fails to inhibit the leukocyte recruitment for an extended time following inflammatory stimulus. *Pharm. Biol.* **2015**, *53*, 72–77. [CrossRef] [PubMed]

110. Gonzalez-Motos, V.; Kropp, K.A.; Viejo-Borbolla, A. Chemokine binding proteins: An immunomodulatory strategy going viral. *Cytokine Growth Factor Rev.* **2016**, *30*, 71–80. [CrossRef] [PubMed]

111. O'Boyle, G.; Mellor, P.; Kirby, J.A.; Ali, S. Anti-inflammatory therapy by intravenous delivery of non-heparan sulfate-binding CXCL12. *FASEB J.* **2009**, *23*, 3906–3916. [CrossRef] [PubMed]

112. Johnson, Z.; Kosco-Vilbois, M.H.; Herren, S.; Cirillo, R.; Muzio, V.; Zaratin, P.; Carbonatto, M.; Mack, M.; Smailbegovic, A.; Rose, M.; et al. Interference with heparin binding and oligomerization creates a novel anti-inflammatory strategy targeting the chemokine system. *J. Immunol.* **2004**, *173*, 5776–5785. [CrossRef] [PubMed]

113. Severin, I.C.; Gaudry, J.-P.; Johnson, Z.; Kungl, A.; Jansma, A.; Gesslbauer, B.; Mulloy, B.; Power, C.; Proudfoot, A.E.I.; Handel, T. Characterization of the chemokine CXCL11-heparin interaction suggests two different affinities for glycosaminoglycans. *J. Biol. Chem.* **2010**, *285*, 17713–17724. [CrossRef] [PubMed]

114. Gschwandtner, M.; Strutzmann, E.; Teixeira, M.M.; Anders, H.J.; Diedrichs-Möhring, M.; Gerlza, T.; Wildner, G.; Russo, R.C.; Adage, T.; Kungl, A.J. Glycosaminoglycans are important mediators of neutrophilic inflammation in vivo. *Cytokine* **2017**, *91*, 65–73. [CrossRef] [PubMed]

115. Gschwandtner, M.; Trinker, M.U.; Hecher, B.; Adage, T.; Ali, S.; Kungl, A.J. Glycosaminoglycan silencing by engineered CXCL12 variants. *FEBS Lett.* **2015**, *589*, 2819–2824. [CrossRef] [PubMed]

116. Gerlza, T.; Winkler, S.; Atlic, A.; Zankl, C.; Konya, V.; Kitic, N.; Strutzmann, E.; Knebl, K.; Adage, T.; Heinemann, A.; et al. Designing a mutant CCL2–HSA chimera with high glycosaminoglycan-binding affinity and selectivity. *Protein Eng. Des. Sel.* **2015**, *28*, 231–240. [CrossRef] [PubMed]

117. Bedke, J.; Nelson, P.J.; Kiss, E.; Muenchmeier, N.; Rek, A.; Behnes, C.-L.; Gretz, N.; Kungl, A.J.; Gröne, H.-J. A novel CXCL8 protein-based antagonist in acute experimental renal allograft damage. *Mol. Immunol.* **2010**, *47*, 1047–1057. [CrossRef] [PubMed]

118. Vanheule, V.; Janssens, R.; Boff, D.; Kitic, N.; Berghmans, N.; Ronsse, I.; Kungl, A.J.; Amaral, F.A.; Teixeira, M.M.; Van Damme, J.; et al. The positively charged COOH-terminal glycosaminoglycan-binding CXCL9 (74–103) peptide inhibits CXCL8-induced neutrophil extravasation and monosodium urate crystal-induced gout in mice. *J. Biol. Chem.* **2015**, *290*, 21292–21304. [CrossRef] [PubMed]

119. Greenacre, S.A.B.; Rocha, F.A.C.; Rawlingson, A.; Meinerikandathevan, S.; Poston, R.N.; Ruiz, E.; Halliwell, B.; Brain, S.D. Protein nitration in cutaneous inflammation in the rat: Essential role of inducible nitric oxide synthase and polymorphonuclear leukocytes. *Br. J. Pharmacol.* **2002**, *136*, 985–994. [CrossRef] [PubMed]

120. Souza, J.M.; Peluffo, G.; Radi, R. Protein tyrosine nitration—Functional alteration or just a biomarker? *Free Radic. Biol. Med.* **2008**, *45*, 357–366. [CrossRef] [PubMed]

121. Hammond, M.E.W.; Shyamala, V.; Siani, M.A.; Gallegos, C.A.; Feucht, P.H.; Abbott, J.; Lapointe, G.R.; Moghadam, M.; Khoja, H.; Zakel, J.; et al. Receptor recognition and specificity of interleukin-8 is determined by residues that cluster near a surface-accessible hydrophobic pocket. *J. Biol. Chem.* **1996**, *271*, 8228–8235. [CrossRef] [PubMed]

122. Clark-Lewis, I.; Dewald, B.; Loetscher, M.; Moser, B.; Baggiolini, M. Structural requirements for interleukin-8 function identified by design of analogs and CXC chemokine hybrids. *J. Biol. Chem.* **1994**, *269*, 16075–16081. [PubMed]

123. Alvarez, B.; Ferrer-Sueta, G.; Freeman, B.A.; Radi, R. Kinetics of peroxynitrite reaction with amino acids and human serum albumin. *J. Biol. Chem.* **1999**, *274*, 842–848. [CrossRef] [PubMed]

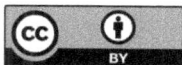

International Journal of
Molecular Sciences

MDPI

Article

Structural Basis of Native CXCL7 Monomer Binding to CXCR2 Receptor N-Domain and Glycosaminoglycan Heparin

Aaron J. Brown, Krishna Mohan Sepuru and Krishna Rajarathnam *

Department of Biochemistry and Molecular Biology, and Sealy Center for Structural Biology and Molecular Biophysics, The University of Texas Medical Branch, Galveston, TX 77555, USA; aj3brown@utmb.edu (A.J.B.); kmsepuru@utmb.edu (K.M.S.)
* Correspondence: krrajara@utmb.edu; Tel.: +1-409-772-2238

Academic Editor: Martin J. Stone
Received: 13 January 2017; Accepted: 21 February 2017; Published: 26 February 2017

Abstract: CXCL7, a chemokine highly expressed in platelets, orchestrates neutrophil recruitment during thrombosis and related pathophysiological processes by interacting with CXCR2 receptor and sulfated glycosaminoglycans (GAG). CXCL7 exists as monomers and dimers, and dimerization (~50 μM) and CXCR2 binding (~10 nM) constants indicate that CXCL7 is a potent agonist as a monomer. Currently, nothing is known regarding the structural basis by which receptor and GAG interactions mediate CXCL7 function. Using solution nuclear magnetic resonance (NMR) spectroscopy, we characterized the binding of CXCL7 monomer to the CXCR2 N-terminal domain (CXCR2Nd) that constitutes a critical docking site and to GAG heparin. We found that CXCR2Nd binds a hydrophobic groove and that ionic interactions also play a role in mediating binding. Heparin binds a set of contiguous basic residues indicating a prominent role for ionic interactions. Modeling studies reveal that the binding interface is dynamic and that GAG adopts different binding geometries. Most importantly, several residues involved in GAG binding are also involved in receptor interactions, suggesting that GAG-bound monomer cannot activate the receptor. Further, this is the first study that describes the structural basis of receptor and GAG interactions of a native monomer of the neutrophil-activating chemokine family.

Keywords: chemokine; CXCL7; NAP-2; CXCR2; glycosaminoglycan; heparin; NMR; monomer

1. Introduction

Chemokines, a large family of signaling proteins, mediate diverse biological functions, including inflammation, development and tissue repair [1–3]. Chemokines mediate their function by activating seven transmembrane G-protein coupled receptors (GPCRs) and binding sulfated glycosaminoglycans (GAGs) that regulate receptor function [4–6]. Another key feature of chemokines is their ability to reversibly exist as monomers and dimers and sometimes as higher order oligomers. Humans express ~50 different chemokines, which are classified on the basis of conserved cysteines near the N-terminus as CXC, CC, CX_3C and XC. Chemokine CXCL7 (also known as NAP-2), released by activated platelets, plays a prominent role in recruiting neutrophils to the injury site during thrombosis [7–9]. CXCL7 belongs to a subset of CXC neutrophil-activating chemokines (NACs) that are characterized by an N-terminal "ELR" motif and function as potent agonists for the CXCR2 receptor [10]. Other members of ELR-chemokines include CXCL1, CXCL2, CXCL3, CXCL5, CXCL6 and CXCL8 (Figure 1).

```
                  5    10   15   20   25   30   35   40   45   50   55   60   65   70
CXCL7  --------AELRCMCIKTTSG-IHPKNIQSLEVIGKGTHCNQVEVIATLKDGRKICLDPDAPRIKKIVQKKLAGDESAD
CXCL1  ----ASVATELRCQCLQTLQG-IHPKNIQSVNVKSPGPHCAQTEVIATLKNGRKACLNPASPIVKKIIEKMLNSDKSN-
CXCL2  ----APLATELRCQCLQTLQG-IHLKNIQSVKVKSPGPHCAQTEVIATLKNGQKACLNPASPMVKKIIEKMLKNGKSN-
CXCL3  ----ASVVTELRCQCLQTLQG-IHLKNIQSVNVRSPGPHCAQTEVIATLKNGKKACLNPASPMVQKIIEKILNKGSTN-
CXCL5  AGPAAAVLRELRCVCLQTTQG-VHPKMISNLQVFAIGPQCSKVEVVASLKNGKEICLDPEAPFLKKVIQKILDGGNKEN
CXCL6  -GPVSAVLTELRCTCLRVTLR-VNPKTIGKLQVFPAGPQCSKVEVVASLKNGKQVCLDPEAPFLKKVIQKILDSGNKKN
CXCL8  ------SAKELRCQCIKTYSKPFHPKFIKELRVIESGPHCANTEIIVKLSDGRELCLDPKENWVQRVVEKFLKRAENS-
```

Figure 1. Sequence alignment of neutrophil-activating chemokines. The conserved "ELR" motif is shown in green. Basic residues that mediate GAG and receptor interactions and hydrophobic residues that mediate receptor interactions for CXCL7 identified in this study are shown in blue and red, respectively. The corresponding residues in other chemokines are likewise highlighted. Residues K9 and R54 shown to be involved in binding only in CXCL7 are italicized and underlined.

Monomer-dimer equilibrium constants have been determined for CXCL1, CXCL5, CXCL7 and CXCL8. Among them, CXCL7 stands out, as it forms a much weaker dimer [11–14]. Whereas the dimerization constant for CXCL7 is ~50 to 100 μM, the values for other chemokines vary around ~1 to 10 μM. We observed that the dimer levels increase with increasing concentration up to a point after which tetramer levels populate, and dimer levels do not go beyond ~50% at any given condition (Table S1). The structure of CXCL7 determined by crystallography corresponded to the tetrameric state [15], which is not surprising, as crystallography by its very nature results in the higher oligomeric state. The solution structure of a CXCL7 monomer determined in the presence of 2-chloroethanol that is known to disrupt intermolecular dimer and tetramer interactions has been reported, but its coordinates are not available in the public domain [16].

Receptor binding and activity measurements have shown that CXCL7 binds CXCR2 with nanomolar (nM) affinity, indicating that the monomer is a potent agonist [17]. Presently, nothing is known regarding the structural basis or molecular mechanisms by which the CXCL7 monomer interacts with the receptor. Knowledge of the GAG interactions is also essential as GAG interactions regulate receptor function. Using solution nuclear magnetic resonance (NMR) spectroscopy, we characterized the binding of the native CXCL7 monomer to the CXCR2 N-terminal domain (N-domain) that functions as a critical ligand binding site and heparin that serves as a representative and well-studied, sulfated GAG. Towards this end, we first assigned the chemical shifts of the native monomer that are essential for characterizing receptor and GAG interactions and also developed a chemical shift-based structural model of the CXCL7 monomer. We observed that receptor binding is largely mediated by hydrophobic interactions, that electrostatic and H-bonding interactions also play a role and that the CXCR2 N-domain binds a groove comprising the N-loop and adjacent β-strand residues. On the other hand, heparin binding is predominantly mediated by electrostatic interactions. We also observe that heparin adopts different binding geometries and that the binding interface is highly plastic. Most interestingly, our data indicate that GAG-bound CXCL7 monomer cannot bind the receptor. Further, to our knowledge, this is the first study characterizing the GAG and receptor interactions of a native neutrophil activating chemokine monomer.

2. Results

2.1. CXCL7 Monomer Chemical Shift Assignments

Chemical shifts are exquisitely sensitive to local changes in the electronic environment and, as such, serve as useful probes for mapping the binding interface of macromolecular interactions. The binding interface is inferred from binding-induced chemical shifts obtained from heteronuclear single quantum coherence (HSQC) titrations of an unlabeled ligand to a ^{15}N-labeled protein. Therefore, knowledge of the native CXCL7 monomer chemical shifts is essential to describe the molecular basis of receptor and GAG interactions. We first characterized how monomer/dimer/tetramer levels vary as a function of buffer, temperature and pH from relative peak intensities in the 2D HSQC spectra. A summary of the distribution is shown in Table S1. Our data indicate that pH had the highest impact, with the monomer dominating at lower pH and tetramer dominating at higher pH. The dimer was always observed in the presence of monomer or tetramer and was not prevalent at any pH. Other variables such as temperature, ionic strength and buffer condition had much less effect. On the basis of these experiments, we settled on a 300-μM sample at pH 4.0 for monomer assignments. Under these experimental conditions, the protein exists as 95% monomer with the remaining 5% as dimer. The HSQC spectrum under these conditions is shown in Figure 2A. A table of the chemical shifts is also shown (Table S2). As we carried out receptor and GAG interactions at pH ≥6 that better reflects physiological conditions, chemical shifts at these pH are needed. We recorded HSQC spectra as a function of pH from 4.0 to 7.5 that allowed assigning monomer chemical shifts at the higher pH despite elevated dimer levels (Figure S1). The backbone assignments at pH 6.0 were also confirmed using triple resonance experiments. Interestingly, HSQC spectra collected as a function of pH also identified several intramolecular interactions. The M6 amide proton is significantly downfield shifted at higher pH (Figure 2B), and the corresponding residue in various human and murine chemokines is also downfield shifted [13,18–23]. On the basis of previous mutagenesis studies in CXCL8 and CXCL1, the chemical shift profile of M6 can be attributed to an intramolecular H-bond between the E35 side chain carboxylate and M6 amide proton [24]. The K17 amide proton is likewise downfield shifted (Figure 2C), which can be attributed to H-bonding to the imidazole group of H15 [25]. The corresponding residue in other NACs has also been shown to be downfield shifted. Mutagenesis studies in related NACs have also shown that these interactions are critical for receptor function [26,27]. Further, we also observed significant chemical shift changes for C7, and most interestingly, two distinct peaks at pH 5.0 and a distinct shoulder could also be observed at higher pH. Structures have shown that the disulfides are dynamic and that the disulfides, in addition to structure, also play crucial roles in receptor function [28].

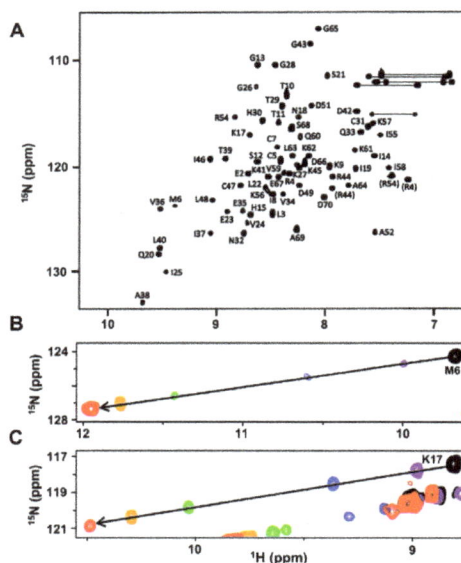

Figure 2. NMR characteristics of the CXCL7 monomer. (**A**) The HSQC spectrum shows excellent chemical shift dispersion indicating a well-folded single species at pH 4.0. The folded arginine side chain peaks are indicated in closed brackets; (**B**,**C**) Large chemical shift changes observed as a function of pH are shown for M6 and K17. The transition is from pH 4.2 (black), 4.4 (purple), 5.0 (blue), 5.5 (green) 6.0 (orange) to 7.0 (red).

2.2. Structural Model of the Native Monomer

A structure of the ethanol-induced monomer of CXCL7 has been previously reported, but its coordinates are not available in the protein data bank [16]. Generally, nuclear Overhauser effect (NOE)-driven structures require a sufficient number of long-range NOEs to describe different structural elements, their relative orientation and the global fold. We could not obtain sufficient unambiguous long range NOEs to generate a structure. In particular, NOEs between the β-strands and the helix could not be unambiguously assigned. As our objective was to characterize the binding of the monomer, and not to determine the monomer structure per se, we generated a chemical shift-based structure.

It is now well established that ^{1}H, ^{15}N, Cα and Cβ chemical shifts can give an accurate structural model provided related structures are available. We first used our chemical shifts to predict the secondary structure and backbone torsion angles using TALOS-N [29,30]. Secondary structure prediction indicated three β-strands, an α-helix, as well as a structured N-loop commonly observed in chemokines. Predicted torsion angles were also well within favorable limits for a folded protein. We then generated a de novo monomer structure using CS-ROSETTA. The resulting structure was a well-folded protein with all the major chemokine structural motifs (Figure 3A). The torsion angles and intramolecular H-bonds were analyzed, and the torsion angles for 67 residues fall within favorable limits with the remaining three falling within acceptable limits.

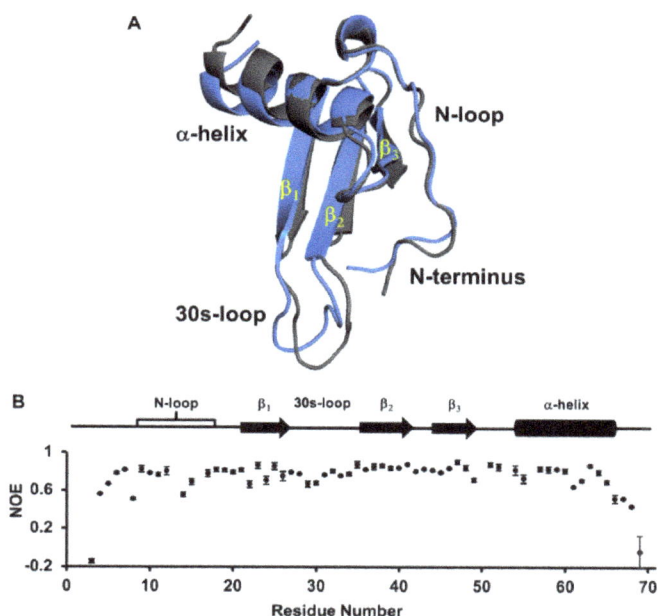

Figure 3. Structural features of the CXCL7 monomer. (**A**) Ribbon diagram of the CS-based CXCL7 monomer (blue) overlaid on a monomer of the tetramer (gray). Major structural regions are labeled; (**B**) Heteronuclear NOE data of the native CXCL7 monomer are shown. Secondary structural elements are given for reference.

We next compared our structure to the previously described monomer units of the tetramer crystal structure. Superimposition of the monomer units from the tetramer reveals a backbone root-mean-square deviation (RMSD) of 0.32 Å for structured β-strands and α-helix (Q20-G26, V34-L40 and R44-A64). Our structure showed a backbone RMSD of 0.82 Å compared to the monomer units of the tetramer over the same regions, and differences in these regions are mainly due to extended β-strands and a slight change in the orientation of the helix. The largest differences between our monomer and the tetramer structure were observed for the N-terminus and 30s-loop residues, which can be attributed to their conformational flexibility [16,31,32] (Figure 3A). In general, we observed that the more dynamic a region, the greater the difference in its backbone RMSD. We further examined the N-loop and helical regions as these are potentially involved in GAG and receptor interactions. Overall, the N-loop and helix closely resemble those of the crystal structure, with an average backbone RMSD of 0.64 Å. Our CS-based structure has a helix that spans from residues 54 to 64, similar to that observed in the tetramer. It is interesting that residues 65 to 70 are also unstructured in the tetramer, as C-terminal residues adopt a more defined helical structure in other NAC dimers. For instance, in CXCL8, the last six residues (66 to 72) are unstructured in the monomer, whereas the helix extends up to residue 70 in the dimer structures [19,22]. Similarly, only the last two or three residues are unstructured in the CXCL1 and CXCL5 dimer structures [13,18,23]. A shorter helix in CXCL7 could in part explain weak dimerization, as the corresponding residues in other NAC structures are involved in favorable interactions across the dimer interface.

To better understand the dynamic properties of the native monomer, we also carried out backbone ^{1}H-^{15}N-heteronuclear relaxation measurements. Heteronuclear NOEs are sensitive to motions in the picosecond-nanosecond timescale. Structured residues tend to have high NOE values (~0.8), and less structured or dynamic residues have lower NOE values. Our data indicated that the N-terminal residues preceding the CXC motif, C-terminal residues 66 to 70, and parts of the N-loop are dynamic, while the rest of the protein appears highly ordered (Figure 3B). Comparison of our data to the previously reported relaxation data of CXCL7 in the presence of chloroethanol shows striking differences for the 30s-loop residues. Heteronuclear NOE measurements in the presence of 2-chloroethanol indicate a highly dynamic 30s-loop, especially residues Q33, V34 and E35, showing very low NOE values observed for the very terminal residues, whereas our values are similar to those of structured residues [16,31,32]. These observations suggest that chloroethanol influences dynamic properties, and so, these data may not fully reflect the dynamics of the native protein.

2.3. CXCL7:CXCR2 N-Domain Interactions

Currently, nothing is known regarding the structural basis of how CXCL7 binds the CXCR2 receptor. Previous studies have indicated a two-site binding model for chemokine-receptor activation [33–35]. Site-I, which functions as a critical docking site, involves interactions between the chemokine N-loop region and receptor N-terminal domain. Site-II functions as the activating site and involves interactions between the chemokine N-terminal domain and receptor extracellular/transmembrane residues. As characterizing the structural basis of binding to the whole receptor is experimentally challenging, albeit possible [36], we used a divide and conquer approach to characterize the Site-I binding of CXCL7 to a CXCR2 N-terminal domain peptide. Such an approach has been extensively used to characterize Site-I interactions for a number of chemokines using different biophysical techniques including solution NMR spectroscopy [37–45].

We characterized native chemokine monomer binding to the CXCR2 N-terminal domain (CXCR2Nd) at pH 6.0 using 2D-HSQC NMR titration experiments. Significant CSP was observed for hydrophobic residues M6, G13, I14, I46 and A52, polar residues C7, T10, T11, N18, Q20 and C47 and charged residues K17, E23, D49, R54 and the R44 side chain (Figure 4). Most of these residues constitute a continuous surface primarily along the N-loop and adjacent β-strand. The perturbation of cysteines is likely due to indirect interactions, as these residues are buried and so cannot be involved in direct interactions. Residues Q20 and E23 are located on the opposite face from the other residues, suggesting their perturbations are also due to indirect interactions.

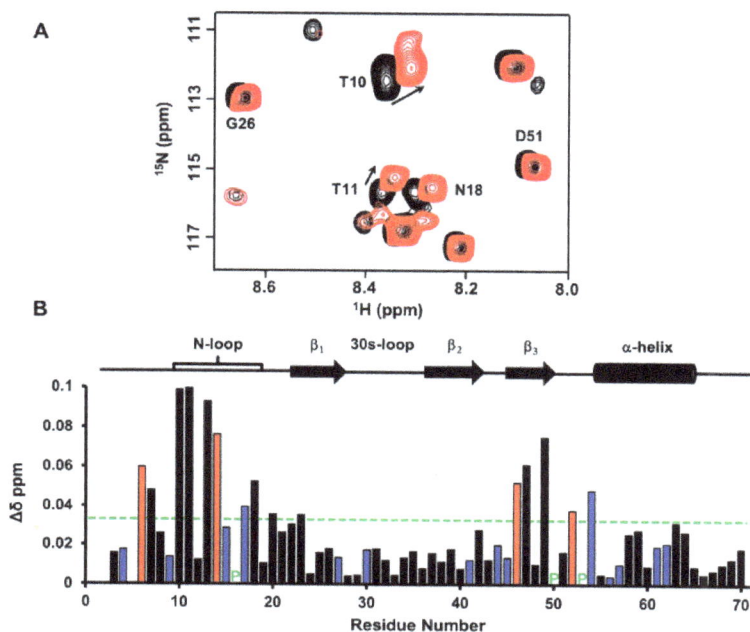

Figure 4. CXCL7 monomer binding to CXCR2 N-domain. (**A**) Portion of the 2D HSQC spectrum showing the overlay of CXCL7 in the free (back) and in the presence of CXCR2 N-domain at a 1:3.5 molar ratio (red). Residues showing significant perturbations are labeled and arrows indicate the direction of the peak movement; (**B**) Histogram plot of binding-induced chemical shift changes in the CXCL7 monomer as a function of amino acid sequence. Basic residues are shown in blue. Hydrophobic residues with significant CSP are shown in red. Prolines are indicated by a green 'P'. Residues that show CSP above the threshold (dashed line) are considered involved in binding. Secondary structural elements are given for reference.

To gain further insight into the binding, we generated a model for the CXCR2Nd-CXCL7 monomer complex using high ambiguity-driven biomolecular docking (HADDOCK)-based calculations that utilize CSP data as ambiguous interaction restraints along with shape complementarity and energetics to drive the docking process. Modeling revealed a single binding mode with the N-domain nestled along a groove between the N-loop and the β_3-strand. Binding in our model is principally mediated by packing interactions between CXCL7 residues I8, T11, I14 and I46 and CXCR2 residues L28, L29 and A31 (Figure 5). Comparison of the chemokine sequences reveals that these residues are highly conserved (Figure 1), further indicating that they are critical to receptor binding. These observations also suggest that the CSP of M6, T10 and A52 are due to indirect interactions. In addition, we observe several transient interactions for charged and polar residues in many, but not all, of the models. These include an aromatic π-stacking interaction between CXCL7 H15 and CXCR2 F27 and an H-bonding interaction between CXCL7 K17 side chain NH_3^+ and CXCR2 S22 side chain hydroxyl groups. CXCL7 R54 is also involved in binding, forming either an H-bond between its guanidine side chain and CXCR2 P28 backbone carbonyl or a cation-π interaction with CXCR2 F27 (Figure 5). The remaining residues were not involved in direct binding interactions, indicating that their CSPs are likely due to binding-induced structural changes. Interestingly, H-bonding interactions were observed between the CXCL7 K9 side chain NH_3^+ and the CXCR2 D30 carboxylate, though K9 showed no chemical shift perturbation. It is likely that the absence of chemical shift changes is due to cancellation between contributions from direct and indirect interactions of similar magnitude but opposite sign. Lack of CSP of lysine residues involved in GAG binding has been previously observed in other chemokines [46–49]. Our docking model and CSP data collectively indicate that hydrophobic packing, guided by H-bonding and ionic interactions, mediates Site-I binding.

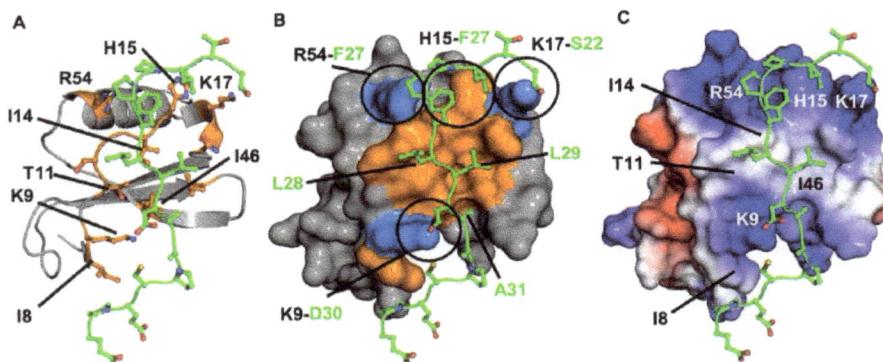

Figure 5. Model of the CXCL7-CXCR2 N-domain complex. (**A**) The ribbon diagram highlights the important binding residues on CXCL7 (orange). The receptor peptide is shown in green; (**B**) A surface filling model of the complex in the same orientation as shown in (**A**), highlighting residues involved in packing (orange) and ionic (blue) interactions. Several intermolecular interactions are circled and CXCL7 and receptor residues are labeled in black and green, respectively; (**C**) A schematic of the electrostatic surface in the same orientation as shown in (**A**,**B**) highlighting the hydrophobic pocket and the flanking basic residues. Important CXCL7 residues are labeled for reference.

2.4. CXCL7 Monomer-Heparin dp8 Interactions

CSP analysis showed significant perturbation for residues in the N-loop, β_3-strand and the α-helix (Figure 6). As basic residues are known to mediate GAG binding, we focused on residues K9, H15 and K17 from the N-loop, R44 from the β_3-strand and R54, K56 and K57 from the helix. Peaks corresponding to residues H15 and K17 are broadened out in the free protein, but appear during the GAG titration, indicating that they are dynamic in the free form and become structured upon binding. We could measure the CSP for K17 as the peak appears early in the titration, but not for H15, as it appears late in the titration. CSPs of hydrophobic and acidic residues, which are located either proximal to basic residues or on the C-terminal helix (residues L63 to E67), are likely due to indirect interactions. Chemical shifts reveal that helical residues L63 to E67 are unstructured in the free form, and the observation that the shifts move upfield in the bound form suggests that GAG binding stabilizes and promotes the formation of the helix. Further, as we are able to simultaneously track the peaks corresponding to monomer and homodimer, we note that the equilibrium does not shift upon GAG binding and that monomer continues to dominate, indicating the monomer and dimer have similar affinities to heparin dp8.

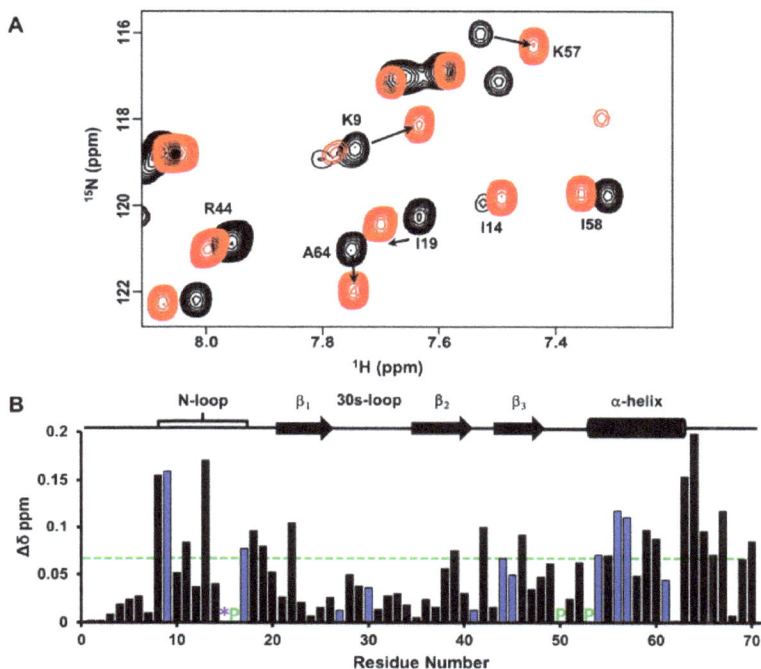

Figure 6. CXCL7 monomer binding to heparin dp8. (**A**) Portion of the HSQC spectrum showing the overlay of CXCL7 in the free (black) and in the presence of heparin dp8 at a 1:4 molar ratio (red). Residues that show significant perturbation are labeled; (**B**) Histogram plot of binding-induced chemical shift changes in CXCL7 monomer as a function of amino acid sequence. Residues that show CSP above the threshold (dashed line) are considered perturbed. Basic residues Arg, Lys and His are shown in blue. Residue H15 is broadened out in the free spectra and is represented by a "*". Prolines are shown by a green "P". Secondary structural elements are given for reference.

To gain insight into the binding geometry, we generated models of the dp8-bound structures using HADDOCK. All significantly perturbed residues, including hydrophobic and negatively charged residues, were used as restraints in generating the models. However, all of the models showed interactions with only basic residues indicating that the CSP of non-basic residues must be due to indirect interactions. Docking models resulted in several families, and interestingly, no one family could satisfy all of the residues that were perturbed in NMR CSP measurements. Models indicate that all binding geometries share a common core consisting of H15 and K17 of the N-loop and R54 of the α-helix. Whereas residues corresponding to H15 and K17 are highly conserved, R54 is unique and only present in CXCL7 (Figure 1). The GAG chain adopts three different orientations about this core due to selective binding to the peripheral residues K9, R44 or K57, defined as Models A, B and C, respectively (Figure 7). Structures failed to show interactions for K56, which is oriented away from the N-loop and towards the dimer interface, indicating that its CSP perturbations are due to indirect interactions. The same is true of the C-terminal residues L63 to E67, further supporting that their CSPs are due to structural changes. These data collectively indicate that the binding interface is plastic and that multiple binding geometries mediate monomer-GAG interactions. Additional docking experiments excluding one of the peripheral residues K9, R44 or K57 resulted in the two remaining geometries with no additional new geometries (Figure 7).

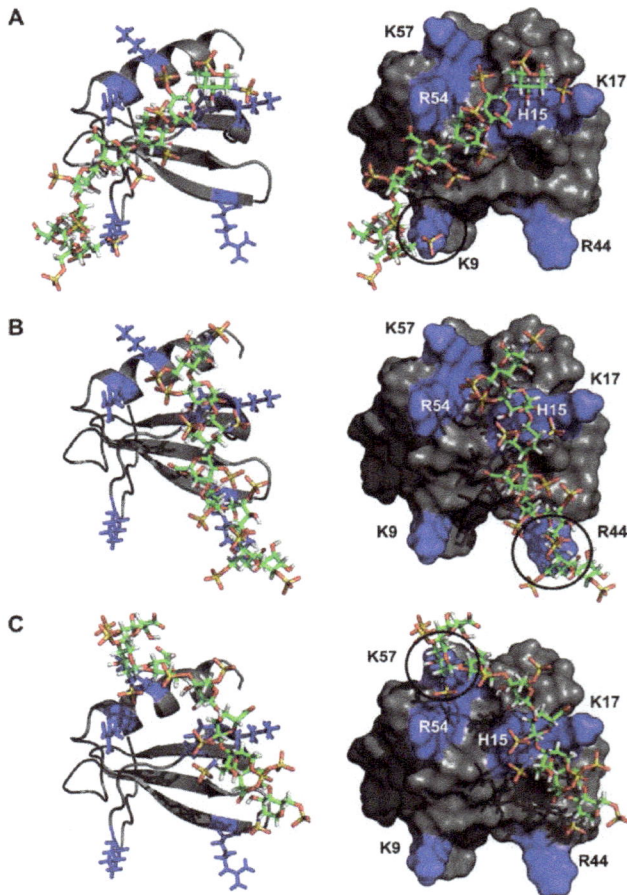

Figure 7. Models of the CXCL7-GAG heparin complexes. Different binding geometries that arise due to differences in peripheral interactions are shown in panels **A**, **B**, and **C**, respectively. The left column shows the ribbon diagram of the CXCL7 monomer, with GAG and positively-charged side chains shown as sticks. The right column shows the surface plots. Arg, Lys and His residues are highlighted in blue and labeled. Black circles highlight peripheral residues that mediate the binding geometry.

The only previous monomer-GAG characterization is for CXCL8 using an engineered monomer [46]. Interestingly, the binding interactions for the CXCL8 monomer were more stringent, with a single binding geometry similar to that observed in Model A. The more stringent geometry is mediated by a much larger core domain involving six residues in contrast to only three in CXCL7. Additional core residues in CXCL8 include the C-terminal helical residues R60, K64, K67 and R68 (corresponding to K57, K61, A64 and G65 in CXCL7). The smaller core in CXL7 appears to grant more degrees of freedom, allowing the GAG to adopt a range of geometries up to 180° about the core. Another key difference is K11 in CXCL8, the residue corresponding to K9 in CXCL7, which shows no interactions, and instead, K15 (equivalent to G13 in CXCL7), a residue unique to CXCL8, mediates binding. These data collectively indicate that both conserved and specific residues play differential roles in mediating GAG interactions and binding geometry in a chemokine-specific manner.

3. Discussion

CXCL7 plays a critical role in recruiting neutrophils to a variety of tissues, and dysregulation in this process has been implicated in inflammatory diseases, such as rheumatoid arthritis, acute lung injury and COPD [50–52], as well as a variety of cancers [53,54]. One of its primary functions involves neutrophil-platelet crosstalk during vascular injury, as it is released at relatively high concentrations from activated platelets and provides cues for directed neutrophil migration to the injury site [7]. However, nothing is known regarding the molecular level interactions between CXCL7 and its target receptor CXCR2 and GAGs.

As a member of the neutrophil activating chemokine family, CXCL7 shares several properties, such as a similar tertiary structure and activation of CXCR2 via the conserved 'ELR' motif. However, CXCL7 is unique, as it alone forms a weak dimer and also a tetramer at high concentrations, whereas other members form stronger dimers and no tetramers. Previous NMR studies have characterized binding interactions for native CXCL1, CXCL5 and CXCL8 dimers and engineered CXCL1 and CXCL8 monomers, as only dimers could be studied at concentrations used for NMR [37,39,46,48,49]. In this study, for the very first time, we have successfully characterized the binding interactions of an NAC monomer. By exploiting the weaker dimerization propensity and carefully varying solution conditions and protein concentration, we could assign the monomer chemical shifts that allowed mapping the binding interactions and generating structural models.

In addition to the ligand structure, knowledge of the receptor and ligand-receptor complex structures is also essential to fully describe residue-specific relationships between structural features, conformational changes and function. In recent years, structures of the free CXCR1 receptor and of other chemokine receptors bound with an antagonist and small molecule inhibitors have been reported [55,56]. However, structures of CXCR2 or the agonist-CXCR2 complex are not available. Therefore, our approach using the isolated N-domain and NMR chemical shift perturbation experiments can provide critical structural information that is otherwise difficult to obtain. Further, NMR CSP-based methods have been shown to be extremely useful for describing residue-specific GAG interactions, as protein-GAG complexes are notoriously difficult to crystallize. The CXCL7 monomer chemical shift assignments were previously reported in the presence of 2-chloroethanol [16,57]. Our chemical shifts were similar, but not identical, and interestingly, our heteronuclear relaxation data of the monomer showed a structured 30s-loop, whereas previous studies carried out in the presence of chloroethanol showed substantial dynamics similar to those observed for terminal residues. These observations highlight that dynamic studies carried out in the presence of reagents that disrupt native H-bonding interactions must be interpreted with caution.

Our NMR and modeling studies suggest that the N-loop and adjacent β-strand residues of CXCL7 mediate CXCR2 Site-I interactions. The binding mode and the nature of these interactions are similar to that observed for other CXCR2-activating chemokines CXCL1, CXCL5 and CXCL8 [37,39,49,58]. Binding is principally mediated by hydrophobic packing interactions that are conserved across the NAC family (Figure 1). However, charged residues unique to CXCL7, such as K9 and R54, also mediate binding, suggesting that such interactions fine-tune receptor activation and confer chemokine-specific function to what at first glance seems a redundant chemokine system. High resolution X-ray or NMR structures are essential to confirm and better describe the binding interactions at a single residue level.

Another important aspect of CXCL7 function is its interaction with GAGs. It is now well established that GAG binding plays a pivotal role in regulating chemokine signaling and establishing chemotactic/haptotactic gradients. Chemokines in solution form chemotactic and in GAG-bound form haptotactic gradients, but whether it is the GAG-bound or free chemokine that activates the receptor is not well understood. Our results indicate that GAG binding to the CXCL7 monomer is highly plastic and that GAG adopts multiple geometries. Independent of the binding models, a number of residues that mediate GAG interactions are also involved in receptor interactions indicating that the GAG-bound CXCL7 monomer cannot bind the receptor (Figure 8). Both monomer and dimer bound heparin dp8 with similar affinity and hence had no effect on the monomer-dimer equilibrium.

However, though the dimer levels of the free chemokine are not dominant and the tetramer is favored at higher concentrations, the dimeric form, compared to the monomer, is favored on binding longer GAGs. During active neutrophil recruitment and tissue injury, it is very likely that local concentrations can vary by orders of magnitude, and so, it is possible that the levels of different oligomeric states and their GAG interactions are highly coupled and regulate in vivo function. We conclude that GAG interactions provide spatial and temporal control of receptor activity by modulating the amount of free chemokine and that the interplay between monomer-receptor and monomer-GAG plays an important role in mediating neutrophil recruitment in response to vascular injury.

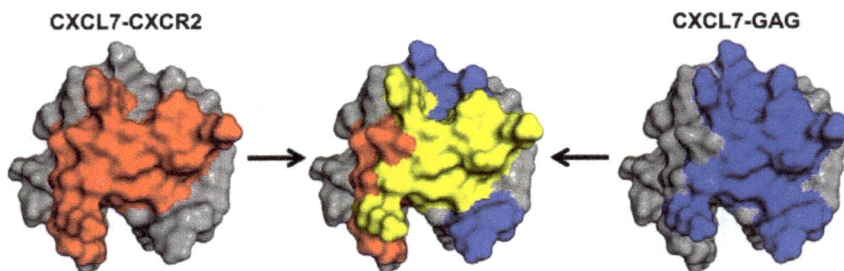

Figure 8. Overlap between GAG and CXCR2 binding domains. A schematic showing the CXCR2 binding domain (red), GAG binding domain (blue) and the overlap between the two domains (yellow).

4. Materials and Methods

4.1. Reagents and Protein Expression

CXCL7 was expressed in *Escherichia coli* cultured in either LB or ^{15}N/^{13}C enriched minimal medium and purified using a combination of nickel column and reverse phase high-performance liquid chromatography as described previously [44]. Purified protein was then lyophilized and stored at −20 °C until further use. The recombinant CXCR2 N-domain (residues 1 to 43) peptide was expressed using the same protocol as described above. Heparin dp8 oligosaccharide was purchased from Iduron. According to the manufacturer, the oligosaccharides were purified using high resolution gel filtration chromatography, consist mainly of the disaccharide unit IdoA,2S-GlcNS,6S (~75%), show some variation in sulfation pattern and contain uronic acid at the non-reducing end and a C4-C5 double bond as a result of the heparinase endolytic action.

4.2. Chemical Shift Assignments of the CXCL7 Monomer

NMR spectra were acquired using Bruker Avance III 600- and 800-MHz spectrometers equipped with cryoprobes and processed and analyzed using either Bruker Topspin 3.2 or Sparky programs [59]. Monomer chemical shift assignments were determined at 30 °C using a 300-μM protein sample in 50 mM phosphate, pH 4.0, containing 1 mM 2,2-dimethyl-2-silapentansesulfonic acid (DSS), 1 mM sodium azide and 10% D_2O. The ^{1}H and ^{15}N chemical shifts were assigned using 3D ^{1}H-^{15}N heteronuclear NOESY and TOCSY experiments with mixing times of 150 and 80 ms, respectively. The carbon chemical shifts assigned from HNCA and CBCACONH experiments at pH 6.0 also helped in resolving some of the ambiguous assignments. The chemical shifts are shown in the Supplementary Material (Table S2). ^{1}H-^{15}N HSQC spectra collected from pH 4.0 to 7.5 in 0.5 increments were used to assign the backbone chemical shifts over this pH range.

4.3. NMR Titrations

Binding interactions of CXCR2 N-terminal domain and heparin dp8 to WT CXCL7 were characterized using solution NMR spectroscopy. A series of ^{1}H-^{15}N HSQC spectra were collected upon titrating either CXCR2 N-domain peptide or heparin to WT CXCL7 until no change in the chemical shifts were observed. The protein concentrations selected were high enough to obtain good quality spectra in a reasonable period. In the case of CXCR2 N-domain, we titrated 320 μM CXCR2 N-domain to 77 μM WT CXCL7 in 50 mM phosphate buffer at pH 6.0 and 35 °C. The final molar ratio of CXCL7:CXCR2 N-domain was 1:3.5. For CXCL7-GAG interactions, we titrated 10 mM heparin dp8 to a 50-μM sample in 50 mM phosphate pH 7.4 at 35 °C. The final molar ratio for CXCL7:octasaccharide was 1:4. For all titrations, chemical shift perturbations were calculated as a weighted average of changes in the ^{1}H and ^{15}N chemical shifts as described [58].

4.4. Model of the Monomer Structure

The monomer structure was generated using CS-ROSETTA, a robust tool for generating de novo structures from NMR chemical shifts [60,61]. The program uses the PDB database to select protein fragments based on the given backbone Cα, Cβ, N and NH chemical shifts and then assembles and relaxes these fragments into a converged structure using a ROSETTA Monte Carlo approach. Disulfide bonds were absent in the initial structure and subsequently added using PyMol. The structure was subjected to constrained energy minimization to allow the disulfides to adopt proper geometry, followed by global energy minimization and structural analysis using the AMBER 12 suite and VADAR [62,63].

4.5. Molecular Docking Using HADDOCK

Molecular docking of CXCR2Nd and heparin to the CXCL7 monomer was carried out using the high ambiguity-driven biomolecular docking (HADDOCK) approach as described previously [46, 48,64,65]. The CXCL7 monomer structure determined using CS-Rosetta, the unstructured CXCR2 N-terminal peptide generated in Pymol and the NMR structure of heparin (PDB ID: 1HPN) [66] were used for docking. Ambiguous interaction restraints (AIRs) were selected based on NMR chemical shift perturbation results. The pair-wise "ligand interface RMSD matrix" over all structures was calculated, and the final structures were clustered using an RMSD cut-off value of 7.5 Å for CXCR2Nd and 4 Å for heparin. The clusters were then prioritized using RMSD and the "HADDOCK score" (weighted sum of a combination of energy terms).

Supplementary Materials: Supplementary materials can be found at www.mdpi.com/1422-0067/18/3/508/s1.

Acknowledgments: This work was supported by a grant from the National Institutes of Health P01 HL107152 to Krishna Rajarathnam and the National Institute of General Medical Sciences Houston Area Molecular Biophysics Training Grants 2T32 GM008280 to Aaron J. Brown. The authors also acknowledge the Sealy Center for Structural Biology and Molecular Biophysics at the University of Texas Medical Branch at Galveston for providing research resources.

Author Contributions: Krishna Rajarathnam and Aaron J. Brown designed the research and wrote the paper; Aaron J. Brown performed the experiments; and Aaron J. Brown and Krishna Mohan Sepuru analyzed the data. All authors reviewed the results and approved the final version of the manuscript.

Conflicts of Interest: The authors declare no conflict of interest.

Abbreviations

CXCL	CXC ligand
CXCR2	CXC chemokine receptor 2
CXCL7/NAP-2	Neutrophil-activating peptide 2
GAG	Glycosaminoglycan
CXCR2Nd	CXCR2 N-terminal domain
GPCR	G-protein coupled receptor
NAC	Neutrophil activating chemokine
NMR	Nuclear magnetic resonance
HSQC	Heteronuclear single quantum coherence
CSP	Chemical shift perturbation
NOE	Nuclear Overhauser effect
AIR	Ambiguous interaction restraints

References

1. Griffith, J.W.; Sokol, C.L.; Luster, A.D. Chemokines and chemokine receptors: Positioning cells for host defense and immunity. *Annu. Rev. Immunol.* **2014**, *32*, 659–702. [CrossRef] [PubMed]
2. Bonecchi, R.; Galliera, E.; Borroni, E.M.; Corsi, M.M.; Locati, M.; Mantovani, A. Chemokines and chemokine receptors: An overview. *Front. Biosci.* **2009**, *14*, 540–551. [CrossRef]
3. Raman, D.; Sobolik-Delmaire, T.; Richmond, A. Chemokines in health and disease. *Exp. Cell Res.* **2011**, *317*, 575–589. [CrossRef] [PubMed]
4. Salanga, C.L.; Handel, T.M. Chemokine oligomerization and interactions with receptors and glycosaminoglycans: The role of structural dynamics in function. *Exp. Cell Res.* **2011**, *317*, 590–601. [CrossRef] [PubMed]
5. Fernandez, E.J.; Lolis, E. Structure, function, and inhibition of chemokines. *Annu. Rev. Pharmacol. Toxicol.* **2002**, *42*, 469–499. [CrossRef] [PubMed]
6. Monneau, Y.; Arenzana-Seisdedos, F.; Lortat-Jacob, H. The sweet spot: How gags help chemokines guide migrating cells. *J. Leukoc. Biol.* **2016**, *99*, 935–953. [CrossRef] [PubMed]
7. Ghasemzadeh, M.; Kaplan, Z.S.; Alwis, I.; Schoenwaelder, S.M.; Ashworth, K.J.; Westein, E.; Hosseini, E.; Salem, H.H.; Slattery, R.; McColl, S.R.; et al. The CXCR1/2 ligand NAP-2 promotes directed intravascular leukocyte migration through platelet thrombi. *Blood* **2013**, *121*, 4555–4566. [CrossRef] [PubMed]
8. Sreeramkumar, V.; Adrover, J.M.; Ballesteros, I.; Cuartero, M.I.; Rossaint, J.; Bilbao, I.; Nácher, M.; Pitaval, C.; Radovanovic, I.; Fukui, Y.; et al. Neutrophils scan for activated platelets to initiate inflammation. *Science* **2014**, *346*, 1234–1238. [CrossRef] [PubMed]
9. Von Hundelshausen, P.; Petersen, F.; Brandt, E. Platelet-derived chemokines in vascular biology. *Thromb. Haemost.* **2007**, *97*, 704–713. [CrossRef] [PubMed]
10. Stillie, R.; Farooq, S.M.; Gordon, J.R.; Stadnyk, A.W. The functional significance behind expressing two IL-8 receptor types on pmn. *J. Leukoc. Biol.* **2009**, *86*, 529–543. [CrossRef] [PubMed]
11. Rajarathnam, K.; Kay, C.M.; Dewald, B.; Wolf, M.; Baggiolini, M.; Clark-Lewis, I.; Sykes, B.D. Neutrophil-activating peptide-2 and melanoma growth-stimulatory activity are functional as monomers for neutrophil activation. *J. Biol. Chem.* **1997**, *272*, 1725–1729. [CrossRef] [PubMed]
12. Yang, Y.; Mayo, K.H.; Daly, T.J.; Barry, J.K.; La Rosa, G.J. Subunit association and structural analysis of platelet basic protein and related proteins investigated by 1H NMR spectroscopy and circular dichroism. *J. Biol. Chem.* **1994**, *269*, 20110–20118. [PubMed]
13. Sepuru, K.M.; Poluri, K.M.; Rajarathnam, K. Solution structure of CXCL5—A novel chemokine and adipokine implicated in inflammation and obesity. *PLoS ONE* **2014**, *9*, e93228. [CrossRef] [PubMed]
14. Lowman, H.B.; Fairbrother, W.J.; Slagle, P.H.; Kabakoff, R.; Liu, J.; Shire, S.; Hébert, C.A. Monomeric variants of IL-8: Effects of side chain substitutions and solution conditions upon dimer formation. *Protein Sci.* **1997**, *6*, 598–608. [CrossRef] [PubMed]
15. Malkowski, M.G.; Wu, J.Y.; Lazar, J.B.; Johnson, P.H.; Edwards, B.F. The crystal structure of recombinant human neutrophil-activating peptide-2 (M6L) at 1.9-a resolution. *J. Biol. Chem.* **1995**, *270*, 7077–7087. [PubMed]

16. Young, H.; Roongta, V.; Daly, T.J.; Mayo, K.H. NMR structure and dynamics of monomeric neutrophil-activating peptide 2. *Biochem. J.* **1999**, *338*, 591–598. [CrossRef] [PubMed]

17. Ahuja, S.K.; Murphy, P.M. The CXC chemokines growth-regulated oncogene (GRO)α, GROβ, GROγ, neutrophil-activating peptide-2, and epithelial cell-derived neutrophil-activating peptide-78 are potent agonists for the type B, but not the type A, human interleukin-8 receptor. *J. Biol. Chem.* **1996**, *271*, 20545–20550. [CrossRef] [PubMed]

18. Fairbrother, W.J.; Reilly, D.; Colby, T.J.; Hesselgesser, J.; Horuk, R. The solution structure of melanoma growth stimulating activity. *J. Mol. Biol.* **1994**, *242*, 252–270. [CrossRef] [PubMed]

19. Rajarathnam, K.; Clark-Lewis, I.; Sykes, B.D. 1H NMR solution structure of an active monomeric interleukin-8. *Biochemistry* **1995**, *34*, 12983–12990. [CrossRef] [PubMed]

20. Shao, W.; Jerva, L.F.; West, J.; Lolis, E.; Schweitzer, B.I. Solution structure of murine macrophage inflammatory protein-2. *Biochemistry* **1998**, *37*, 8303–8313. [CrossRef] [PubMed]

21. Qian, Y.Q.; Johanson, K.O.; McDevitt, P. Nuclear magnetic resonance solution structure of truncated human GROβ and its structural comparison with CXC chemokine family members GROα and IL-8. *J. Mol. Biol.* **1999**, *294*, 1065–1072. [CrossRef] [PubMed]

22. Clore, G.M.; Appella, E.; Yamada, M.; Matsushima, K.; Gronenborn, A.M. Three-dimensional structure of interleukin 8 in solution. *Biochemistry* **1990**, *29*, 1689–1696. [CrossRef] [PubMed]

23. Kim, K.S.; Clark-Lewis, I.; Sykes, B.D. Solution structure of GRO/melanoma growth stimulatory activity determined by 1H NMR spectroscopy. *J. Biol. Chem.* **1994**, *269*, 32909–32915. [PubMed]

24. Rajarathnam, K.; Clark-Lewis, I.; Dewald, B.; Baggiolini, M.; Sykes, B.D. 1H NMR evidence that Glu-38 interacts with the N-terminal functional domain in interleukin-8. *FEBS Lett.* **1996**, *399*, 43–46. [CrossRef]

25. Baldwin, E.T.; Weber, I.T.; St Charles, R.; Xuan, J.C.; Appella, E.; Yamada, M.; Matsushima, K.; Edwards, B.F.; Clore, G.M.; Gronenborn, A.M. Crystal structure of interleukin 8: Symbiosis of NMR and crystallography. *Proc. Natl. Acad. Sci. USA* **1991**, *88*, 502–506. [CrossRef] [PubMed]

26. Hesselgesser, J.; Chitnis, C.E.; Miller, L.H.; Yansura, D.G.; Simmons, L.C.; Fairbrother, W.J.; Kotts, C.; Wirth, C.; Gillece-Castro, B.L.; Horuk, R. A mutant of melanoma growth stimulating activity does not activate neutrophils but blocks erythrocyte invasion by malaria. *J. Biol. Chem.* **1995**, *270*, 11472–11476. [CrossRef] [PubMed]

27. Baly, D.L.; Horuk, R.; Yansura, D.G.; Simmons, L.C.; Fairbrother, W.J.; Kotts, C.; Wirth, C.M.; Gillece-Castro, B.L.; Toy, K.; Hesselgesser, J.; et al. A His19 to ALA mutant of melanoma growth-stimulating activity is a partial antagonist of the CXCR2 receptor. *J. Immunol.* **1998**, *161*, 4944–4949. [PubMed]

28. Rajarathnam, K.; Sykes, B.D.; Dewald, B.; Baggiolini, M.; Clark-Lewis, I. Disulfide bridges in interleukin-8 probed using non-natural disulfide analogues: Dissociation of roles in structure from function. *Biochemistry* **1999**, *38*, 7653–7658. [CrossRef] [PubMed]

29. Shen, Y.; Delaglio, F.; Cornilescu, G.; Bax, A. Talos+: A hybrid method for predicting protein backbone torsion angles from NMR chemical shifts. *J. Biomol. NMR* **2009**, *44*, 213–223. [CrossRef] [PubMed]

30. Shen, Y.; Bax, A. Protein backbone and sidechain torsion angles predicted from NMR chemical shifts using artificial neural networks. *J. Biomol. NMR* **2013**, *56*, 227–241. [CrossRef] [PubMed]

31. Herring, C.A.; Singer, C.M.; Ermakova, E.A.; Khairutdinov, B.I.; Zuev, Y.F.; Jacobs, D.J.; Nesmelova, I.V. Dynamics and thermodynamic properties of CXCL7 chemokine. *Proteins* **2015**, *83*, 1987–2007. [CrossRef] [PubMed]

32. Nguyen, L.T.; Kwakman, P.H.; Chan, D.I.; Liu, Z.; de Boer, L.; Zaat, S.A.; Vogel, H.J. Exploring platelet chemokine antimicrobial activity: Nuclear magnetic resonance backbone dynamics of NAP-2 and TC-1. *Antimicrob. Agents Chemother.* **2011**, *55*, 2074–2083. [CrossRef] [PubMed]

33. Rajagopalan, L.; Rajarathnam, K. Structural basis of chemokine receptor function—A model for binding affinity and ligand selectivity. *Biosci. Rep.* **2006**, *26*, 325–339. [CrossRef] [PubMed]

34. Wells, T.N.; Power, C.A.; Lusti-Narasimhan, M.; Hoogewerf, A.J.; Cooke, R.M.; Chung, C.W.; Peitsch, M.C.; Proudfoot, A.E. Selectivity and antagonism of chemokine receptors. *J. Leukoc. Biol.* **1996**, *59*, 53–60. [PubMed]

35. Joseph, P.R.; Sarmiento, J.M.; Mishra, A.K.; Das, S.T.; Garofalo, R.P.; Navarro, J.; Rajarathnam, K. Probing the role of CXC motif in chemokine CXCL8 for high affinity binding and activation of CXCR1 and CXCR2 receptors. *J. Biol. Chem.* **2010**, *285*, 29262–29269. [CrossRef] [PubMed]

36. Kofuku, Y.; Yoshiura, C.; Ueda, T.; Terasawa, H.; Hirai, T.; Tominaga, S.; Hirose, M.; Maeda, Y.; Takahashi, H.; Terashima, Y.; et al. Structural basis of the interaction between chemokine stromal cell-derived factor-1/CXCL12 and its G-protein-coupled receptor CXCR4. *J. Biol. Chem.* **2009**, *284*, 35240–35250. [CrossRef] [PubMed]

37. Joseph, P.R.; Rajarathnam, K. Solution NMR characterization of WT CXCL8 monomer and dimer binding to CXCR1 N-terminal domain. *Protein Sci.* **2015**, *24*, 81–92. [CrossRef] [PubMed]

38. Joseph, P.R.; Sawant, K.V.; Isley, A.; Pedroza, M.; Garofalo, R.P.; Richardson, R.M.; Rajarathnam, K. Dynamic conformational switching in the chemokine ligand is essential for G-protein-coupled receptor activation. *Biochem. J.* **2013**, *456*, 241–251. [CrossRef] [PubMed]

39. Ravindran, A.; Sawant, K.V.; Sarmiento, J.; Navarro, J.; Rajarathnam, K. Chemokine CXCL1 dimer is a potent agonist for the CXCR2 receptor. *J. Biol. Chem.* **2013**, *288*, 12244–12252. [CrossRef] [PubMed]

40. Veldkamp, C.T.; Seibert, C.; Peterson, F.C.; De la Cruz, N.B.; Haugner, J.C., 3rd; Basnet, H.; Sakmar, T.P.; Volkman, B.F. Structural basis of CXCR4 sulfotyrosine recognition by the chemokine SDF-1/CXCL12. *Sci. Signal.* **2008**, *1*, ra4. [CrossRef] [PubMed]

41. Millard, C.J.; Ludeman, J.P.; Canals, M.; Bridgford, J.L.; Hinds, M.G.; Clayton, D.J.; Christopoulos, A.; Payne, R.J.; Stone, M.J. Structural basis of receptor sulfotyrosine recognition by a CC chemokine: The N-terminal region of CCR3 bound to CCL11/eotaxin-1. *Structure* **2014**, *22*, 1571–1581. [CrossRef] [PubMed]

42. Schnur, E.; Kessler, N.; Zherdev, Y.; Noah, E.; Scherf, T.; Ding, F.X.; Rabinovich, S.; Arshava, B.; Kurbatska, V.; Leonciks, A.; et al. NMR mapping of RANTES surfaces interacting with CCR5 using linked extracellular domains. *FEBS J.* **2013**, *280*, 2068–2084. [CrossRef] [PubMed]

43. Fernando, H.; Nagle, G.T.; Rajarathnam, K. Thermodynamic characterization of interleukin-8 monomer binding to CXCR1 receptor N-terminal domain. *FEBS J.* **2007**, *274*, 241–251. [CrossRef] [PubMed]

44. Rajagopalan, L.; Rajarathnam, K. Ligand selectivity and affinity of chemokine receptor CXCR1. Role of N-terminal domain. *J. Biol. Chem.* **2004**, *279*, 30000–30008. [CrossRef] [PubMed]

45. Girrbach, M.; Meliciani, I.; Waterkotte, B.; Berthold, S.; Oster, A.; Brurein, F.; Strunk, T.; Wadhwani, P.; Berensmeier, S.; Wenzel, W.; et al. A fluorescence polarization assay for the experimental validation of an in silico model of the chemokine CXCL8 binding to receptor-derived peptides. *Phys. Chem. Chem. Phys.* **2014**, *16*, 8036–8043. [CrossRef] [PubMed]

46. Joseph, P.R.; Mosier, P.D.; Desai, U.R.; Rajarathnam, K. Solution NMR characterization of chemokine CXCL8/IL-8 monomer and dimer binding to glycosaminoglycans: Structural plasticity mediates differential binding interactions. *Biochem. J.* **2015**, *472*, 121–133. [CrossRef] [PubMed]

47. Sawant, K.V.; Poluri, K.M.; Dutta, A.K.; Sepuru, K.M.; Troshkina, A.; Garofalo, R.P.; Rajarathnam, K. Chemokine CXCL1 mediated neutrophil recruitment: Role of glycosaminoglycan interactions. *Sci. Rep.* **2016**, *6*, 33123. [CrossRef] [PubMed]

48. Sepuru, K.M.; Rajarathnam, K. CXCL1/MGSA is a novel glycosaminoglycan (GAG)-binding chemokine: Structural evidence for two distinct non-overlapping binding domains. *J. Biol. Chem.* **2016**, *291*, 4247–4255. [CrossRef] [PubMed]

49. Sepuru, K.M.; Nagarajan, B.; Desai, U.R.; Rajarathnam, K. Molecular basis of chemokine CXCL5-glycosaminoglycan interactions. *J. Biol. Chem.* **2016**, *291*, 20539–20550. [CrossRef] [PubMed]

50. Di Stefano, A.; Caramori, G.; Gnemmi, I.; Contoli, M.; Bristot, L.; Capelli, A.; Ricciardolo, F.L.; Magno, F.; D'Anna, S.E.; Zanini, A.; et al. Association of increased CCL5 and CXCL7 chemokine expression with neutrophil activation in severe stable COPD. *Thorax* **2009**, *64*, 968–975. [CrossRef] [PubMed]

51. Yeo, L.; Adlard, N.; Biehl, M.; Juarez, M.; Smallie, T.; Snow, M.; Buckley, C.D.; Raza, K.; Filer, A.; Scheel-Toellner, D. Expression of chemokines CXCL4 and CXCL7 by synovial macrophages defines an early stage of rheumatoid arthritis. *Ann. Rheum. Dis.* **2016**, *75*, 763–771. [CrossRef] [PubMed]

52. Bdeir, K.; Gollomp, K.; Stasiak, M.; Mei, J.; Papiewska-Pajak, I.; Zhao, G.; Worthen, G.S.; Cines, D.B.; Poncz, M.; Kowalska, M.A. Platelet-specific chemokines contribute to the pathogenesis of acute lung injury. *Am. J. Respir. Cell Mol. Biol.* **2017**, *56*, 261–270. [CrossRef] [PubMed]

53. Desurmont, T.; Skrypek, N.; Duhamel, A.; Jonckheere, N.; Millet, G.; Leteurtre, E.; Gosset, P.; Duchene, B.; Ramdane, N.; Hebbar, M.; et al. Overexpression of chemokine receptor CXCR2 and ligand CXCL7 in liver metastases from colon cancer is correlated to shorter disease-free and overall survival. *Cancer Sci.* **2015**, *106*, 262–269. [CrossRef] [PubMed]

54. Grépin, R.; Guyot, M.; Giuliano, S.; Boncompagni, M.; Ambrosetti, D.; Chamorey, E.; Scoazec, J.Y.; Negrier, S.; Simonnet, H.; Pagès, G. The CXCL7/CXCR1/2 axis is a key driver in the growth of clear cell renal cell carcinoma. *Cancer Res.* **2014**, *74*, 873–883. [CrossRef] [PubMed]

55. Park, S.H.; Das, B.B.; Casagrande, F.; Tian, Y.; Nothnagel, H.J.; Chu, M.; Kiefer, H.; Maier, K.; de Angelis, A.A.; Marassi, F.M.; et al. Structure of the chemokine receptor CXCR1 in phospholipid bilayers. *Nature* **2012**, *491*, 779–783. [CrossRef] [PubMed]

56. Kufareva, I. Chemokines and their receptors: Insights from molecular modeling and crystallography. *Curr. Opin. Pharmacol.* **2016**, *30*, 27–37. [CrossRef] [PubMed]

57. Mayo, K.H.; Yang, Y.; Daly, T.J.; Barry, J.K.; La Rosa, G.J. Secondary structure of neutrophil-activating peptide-2 determined by 1H-nuclear magnetic resonance spectroscopy. *Biochem. J.* **1994**, *304*, 371–376. [CrossRef] [PubMed]

58. Ravindran, A.; Joseph, P.R.; Rajarathnam, K. Structural basis for differential binding of the interleukin-8 monomer and dimer to the CXCR1 N-domain: Role of coupled interactions and dynamics. *Biochemistry* **2009**, *48*, 8795–8805. [CrossRef] [PubMed]

59. Goddard, T.D.; Kneller, D.G. *Sparky 3*; University of California: San Francisco, CA, USA, 2008.

60. Shen, Y.; Lange, O.; Delaglio, F.; Rossi, P.; Aramini, J.M.; Liu, G.; Eletsky, A.; Wu, Y.; Singarapu, K.K.; Lemak, A.; et al. Consistent blind protein structure generation from NMR chemical shift data. *Proc. Natl. Acad. Sci. USA* **2008**, *105*, 4685–4690. [CrossRef] [PubMed]

61. Shen, Y.; Vernon, R.; Baker, D.; Bax, A. De novo protein structure generation from incomplete chemical shift assignments. *J. Biomol. NMR* **2009**, *43*, 63–78. [CrossRef] [PubMed]

62. Case, D.A.; Darden, T.A.; Cheatham, T.E.; Simmerling, C.L.; Wang, J.; Duke, R.E.; Luo, R.; Walker, R.C.; Zhang, W.; Merz, K.M.; et al. *Amber 12*; University of California: San Francisco, CA, USA, 2012.

63. Willard, L.; Ranjan, A.; Zhang, H.; Monzavi, H.; Boyko, R.F.; Sykes, B.D.; Wishart, D.S. Vadar: A web server for quantitative evaluation of protein structure quality. *Nucleic Acids Res.* **2003**, *31*, 3316–3319. [CrossRef] [PubMed]

64. Dominguez, C.; Boelens, R.; Bonvin, A.M. Haddock: A protein–protein docking approach based on biochemical or biophysical information. *J. Am. Chem. Soc.* **2003**, *125*, 1731–1737. [CrossRef] [PubMed]

65. De Vries, S.J.; van Dijk, A.D.; Krzeminski, M.; van Dijk, M.; Thureau, A.; Hsu, V.; Wassenaar, T.; Bonvin, A.M. Haddock versus haddock: New features and performance of haddock2.0 on the capri targets. *Proteins* **2007**, *69*, 726–733. [CrossRef] [PubMed]

66. Mulloy, B.; Forster, M.J.; Jones, C.; Davies, D.B. NMR and molecular-modelling studies of the solution conformation of heparin. *Biochem. J.* **1993**, *293*, 849–858. [CrossRef] [PubMed]

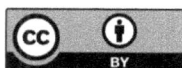

International Journal of
Molecular Sciences

MDPI

Article

Chemokine CXCL7 Heterodimers: Structural Insights, CXCR2 Receptor Function, and Glycosaminoglycan Interactions

Aaron J. Brown, Prem Raj B. Joseph, Kirti V. Sawant and Krishna Rajarathnam *

Department of Biochemistry and Molecular Biology, and Sealy Center for Structural Biology and Molecular Biophysics, The University of Texas Medical Branch, Galveston, TX 77555, USA; aj3brown@utmb.edu (A.J.B.); pbjoseph@utmb.edu (P.R.B.J.); kisawant@utmb.edu (K.V.S.)
* Correspondence: krrajara@utmb.edu; Tel.: +1-409-772-2238

Academic Editor: Martin J. Stone
Received: 28 February 2017; Accepted: 29 March 2017; Published: 1 April 2017

Abstract: Chemokines mediate diverse fundamental biological processes, including combating infection. Multiple chemokines are expressed at the site of infection; thus chemokine synergy by heterodimer formation may play a role in determining function. Chemokine function involves interactions with G-protein-coupled receptors and sulfated glycosaminoglycans (GAG). However, very little is known regarding heterodimer structural features and receptor and GAG interactions. Solution nuclear magnetic resonance (NMR) and molecular dynamics characterization of platelet-derived chemokine CXCL7 heterodimerization with chemokines CXCL1, CXCL4, and CXCL8 indicated that packing interactions promote CXCL7-CXCL1 and CXCL7-CXCL4 heterodimers, and electrostatic repulsive interactions disfavor the CXCL7-CXCL8 heterodimer. As characterizing the native heterodimer is challenging due to interference from monomers and homodimers, we engineered a "trapped" disulfide-linked CXCL7-CXCL1 heterodimer. NMR and modeling studies indicated that GAG heparin binding to the heterodimer is distinctly different from the CXCL7 monomer and that the GAG-bound heterodimer is unlikely to bind the receptor. Interestingly, the trapped heterodimer was highly active in a Ca^{2+} release assay. These data collectively suggest that GAG interactions play a prominent role in determining heterodimer function in vivo. Further, this study provides proof-of-concept that the disulfide trapping strategy can serve as a valuable tool for characterizing the structural and functional features of a chemokine heterodimer.

Keywords: chemokine; heterodimer; CXCL7; CXCR2; glycosaminoglycan; heparin; NMR

1. Introduction

Chemokines, a large family of signaling proteins, mediate diverse biological processes, including innate and adaptive immunity, organogenesis, and tissue repair [1–3]. Common to these functions is the directed trafficking of various cell types through interactions with seven transmembrane G-protein coupled receptors. Chemokine–chemokine receptor interactions form an intricate network of crosstalk, with a given chemokine binding either a single or multiple receptors and a given receptor binding either a single or multiple chemokines [4,5]. Additional layers of complexity arise from chemokines existing in multiple states, from monomers, dimers, and tetramers to oligomers and polymers, and from their interactions with sulfated glycosaminoglycans (GAG) [6–8]. During active inflammation, local chemokine concentrations both in the free and GAG-bound forms could vary by orders of magnitude, which in turn could regulate the steepness and duration of chemotactic and haptotactic gradients [9,10]. Further, several lines of evidence indicate that chemokines also form heterodimers, suggesting yet another layer of complexity in regulating function.

Humans express ~50 different chemokines, which can be classified into subfamilies on the basis of the first two conserved cysteine residues as CXC, CC, CX$_3$C, and XC [11,12]. Despite sequence identity that can be as low as 20%, chemokines share a similar structure at the monomer level. Considering that they are small (~8 to 10 kDa), they show a remarkable array of oligomeric states and binding interfaces. At the simplest level, chemokines share similar dimeric structures within a subfamily. The CXC-family forms globular dimers, with the first β-strand constituting the dimer interface, while the CC-family forms elongated dimers, with the N-loop constituting the dimer interface. However, this classification is not stringent, as some CC chemokines form CXC dimers [13] and some do not form dimers even at mM concentrations [14,15]. Chemokines that form tetramers exhibit both CXC and CC dimer interfaces [16–18]. Some chemokines form elongated polymers that have a completely different interface [19,20]. Further, lymphotactin, the only member of the C family, shows a typical chemokine fold and yet a completely different fold as a function of pH and solution conditions [21]. These properties speak to the inherent plasticity of the chemokine dimer interface. Considering that many chemokines are co-expressed under conditions of insult or co-exist in granules, it follows that chemokines are capable of forming heterodimers.

Functional studies have provided evidence for chemokine "synergy", wherein the presence of multiple chemokines results in enhanced or altered activity [22–25]. Synergy is thought to play an important role at the onset of inflammatory signaling and has been attributed to altered receptor signaling [26] and/or heterodimer formation [27,28]. As an example, the functional potential of chemokine synergy was demonstrated in vivo using peptides that inhibit the CXCL4/CCL5 heterodimer in a mouse atherosclerosis model [29]. Many of the chemokines known to exist in platelets, as well as those that mediate neutrophil recruitment, form heterodimers. Several studies have provided evidence for heterodimers [30–32], but very little is known regarding the structural features, the molecular mechanisms underlying heterodimerization, or how heterodimers interact with their cognate receptors and GAGs. Such knowledge is essential to describe how the interplay between heterodimers, GAGs, and receptors mediates crosstalk between platelets and neutrophils towards the successful resolution of disease.

In this study, we investigated the molecular basis of heterodimer formation for the chemokine CXCL7 with chemokines CXCL1, CXCL4, and CXCL8. These chemokines co-exist in platelet granules, and their release upon platelet activation orchestrates neutrophils to the tissue injury site. CXCL7, CXCL1, and CXCL8, characterized by the conserved N-terminal "ELR" motif, direct neutrophil trafficking by activating the CXCR2 receptor [33]. CXCL4 is not a CXCR2 agonist as it lacks the ELR motif, but it plays an important role in promoting neutrophil adhesion [34]. We show that favorable packing and ionic interactions promote CXCL7-CXCL1 and CXCL7-CXCL4 heterodimers and that repulsive ionic interactions disfavor the CXCL7-CXCL8 heterodimer. Using a "trapped" disulfide-linked CXCL7-CXCL1 heterodimer, we provide definitive insights into GAG and receptor binding interactions. Interestingly, we observed that the trapped heterodimer was as active as the native proteins for CXCR2 function in a Ca^{2+} release assay. Further, GAG heparin interactions of the heterodimer are distinctly different from the CXCL7 monomer, and the GAG-bound heterodimer is unlikely to bind the receptor. Our observation that GAG binding interactions of a heterodimer could be quite different from the monomer suggests that these differences could play important roles in fine-tuning in vivo neutrophil recruitment and function. To our knowledge, this is the very first report of receptor and GAG interactions that could be unambiguously attributed to a chemokine heterodimer.

2. Results

2.1. NMR (Nuclear Magnetic Resonance) Characterization of CXCL7 Heterodimers

CXCL7, compared to CXCL1 and CXCL8, forms weak dimers, and actually forms a tetramer at high concentrations. CXCL4, on the other hand, forms an even stronger tetramer. Tetramer structures of CXCL7 and CXCL4 reveal both CXC and CC type dimer interfaces [16,35]. CXC-type homodimers are stabilized by six H-bonds across the dimer interface β-strands and inter-subunit packing interactions between helical and β-sheet residues [16,17,36–38]. Sequences and the structures reveal that many of the hydrophobic dimer interface residues are conserved and that polar and charged dimer interface residues are not (Figure 1A). Comparing dimer interface residues of CXCL7 to CXCL1, CXCL4, and CXCL8 reveals ~40% to 60% similarity, suggesting that the propensity to form heterodimers could vary between each chemokine pair.

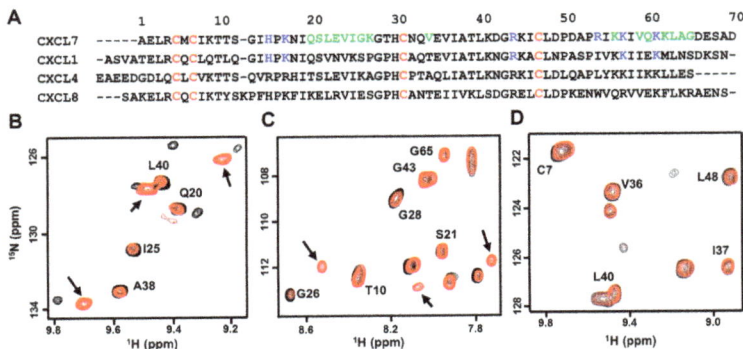

Figure 1. NMR (nuclear magnetic resonance) characterization of CXCL7 heterodimers. (**A**) Sequence alignment of platelet-derived CXC chemokines. GAG (glycosaminoglycans)binding residues identified from this study are in blue, dimer interface residues for CXCL7 are in green, and conserved Cys residues are in red; (**B–D**) Sections of the ¹H–¹⁵N HSQC (heteronuclear single quantum coherence) spectra showing the overlay of CXCL7 in the free (black) and in the presence of CXCL1 (**B**, red), CXCL4 (**C**, red), and CXCL8 (**D**, red). Arrows indicate new peaks corresponding to the heterodimer. No new peaks were observed in the case of the CXCL8 titration.

Solution nuclear magnetic resonance (NMR) spectroscopy is ideally suited for characterizing CXCL7 heterodimers compared to other techniques. We recently assigned the chemical shifts of the CXCL7 monomer and extensively characterized dimerization propensity as a function of solution conditions such as pH and buffer [39]. The heteronuclear single quantum coherence (HSQC) spectrum of ¹⁵N-labeled CXCL7 shows essentially a monomer along with some weak homodimer peaks. On titrating unlabeled CXCL1 or CXCL4 to ¹⁵N-CXCL7, the monomer and homodimer peaks gradually weaken, and new peaks appear that must correspond to the heterodimer (Figure 1B,C). These new peaks are in slow exchange with the CXCL7 monomer and homodimer. No changes were observed on titrating CXCL8 to ¹⁵N-CXCL7, indicating the absence of heterodimer formation (Figure 1D). We also carried out reverse titrations by titrating unlabeled CXCL7 to ¹⁵N-labeled CXCL1 or CXCL8. Titrating CXCL7 to ¹⁵N-CXCL1 resulted in the disappearance of monomer peaks and the appearance of new peaks confirming heterodimer formation. Conversely, titrating CXCL7 to ¹⁵N-CXCL8 resulted in no spectral changes.

The appearance of a new peak during the course of a titration indicates that the environment of the particular residue in the heterodimer is different compared to the monomer or homodimer. On titrating CXCL1 to ¹⁵N-CXCL7, new peaks are observed that correspond to CXCL7 β₁-strand residues S21, L22, V24, β₂-strand residues V34, E35, V36, and I37, and C-terminal helical residues K56, K62, A64, and G65. These residues are located either at or proximal to the dimer interface. In the reverse titration of adding CXCL7 to ¹⁵N-CXCL1, new peaks corresponding to residues I23 to S30 of the dimer-interface β₁-strand, T38 to L44 of the adjacent β₂-strand, and C-terminal helical residues I58 to S69 are observed. These data collectively indicate that CXCL7-CXCL1 forms a CXC-type heterodimer and that the residues involved in packing interactions that stabilize the homodimers also stabilize the heterodimer. We also explored whether side chain chemical shifts of glutamine and asparagine can serve as probes for heterodimer formation. In CXCL1, a glutamine and an asparagine are located at the CXC dimer interface as well as a pair of glutamines in the CC dimer interface (Figure 2A). Upon titrating CXCL7, chemical shift changes were observed for CXC dimer-interface Q24 and N27 but not for CC dimer-interfaces Q10 and Q13 (Figure 2B), providing further structural evidence for a CXC-type dimer.

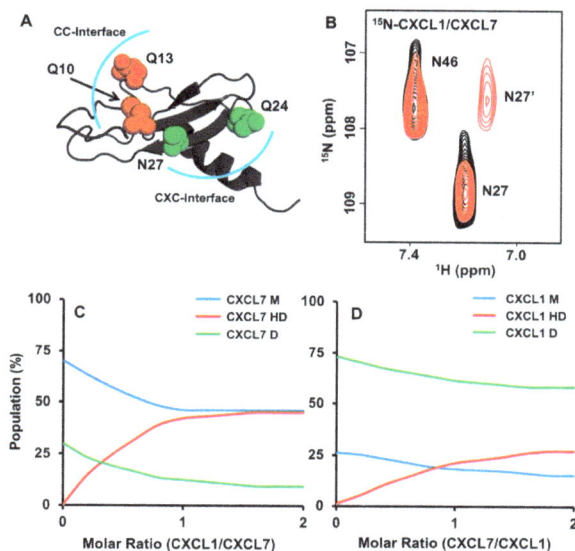

Figure 2. Characterization of the native CXCL7-CXCL1 heterodimer. (**A**) CXC (green) and CC (red) dimer-interface asparagine and glutamine residues are highlighted in the CXCL1 structure. The CXC and CC dimer interfaces are outlined with a blue arc; (**B**) Section of the spectra showing the CXCL1 side chain peaks for N27 and N46 in the free form (black) and in the presence of CXCL7 (red). Of the two peaks, only N27 shows reduced intensity and a new peak corresponding to the heterodimer (labeled as N27'); (**C,D**) Plots showing the relative populations of monomer (M), homodimer (D), and heterodimer (HD) based on NMR peak intensities during the course of the titration. Panel **C** shows the relative populations on adding CXCL1 to ^{15}N-CXCL7, and panel **D** shows the relative populations on adding CXCL7 to ^{15}N-CXCL1.

Peak intensities can provide valuable information on the relative populations of the monomer, homodimer, and heterodimer. We were able to track intensity changes for a number of residues upon titrating CXCL1 into ^{15}N-CXCL7 and vice versa. During the course of the titration, populations of both the CXCL7 monomer and homodimer decrease and populations of the heterodimer increase. On adding excess CXCL1, heterodimer and monomer populations become comparable and the homodimer population becomes negligible (Figure 2C). However, in the case of CXCL1, the heterodimer population continues to increase, but the homodimer levels remain high and the monomer population becomes negligible (Figure 2D). The relative populations from both titrations indicate that the heterodimer is more favored than the CXCL7 homodimer but less favored than the CXCL1 homodimer.

We briefly describe our findings for the CXCL7-CXCL4 heterodimer. Considering that the tetramer structures of CXCL7 and CXCL4 reveal both CXC and CC dimer interfaces [16,17], heterodimerization could occur via one or both interfaces. However, similar to the CXCL7-CXCL1 heterodimer, most of the new peaks lie in proximity to the first and second β-strand residues and none were found close to the N-loop residues, indicating a CXC-type dimer interface. Side chain chemical shifts of Asn and Gln residues of the CXC dimer interface were also perturbed, providing further evidence for a CXC-type dimer.

2.2. Molecular Dynamics of Chemokine Heterodimers

We utilized a molecular dynamics-based approach to gain insight into the molecular basis for heterodimer formation. Energy minimized heterodimer structures were subjected to ~180 ns molecular dynamics (MD) simulations in order to arrive at a stable structure that had minimal fluctuations in backbone root-mean-square deviation (RMSD). To gain insight into the relative stabilities and better understand the structural features that mediate heterodimer formation, we examined several parameters during the course of the simulation; H-bonds and packing interactions of the dimer-interface residues, backbone φ–ψ angles, and charge-charge interactions. The MD simulations collectively indicated that a combination of favorable H-bonding, packing, and electrostatic interactions, similar to what drives any complex formation, dictate heterodimer formation.

In the case of CXCL7-CXCL1, both monomer structures retained their tertiary fold. The H-bond network across the dimer interface β-strands remained intact for the CXCL7 residues L22 and V24 to CXCL1 residues V26 and V28, while peripheral H-bonds between CXCL7 G26 and Q20 to CXCL1 Q24 and S30 are transient throughout the run (Figure 3B). Backbone φ–ψ angles fall in the allowed region of the Ramachandran plot throughout the simulation. The dimer interface is stabilized by a number of favorable intermolecular packing interactions ? between M66 and L67 of CXCL1 and V24, G26, K56, and V59 of CXCL7 and between K62 and L63 of CXCL7 and V28, S30, V40, and I63 of CXCL1 (Figure 3C,D). Further, as is the case for the respective homodimer structures, the relative orientation of the helices remained parallel and in register (Figure 3A).

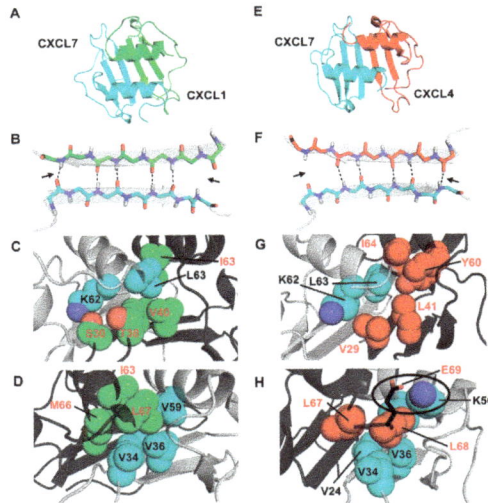

Figure 3. Structural features of the CXCL7 heterodimers. (**A,E**) Snap shots of the structural models of CXCL7-CXCL1 and CXCL7-CXCL4 heterodimers from the last 5 ns of the MD (molecular dynamics) simulations; (**B,F**) A schematic showing the β$_1$-strand dimer interface H-bonds (dashed line) from the final 5 ns of the MD run. Arrows indicate transient H-bonds; (**C,D**) Packing interactions involving CXCL7 helical (cyan) and CXCL1 β-sheet residues (green) and CXCL1 helical (green) and CXCL7 β-sheet (cyan) residues; (**G,H**) Packing interactions involving CXCL7 helical (cyan) and CXCL4 β-sheet (red) residues and the CXCL4 helical (red) and CXCL7 β-sheet (cyan) residues. The circle highlights the potential ionic interaction between CXCL4 E69 and CXCL7 K56. Nitrogen atoms are shown in the conventional dark blue and oxygen in light red.

For the CXCL7-CXCL4 heterodimer, the final MD structure revealed that the monomer structures maintained their tertiary fold (Figure 3E). The dimer interface H-bonds across the β_1-strands remain intact for CXCL7 residues L22 and V24 to CXCL4 residues L27 and V29, whereas the edge H-bonds (between CXCL7 Q20 and CXCL4 K31 and between CXCL7 G26 and CXCL4 T25) are transient (Figure 3F). The dimer is stabilized by favorable packing interactions between K62 and L63 of CXCL7 and V29, L41, Y60, and I64 of CXCL4 and between L67 and L68 of CXCL4 and V24, V34, V36, K56, V59, and L63 of CXCL7 (Figure 3G,H). Many of these residues are similar in the corresponding homodimers indicating conserved interactions (Figure 1A). However, there are unique structural differences in the heterodimer. For instance, E69 of CXCL4 (corresponding to A64 in CXCL7) is involved in ionic interactions with K56 from the opposite helix in CXCL7 (Figure 3H), and CXCL4 L67 and L68 are involved in additional packing interactions with CXCL7 L63 and V59. These new interactions result in the realignment of the helix and partial unwinding of the terminal helical residues.

For the CXCL7-CXCL8 heterodimer, despite favorable H-bonding and packing interactions, there was significant disruption of the tertiary fold due to unfavorable ionic interactions. The structure reveals that CXCL7 K27 and CXCL8 R68 are positioned across the dimer interface, resulting in electrostatic repulsion. In the CXCL8 homodimer, R68 is involved in favorable ionic interactions with E29 across the dimer interface. This swap from favorable to unfavorable interactions provides a molecular basis as to why CXCL7-CXCL8 fails to form a heterodimer.

2.3. Design and Characterization of a Trapped Heterodimer

Characterizing the structural and functional features of the native heterodimer is challenging due to contributions from two native homodimers and two native monomers. In principle, the solution contains as many as ten species; two monomers in the free and bound form, two dimers in the free and bound form, and heterodimers in the free and bound form. NMR experiments reduce this complexity by selectively labeling one of the monomers of the heterodimer, which simplifies the spectra to six species. In reality, we observe three sets of peaks due to fast exchange between the free and the bound form. Nevertheless, interpretation of such spectra is still challenging due to challenges in unambiguously assigning the chemical shifts of the newly formed heterodimer and tracking chemical shift perturbations (CSPs) of multiple species. This was evident when we initially attempted to characterize GAG binding to a wild type (WT) heterodimer mixture of ^{15}N-CXCL7/CXCL1 or CXCL7/^{15}N-CXCL1 at a 1:1 molar ratio. In order to overcome these limitations, we designed a disulfide-linked "trapped" CXCL7-CXCL1 heterodimer.

We used our heterodimer structural models from MD simulations to examine potential mutation sites in the CXCL7-CXCL1 heterodimer. To ensure formation of only the disulfide-linked heterodimer and no disulfide-linked homodimers, we looked for residues that are away from the two-fold symmetry axis. Other criteria that we considered were that these residues should minimally contribute to dimerization and/or influence the native fold. Our analysis pinpointed the solvent exposed β_1-strand residues as likely candidates (Figure 4A,B). From this group, we chose the pair S21 from CXCL7 and K29 from CXCL1. The individual cysteine mutants (CXCL7 S21C and CXCL1 K29C) were recombinantly expressed and purified, and the trapped heterodimer was allowed to form by simple mixing of the proteins. We confirmed trapped heterodimer formation using SDS-PAGE, mass spectrometry, and NMR spectroscopy. Bands corresponding to the heterodimer were observed only under non-reducing conditions, indicating a disulfide-linked heterodimer (Figure 4C). The NMR spectra of the trapped heterodimer showed well-dispersed peaks characteristic of a single folded protein (Figure 5A,B). We also compared NMR spectra of the trapped heterodimer to the WT heterodimer (Figure 5C). The spectra were essentially similar except for residues in and around the mutation, indicating that the introduction of the disulfide does not perturb the native fold and that the trapped heterodimer retains the structural characteristics of the native heterodimer.

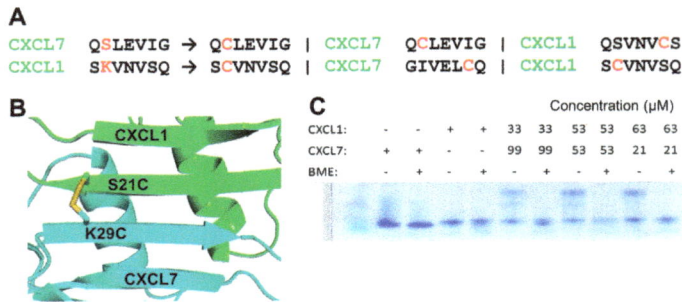

Figure 4. Characterization of the CXCL7-CXCL1 trapped heterodimer. (**A**) Trapping strategy showing cysteine mutations (in red) that will result only in a trapped heterodimer. Cysteines are too far away in the homodimer for disulfide formation; (**B**) A schematic of the heterodimer showing the location of the disulfide across the heterodimer interface and away from the two fold symmetry axis. CXCL7 is in cyan and CXCL1 is in green. (**C**) SDS-PAGE gel showing the formation of the disulfide bond. The higher molecular weight heterodimer band is observed only under non-reducing conditions. BME stands for β-mercaptoethanol.

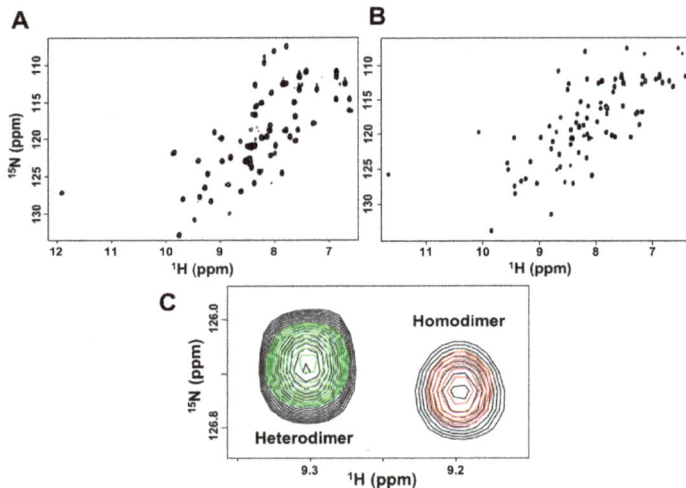

Figure 5. NMR structural features of the trapped heterodimer. ^{1}H-^{15}N HSQC spectra of the (**A**) ^{15}N-CXCL7:CXCL1 and (**B**) ^{15}N-CXCL1:CXCL7 trapped heterodimer. Spectra demonstrate a properly folded heterodimer with no evidence of monomer or homodimer; (**C**) The structure of the trapped heterodimer is similar to the native heterodimer. A section of the HSQC spectra of CXCL7 (red), trapped heterodimer (green), and a mixture of CXCL7 and CXCL1 in which both native heterodimer and native homodimer are present (black). Trapped heterodimer alone exists as a single species, free CXCL7 exists as monomers and homodimers, and native heterodimer is present along with native monomer and homodimer (Figure 2C). The trapped and native heterodimers have similar chemical shifts, as is evident from superimposed peaks. Please note the absence of a green peak superimposed on the homodimer peak. The peak corresponding to the monomer is not shown as it resonates outside of the displayed spectral window.

Knowledge of the chemical shifts is essential for NMR characterization of trapped heterodimer GAG interactions. Towards this, we carried out ^{15}N-edited NOESY and TOCSY experiments on ^{15}N-CXCL7-CXCL1 and ^{15}N-CXCL1-CXCL7 trapped heterodimer samples. We were able to assign the backbone ^{1}H and ^{15}N chemical shifts of all CXCL1 residues and ~80% of CXCL7 residues. Some of the CXCL7 residues could not be assigned due to overlap or lack of sequential nuclear Overhauser effects (NOEs), but this was not limiting as most of the unassigned residues play no role in GAG interactions.

2.4. Heterodimer-GAG Interactions

We characterized the binding interactions of GAG heparin octasaccharide (dp8) by individual titrations to ^{15}N-CXCL7-CXCL1 and ^{15}N-CXCL1-CXCL7 trapped heterodimer samples. In the ^{15}N-CXCL7-CXCL1 trapped heterodimer, significant perturbations were observed for N-loop, β_3-strand, and α-helical residues. Of particular interest are the basic residues H15 and K17 of the N-loop, R44 and K45 from the β_3-strand, and K56 and K57 from the helix (Figure 6A). CSPs for hydrophobic or acidic residues located proximal to these basic residues are likely due to indirect interactions. In the case of the ^{15}N-CXCL1-CXCL7 trapped heterodimer, significant perturbations were observed for residues in the N-loop, β_3-strand, and α-helix. These include the basic residues H19 and K21 of the N-loop, K45 and R48 of the 40s loop and β_3-strand, and K61, K65, and K71 of the α-helix (Figure 6B).

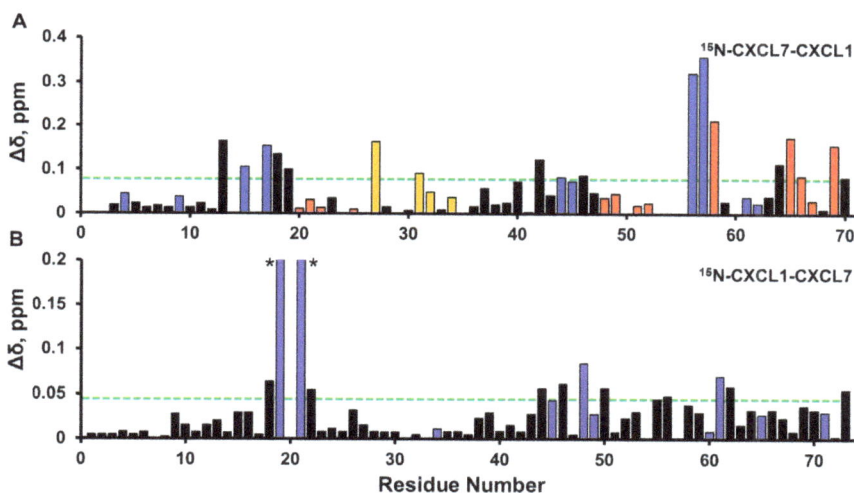

Figure 6. Histogram plots of chemical shift changes on heparin binding to trapped heterodimer. Heparin binding-induced chemical shift changes in CXCL7 (**A**) and CXCL1 (**B**) of the CXCL7-CXCL1 trapped heterodimer. Residues that show CSP above the threshold (dashed line) are considered involved in binding. Basic residues Arg, Lys, and His are shown in blue. CXCL7 residues that show sigmoidal binding profiles are shown in red, and CXCL7 residues showing normal hyperbolic profiles are shown in gold. Residues H19 and K21 (highlighted by *) show much higher CSPs (0.26 and 0.71 ppm, respectively).

Interestingly, the CSP profiles of CXCL1 versus CXCL7 residues were strikingly different (Figure 7A,B). Whereas all CXCL1 residues showed similar hyperbolic profiles, CXCL7 showed three distinctly different profiles. A subset of residues showed hyperbolic profiles (Figure 7C), a subset showed an initial delay in perturbation followed by a hyperbolic profile (Figure 7D), and a subset showed sigmoidal like profiles (Figure 7E). We define these residues as belonging to Set-I, Set-II, and Set-III, respectively.

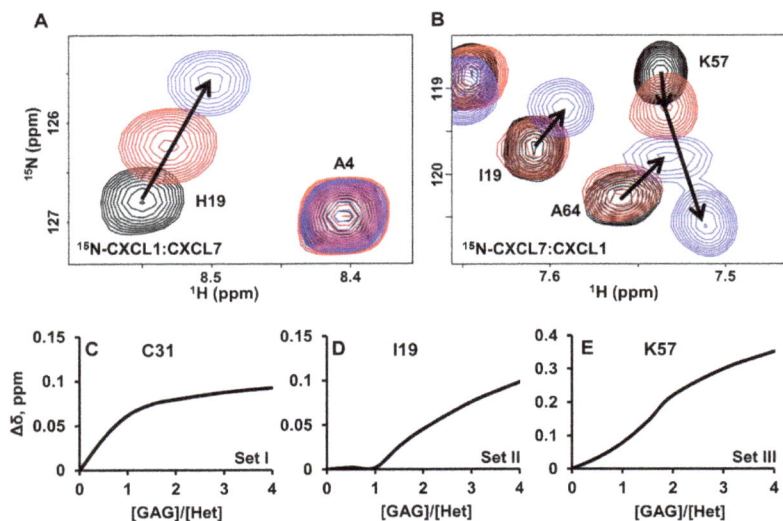

Figure 7. NMR characteristics of trapped heterodimer-heparin interactions. Sections of the ^{1}H-^{15}N HSQC spectra showing the overlay of CXCL7-CXCL1 trapped heterodimer in the free (black) and heparin dp8 bound form at 1:1 (red) and 1:4 (blue) molar ratios. Arrows indicate the direction of movement. (**A**) For CXCL1, only linear chemical shifts are observed; (**B**) In the case of CXCL7, both non-linear chemical shifts (K57) and delayed linear chemical shifts (I19 and A64) are observed; (**C–E**) Plots of binding-induced chemical shift changes on adding heparin. For CXCL7, (**C**) hyperbolic, (**D**) hyperbolic after a delay, and (**E**) sigmoidal profiles are observed.

Set-I residues include K27 and C31 to V34 of the 30s-loop and K56 of the helix (Figure 6A). These residues lie along the dimer interface across from the CXCL1 β-sheet and the helical residues. Considering that these residues show hyperbolic perturbation profiles similar to CXCL1 residues, it is likely that their CSPs are due to indirect interactions of dp8 binding to CXCL1. For example, our structural model reveals that the CXCL7 K27 side chain is oriented towards the CXCL1 helix, likely making it sensitive to any structural changes in the CXCL1 helix, such as those often associated with dp8 binding.

Set-II residues include G13 to I19 of the N-loop, D42 to I46 of the β₃-strand, and V59 to A64 of the helix (Figure 6A). These residues are located away from the dimer interface and are not influenced by CXCL1 binding. These perturbations can thus be attributed to direct dp8 binding to CXCL7.

Set-III residues include Q20 to I25 of the β₁-strand, K57, I58, and G65 to A69 of the helix, and L48 to A52 that precede the helix (Figure 6A). In addition to sigmoidal binding profiles, these peaks showed non-linear chemical shift perturbations (Figure 7B). These residues are located at the crossroad between the CXCL7-GAG binding interface and the dimer interface. Therefore, their perturbations are likely a composite of both CXCL1 and CXCL7 dp8-binding. Residues K56, K57, and I58 are prominent examples. The K56 side chain is pointed towards the dimer interface, while K57 points out towards the N-loop. K56 shows a linear perturbation similar to CXCL1 residues, suggesting that its perturbation is due to direct or indirect interactions from dp8 binding to CXCL1. The initial perturbation of residues K57 and I58 can thus be attributed to a proximity effect of K56. However, the perturbation profile of K57 and I58 is altered upon further addition of dp8, indicating that these changes must be due to direct dp8 binding to CXCL7. Thus the sigmoidal profiles are a composite of CXCL1 and CXCL7 binding (Figure 7B,E). These data collectively indicate two independent binding sites, with one heparin binding one monomer and the second heparin binding the other monomer of the heterodimer, and that heparin first binds to CXCL1, due to higher affinity, and then to CXCL7.

As discussed above, characterizing GAG binding to the WT heterodimer is challenging. However, using the trapped heterodimer titration spectrum as a template, we explored whether we could characterize heparin binding to the native heterodimer. Indeed, we were able to track heparin binding to a few well-dispersed heterodimer peaks. For instance, upon titration, we observed a heterodimer peak, which showed significant CSP, a non-linear sigmoidal profile, and similar chemical shifts as K57 and I58 in the trapped heterodimer. Additionally, heterodimer peaks that could be assigned to Q20, L48, and G65 showed sigmoidal profiles similar to what was observed in the trapped heterodimer. These observations provide compelling evidence that binding interactions of the trapped heterodimer capture the complexity of the native heterodimer.

To gain insight into the binding geometries, we generated models of the GAG heparin dp8 bound CXCL1-CXCL7 heterodimer complex using HADDOCK-based docking. We performed two independent runs. In run-I, restraints were given between one dp8 and CXCL7 and between another dp8 and CXCL1. In run-II, restraints were given between two GAGs and both monomers of the heterodimer. Both runs showed essentially the same binding geometry, with one GAG binding to each monomer of the heterodimer (Figure 8A). In CXCL7, the GAG-binding interface spans the β_3-strand, the N-loop, and the helix and is mediated by H15 and K17 of the N-loop, R44 of the β_3-strand, and R54, K57, and K61 of the helix (Figure 8B). In CXCL1, the GAG-binding interface also spans the β_3-strand, the N-loop, and the helix and is mediated by H19 and K21 of the N-loop, R48 of the β_3-strand, and K61 and K65 of the helix (Figure 8C). CXCL1 K45 and CXCL7 K27 were not involved in binding, though both showed significant CSP, indicating that their CSP is most likely due to indirect interactions. We also carried out modeling of one GAG to either CXCL1 or CXCL7 and observed the same binding interactions as observed for two GAGs. Our models provide the structural basis for stepwise and non-overlapping binding geometry, which is consistent with the NMR titrations. Further, the GAG-binding geometry is distinct from that observed in the CXCL1 dimer, wherein GAG binds across the β-sheet dimer interface [40]. Considering that previous studies have established that the N-loop residues in CXCL7 and CXCL1 are involved in receptor binding, the models also suggest that GAG-bound heterodimer cannot bind the receptor [39,41].

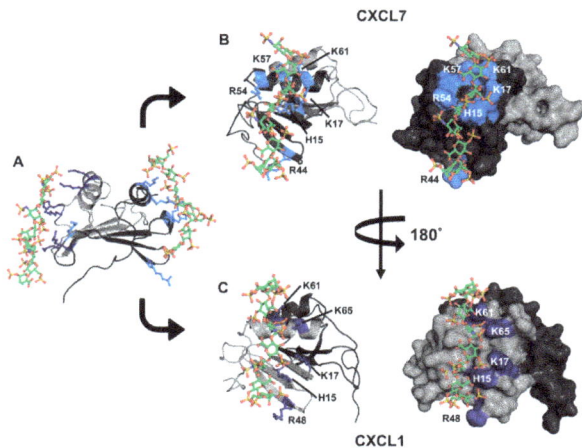

Figure 8. A model of the heparin-bound CXCL7-CXCL1 heterodimer complex. (**A**) Ribbon diagram showing that heparin binds to both monomers of the heterodimer. CXCL7 is shown in dark gray and CXCL1 light gray; (**B,C**) Cartoon and surface plots showing side views of the CXCL7 and CXCL1 monomer faces interacting with heparin dp8, respectively. The basic residues involved in binding are labeled and shown in blue.

2.5. Heterodimer Receptor Binding Activity

We characterized receptor activity by measuring Ca^{2+} release using HL60 cells stably transfected with the CXCR2 receptor [41]. We compared the receptor activities of WT CXCL1, WT CXCL7, a mixture of both chemokines (CXCL7 and CXCL1), and our trapped heterodimer (CXCL7-CXCL1). The trapped heterodimer was as potent as the WT chemokines, and the activity of the mixture of CXCL1 and CXCL7 (that corresponds to the native heterodimer) was no different from the trapped heterodimer or WT proteins (Figure 9). These data indicate that there is no synergy and that essentially one of the monomers of the heterodimer binds and activates the receptor. Previous studies using a trapped homodimer for CXCL1 and CXCL8 have also shown that the activity of the homodimer was no different from the monomer [41–43].

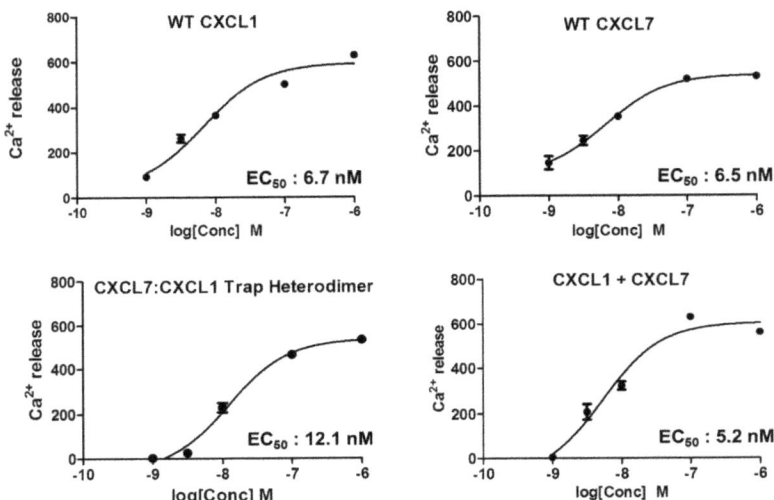

Figure 9. CXCR2 activity of the heterodimer. A plot showing the activity curves for WT CXCL1, WT CXCL7, 1:1 CXCL7/CXCL1 mixture, and the trapped CXCL7-CXCL1 heterodimer. The EC_{50} values indicate that the heterodimer binds and activates the receptor like the WT proteins.

3. Discussion

Animal model and in vitro studies have shown enhanced or altered activity for a wide variety of CXC, CC, and CXC/CC chemokine pairs [22–25,44–46]. For instance, high levels of CXCL1 (KC) and CXCL2 (MIP-2) have been observed in a number of murine disease models: virus-infected epithelial cells release multiple chemokines that direct neutrophil chemotaxis; peptides that inhibit CCL5/CXCL4 heterodimer formation alleviate atherosclerosis in a mouse model; and the CXCL7/CXCL4 pair compared to CXCL7 alone shows differential activity for neutrophil adhesion and transendothelial migration [29,47–49]. However, whether altered activity is due to non-additive receptor activity of two chemokines or to distinct heterodimer receptor activity is unknown.

Knowledge of the structural basis and molecular mechanisms by which chemokines form heterodimers is essential to understanding how heterodimers mediate function. In this study, using solution NMR spectroscopy, we were able to describe the structural features and molecular basis by which CXCL7 is able to form heterodimers with some chemokines but not with others. Further, using NMR spectroscopy, we were able to describe the molecular basis of heparin GAG binding to the CXCL7-CXCL1 heterodimer. NMR detects direct binding and does not require exogenous tagging, as do the fluorescence-based FRET/BRET methods, and so does not suffer from potential artifacts.

Int. J. Mol. Sci. **2017**, *18*, 748

Popular techniques for distinguishing between monomers and dimers such as gel filtration and native gel electrophoresis cannot distinguish between heterodimers and homodimers due to their similar size and molecular weight. Mass spectrometry and co-immunoprecipitation techniques have been used to detect chemokine heterodimers [30,50,51], but these techniques do not provide any insight into the molecular basis of heterodimer formation. NMR chemical shifts of the backbone amide (^{1}H and ^{15}N) are sensitive to secondary, tertiary, and quaternary structures. Therefore, under ideal conditions, NMR could distinguish heterodimers from homodimers and monomers. Previous NMR studies have shown heterodimer formation between CXCL4 and CXCL8 [32] and that the CCL2-CCL8 heterodimer is favored compared to the CCL2 homodimer [50] but did not describe the structural features of the heterodimer. This is challenging and requires chemical shift assignments not only of the monomer but also of the heterodimer.

The role of in vivo heterodimer function is dependent on receptor and GAG interactions. GAG interactions play multiple roles that include determining the makeup of the chemotactic/haptotactic gradients, influencing whether it is the free or GAG-bound chemokine that activates the receptor, and regulating the levels of the free monomer and homodimer. Further, free and GAG-bound heterodimer levels depend on the GAG affinities, the equilibrium constants (K_d) of the heterodimer and of the two homodimers, and the relative amounts of the two chemokines. Using trapped dimers, it has been shown that the dimer could be as active as the monomer for CXCR2 function in cellular assays [41]. However, the in vivo recruitment activity of the monomers and dimers is distinctly different, indicating that the monomer-dimer equilibrium and GAG binding are coupled and regulate in vivo recruitment [8,52,53]. Therefore, any novel activity of the heterodimer can be inferred only under conditions in which the heterodimer dominates and in which its activity is different from monomers and dimers, and this becomes challenging if its levels are not high and/or its activity is not very different from monomers and homodimers.

In this study, using a disulfide-trapping strategy, we characterized heparin dp8 binding and CXCR2 activity of the CXCL7-CXCL1 heterodimer. We observed that the calcium release activity of the trapped CXCL7-CXCL1 heterodimer, which functions as a readout for the G-protein signaling pathway, was no different compared to the WT proteins. However, chemokine engagement of the CXCR2 receptor activates G-protein and β-arrestin signaling pathways and β-arrestin mediated endocytosis. Several studies have shown that a given chemokine-receptor pair, or multiple chemokines that target a single receptor, can have large differences in G-protein or β-arrestin mediated signaling or receptor internalization activities. Future functional studies of both G-protein and β-arrestin signaling and internalization activities are required to completely understand how heterodimers differ from monomers and homodimers in eliciting receptor function.

To our knowledge, this is the very first study that describes the GAG interactions and receptor activity of a heterodimer without interference from the monomers or homodimers. The GAG interactions of the heterodimer were strikingly different from the CXCL7 monomer and CXCL1 homodimer [39,40]. Further, a number of residues implicated in GAG binding also mediate receptor interactions, suggesting that a GAG-bound heterodimer is unlikely to activate the receptor. We conclude that differences in heterodimer-GAG interactions may play a role in fine-tuning chemotactic/haptotactic gradients and also control the amount of free chemokine available to activate the receptor. Finally, our strategy of engineering a disulfide-linked trapped chemokine heterodimer opens up new avenues to characterize in vivo heterodimer function and the role of differential receptor signaling pathways and to elucidate the heterodimer's role for a variety of chemokine pairs in health and disease.

4. Materials and Methods

4.1. Molecular Dynamics Simulations

Initial structures were prepared using NMR or X-ray coordinates available from the protein data bank (PDB). The PDB IDs used were 1NAP (CXCL7) [16], 1MSG (CXCL1) [37], 1PFM (CXCL4) [35], and 1IL8 (CXCL8) [38]. Structures were generated by alignment of homodimer backbones and then removal of one of the monomers of each homodimer using PyMol [54]. In the heterodimer, the monomer structures were adjusted by translational and rotational motions about the two fold symmetry axis to align the hydrogen bond network across the β-strands of the dimer interface. The modelled heterodimer structures were then subjected to constrained energy minimization to eliminate any steric clashes, followed by free minimization using the AMBER 12 suite software and the ff03 force field [55,56]. The energy-minimized structures were subjected to an equilibration protocol in explicit solvent [57], followed by ~180 ns of MD production runs carried out using the PMEMD (Particle mesh Ewald molecular dynamics) module of the AMBER 12 software suite on the Lonestar Dell Linux Cluster at the Texas Advanced Computing Center (Texas Advanced Computing Center, The University of Texas, Austin, TX, USA). The trajectories were analyzed using AMBERtools 12, VMD, and PyMol [54,56,58].

4.2. Expression and Purification of Chemokines

Chemokines were expressed in *Escherichia coli* cultured in either LB or ^{15}N-enriched minimal medium and purified using a combination of nickel column and reverse phase high-performance liquid chromatography, as previously described [59]. The CXCL7-CXCL1 trapped heterodimer was prepared by introducing a disulfide across the dimer interface. CXCL7 S21C and CXCL1 K29C mutants were purified using a Ni-NTA column, cleaved using Factor Xa, and were combined without further purification and left overnight at 35 °C. Heterodimer was purified using high performance liquid chromatography, lyophilized, and stored at −20 °C until further use.

4.3. NMR Spectroscopy

The samples were prepared in a 50 mM sodium phosphate buffer pH 7.4 at 25 °C containing 1 mM 2,2-dimethyl-2-silapentansesulfonic acid (DSS), 1 mM sodium azide, and 10% D_2O. Heterodimer formation between two chemokines can be inferred from changes in the HSQC spectra on titrating an unlabeled chemokine to a ^{15}N-labeled chemokine prepared in the same buffer. Initial ^{15}N-labeled chemokine concentrations varied between 30 and 150 μM. The final molar ratios of labeled to unlabeled chemokine varied from 1:2 to 1:4. For these experiments, titrations were carried out until essentially no change in the spectra was observed. NMR experiments were performed on a Bruker Avance III 600 (with a QCI cryoprobe) or 800 MHz (with a TXI cryoprobe) spectrometer. All spectra were processed and analyzed using Bruker Topspin 3.2 or Sparky software [60].

The ^{1}H and ^{15}N chemical shifts of the trapped CXCL7-CXCL1 heterodimer were assigned using ^{15}N-CXCL1-CXCL7 and ^{15}N-CXCL7-CXCL1 samples prepared in 50 mM phosphate pH 6.0 and 35 °C. The concentrations of ^{15}CXCL7-CXCL1 and CXCL7-^{15}CXCL1 were 300 and 670 μM, respectively, and the assignments were obtained from analysis of ^{1}H-^{15}N heteronuclear NOESY and TOCSY experiments with mixing times of 150 and 80 ms, respectively.

4.4. Heparin-Heterodimer Interactions

The binding of heparin dp8 to the CXCL7-CXCL1 heterodimer was characterized using solution NMR spectroscopy in 50 mM phosphate buffer at pH 6.0 and 30 °C. The protein concentration for the titrations varied between 50 and 70 μM. Heparin dp8 was purchased from Iduron (Manchester, UK) and prepared in the same buffer (10 mM stock), and a series of ^{1}H-^{15}N HSQC spectra were collected upon titrating GAG until no changes in the spectra were observed. The final molar ratio of heterodimer to GAG was 1:4. For the trapped heterodimer, both ^{15}N-CXCL7-CXCL1 and ^{15}N-CXCL1-CXCL7 samples were used. For native heterodimer interactions, a mixture of CXCL7 and CXCL1 at 1:1 molar ratio was used. The final molar ratio of heterodimer to GAG was ~1:3 to 1:4. For all titrations, chemical shift perturbations were calculated as a weighted average of changes in the ^{1}H and ^{15}N chemical shifts, as described previously [61].

4.5. Heterodimer-GAG Docking

Molecular docking of heparin to the CXCL7-CXCL1 heterodimer was carried out using the High Ambiguity Driven biomolecular DOCKing (HADDOCK) approach, as described previously [62–64]. The CXCL7-CXCL1 heterodimer structure from MD studies and the NMR structure of heparin (PDB ID: 1HPN) [65] were used for docking. Ambiguous interaction restraints (AIRs) were selected based on NMR chemical shift perturbation data. The pair-wise "ligand interface RMSD matrix" over all structures was calculated and final structures were clustered using an RMSD cut-off value of 4 Å. The clusters were then prioritized using RMSD and a "HADDOCK score" (weighted sum of a combination of energy terms).

4.6. Receptor Activity of the Heterodimer

The CXCR2 receptor activity of the heterodimer was determined using a Ca^{2+} release assay, as described previously [41]. Ca^{2+} levels were measured using a FlexStation III microplate reader using the Calcium 5 assay kit (FLIPR, Molecular Devices). Differentiated HL60 cells expressing CXCR2 were incubated with varying concentrations of either WT CXCL1, WT CXCL7, a mixture of both WTs, or the trapped CXCL7-CXCL1 heterodimer. Changes in fluorescence of the Calcium 5 dye upon addition of chemokine were measured every 5 s for up to 500 s, and the agonist response was determined from the maximum change in fluorescence. EC_{50} values were calculated based on the response over a range of concentrations.

Acknowledgments: This work was supported by a grant from the National Institutes of Health P01 HL107152 to Krishna Rajarathnam and the National Institute of General Medical Sciences Houston Area Molecular Biophysics Training Grants 2T32 GM008280 to Aaron J. Brown. The authors acknowledge the Sealy Center for Structural Biology and Molecular Biophysics at the University of Texas Medical Branch at Galveston for providing research resources. We also thank Jiqing Sai of Vanderbilt University for the HL60 cells and Heather Lander for editorial assistance.

Author Contributions: Krishna Rajarathnam and Aaron J. Brown designed the research and wrote the paper; Aaron J. Brown performed the experiments; and Aaron J. Brown and Prem Raj B. Joseph analyzed the data. Kirti V. Sawant performed all cellular assays. All authors reviewed the results and approved the final version of the manuscript.

Conflicts of Interest: The authors declare no conflict of interest.

Abbreviations

CXCL	CXC ligand
CXCR2	CXC chemokine receptor 2
CXCL7/NAP2	Neutrophil-activating peptide 2
GAG	Glycosaminoglycan
NAC	CXCR2 N-terminal domain
NMR	Nuclear Magnetic Resonance
HSQC	Heteronuclear single quantum coherence
CSP	Chemical shift perturbation
NOE	Nuclear Overhauser effect
AIR	Ambiguous interaction restraints
Dp8	Heparin octasaccharide

References

1. Raman, D.; Sobolik-Delmaire, T.; Richmond, A. Chemokines in health and disease. *Exp. Cell Res.* **2011**, *317*, 575–589. [CrossRef] [PubMed]
2. Griffith, J.W.; Sokol, C.L.; Luster, A.D. Chemokines and chemokine receptors: Positioning cells for host defense and immunity. *Annu. Rev. Immunol.* **2014**, *32*, 659–702. [CrossRef] [PubMed]
3. Zlotnik, A.; Yoshie, O. The chemokine superfamily revisited. *Immunity* **2012**, *36*, 705–716. [CrossRef] [PubMed]
4. Rajagopalan, L.; Rajarathnam, K. Structural basis of chemokine receptor function—A model for binding affinity and ligand selectivity. *Biosci. Rep.* **2006**, *26*, 325–339. [CrossRef] [PubMed]
5. Stone, M.J.; Hayward, J.A.; Huang, C.; Huma, Z.E.; Sanchez, J. Mechanisms of regulation of the chemokine-receptor network. *Int. J. Mol. Sci.* **2017**, *18*, 342. [CrossRef] [PubMed]
6. Salanga, C.L.; Handel, T.M. Chemokine oligomerization and interactions with receptors and glycosaminoglycans: The role of structural dynamics in function. *Exp. Cell Res.* **2011**, *317*, 590–601. [CrossRef] [PubMed]
7. Monneau, Y.; Arenzana-Seisdedos, F.; Lortat-Jacob, H. The sweet spot: How gags help chemokines guide migrating cells. *J. Leukoc. Biol.* **2016**, *99*, 935–953. [CrossRef] [PubMed]
8. Das, S.T.; Rajagopalan, L.; Guerrero-Plata, A.; Sai, J.; Richmond, A.; Garofalo, R.P.; Rajarathnam, K. Monomeric and dimeric CXCL8 are both essential for in vivo neutrophil recruitment. *PLoS ONE* **2010**, *5*, e11754. [CrossRef] [PubMed]
9. Blanchet, X.; Langer, M.; Weber, C.; Koenen, R.R.; von Hundelshausen, P. Touch of chemokines. *Front. Immunol.* **2012**, *3*, 175. [CrossRef] [PubMed]
10. Massena, S.; Christoffersson, G.; Hjertström, E.; Zcharia, E.; Vlodavsky, I.; Ausmees, N.; Rolny, C.; Li, J.P.; Phillipson, M. A chemotactic gradient sequestered on endothelial heparan sulfate induces directional intraluminal crawling of neutrophils. *Blood* **2010**, *116*, 1924–1931. [CrossRef] [PubMed]
11. Fernandez, E.J.; Lolis, E. Structure, function, and inhibition of chemokines. *Annu. Rev. Pharmacol. Toxicol.* **2002**, *42*, 469–499. [CrossRef] [PubMed]
12. Zlotnik, A.; Yoshie, O. Chemokines: A new classification system and their role in immunity. *Immunity* **2000**, *12*, 121–127. [CrossRef]
13. Hoover, D.M.; Boulegue, C.; Yang, D.; Oppenheim, J.J.; Tucker, K.; Lu, W.; Lubkowski, J. The structure of human macrophage inflammatory protein-3α/CCL20. Linking antimicrobial and CC chemokine receptor-6-binding activities with human β-defensins. *J. Biol. Chem.* **2002**, *277*, 37647–37654. [CrossRef] [PubMed]
14. Li Wang, A.C.; Cao, J.J.; Zheng, H.; Lu, Z.; Peiper, S.C.; Li Wang, P.J. Dynamics study on the anti-human immunodeficiency virus chemokine viral macrophage-inflammatory protein-II (VMIP-II) reveals a fully monomeric protein. *Biochemistry* **1999**, *38*, 442–453. [CrossRef] [PubMed]
15. Rajarathnam, K.; Li, Y.; Rohrer, T.; Gentz, R. Solution structure and dynamics of myeloid progenitor inhibitory factor-1 (MPIF-1), a novel monomeric cc chemokine. *J. Biol. Chem.* **2001**, *276*, 4909–4916. [CrossRef] [PubMed]
16. Malkowski, M.G.; Wu, J.Y.; Lazar, J.B.; Johnson, P.H.; Edwards, B.F. The crystal structure of recombinant human neutrophil-activating peptide-2 (M6L) at 1.9-A resolution. *J. Biol. Chem.* **1995**, *270*, 7077–7087. [PubMed]
17. St Charles, R.; Walz, D.A.; Edwards, B.F. The three-dimensional structure of bovine platelet factor 4 at 3.0-A resolution. *J. Biol. Chem.* **1989**, *264*, 2092–2099. [PubMed]
18. Liang, W.G.; Ren, M.; Zhao, F.; Tang, W.J. Structures of human CCL18, CCL3, and CCL4 reveal molecular determinants for quaternary structures and sensitivity to insulin-degrading enzyme. *J. Mol. Biol.* **2015**, *427*, 1345–1358. [CrossRef] [PubMed]
19. Wang, X.; Watson, C.; Sharp, J.S.; Handel, T.M.; Prestegard, J.H. Oligomeric structure of the chemokine CCL5/RANTES from NMR, MS, and SAXS data. *Structure* **2011**, *19*, 1138–1148. [CrossRef] [PubMed]
20. Liang, W.G.; Triandafillou, C.G.; Huang, T.Y.; Zulueta, M.M.; Banerjee, S.; Dinner, A.R.; Hung, S.C.; Tang, W.J. Structural basis for oligomerization and glycosaminoglycan binding of CCL5 and CCL3. *Proc. Natl. Acad. Sci. USA* **2016**, *113*, 5000–5005. [CrossRef] [PubMed]

21. Tuinstra, R.L.; Peterson, F.C.; Kutlesa, S.; Elgin, E.S.; Kron, M.A.; Volkman, B.F. Interconversion between two unrelated protein folds in the lymphotactin native state. *Proc. Natl. Acad. Sci. USA* **2008**, *105*, 5057–5062. [CrossRef] [PubMed]

22. Von Hundelshausen, P.; Koenen, R.R.; Sack, M.; Mause, S.F.; Adriaens, W.; Proudfoot, A.E.; Hackeng, T.M.; Weber, C. Heterophilic interactions of platelet factor 4 and rantes promote monocyte arrest on endothelium. *Blood* **2005**, *105*, 924–930. [CrossRef] [PubMed]

23. Gijsbers, K.; Gouwy, M.; Struyf, S.; Wuyts, A.; Proost, P.; Opdenakker, G.; Penninckx, F.; Ectors, N.; Geboes, K.; van Damme, J. GCP-2/CXCL6 synergizes with other endothelial cell-derived chemokines in neutrophil mobilization and is associated with angiogenesis in gastrointestinal tumors. *Exp. Cell Res.* **2005**, *303*, 331–342. [CrossRef] [PubMed]

24. Gouwy, M.; Schiraldi, M.; Struyf, S.; van Damme, J.; Uguccioni, M. Possible mechanisms involved in chemokine synergy fine tuning the inflammatory response. *Immunol. Lett.* **2012**, *145*, 10–14. [CrossRef] [PubMed]

25. Proudfoot, A.E.; Uguccioni, M. Modulation of chemokine responses: Synergy and cooperativity. *Front. Immunol.* **2016**, *7*, 183. [CrossRef] [PubMed]

26. Krug, A.; Uppaluri, R.; Facchetti, F.; Dorner, B.G.; Sheehan, K.C.; Schreiber, R.D.; Cella, M.; Colonna, M. Ifn-producing cells respond to CXCR3 ligands in the presence of CXCL12 and secrete inflammatory chemokines upon activation. *J. Immunol.* **2002**, *169*, 6079–6083. [CrossRef] [PubMed]

27. Dudek, A.Z.; Nesmelova, I.; Mayo, K.; Verfaillie, C.M.; Pitchford, S.; Slungaard, A. Platelet factor 4 promotes adhesion of hematopoietic progenitor cells and binds IL-8: Novel mechanisms for modulation of hematopoiesis. *Blood* **2003**, *101*, 4687–4694. [CrossRef] [PubMed]

28. Paoletti, S.; Petkovic, V.; Sebastiani, S.; Danelon, M.G.; Uguccioni, M.; Gerber, B.O. A rich chemokine environment strongly enhances leukocyte migration and activities. *Blood* **2005**, *105*, 3405–3412. [CrossRef] [PubMed]

29. Koenen, R.R.; von Hundelshausen, P.; Nesmelova, I.V.; Zernecke, A.; Liehn, E.A.; Sarabi, A.; Kramp, B.K.; Piccinini, A.M.; Paludan, S.R.; Kowalska, M.A.; et al. Disrupting functional interactions between platelet chemokines inhibits atherosclerosis in hyperlipidemic mice. *Nat. Med.* **2009**, *15*, 97–103. [CrossRef] [PubMed]

30. Carlson, J.; Baxter, S.A.; Dréau, D.; Nesmelova, I.V. The heterodimerization of platelet-derived chemokines. *Biochim. Biophys. Acta* **2013**, *1834*, 158–168. [CrossRef] [PubMed]

31. Nesmelova, I.V.; Sham, Y.; Gao, J.; Mayo, K.H. CXC and CC chemokines form mixed heterodimers: Association free energies from molecular dynamics simulations and experimental correlations. *J. Biol. Chem.* **2008**, *283*, 24155–24166. [CrossRef] [PubMed]

32. Nesmelova, I.V.; Sham, Y.; Dudek, A.Z.; van Eijk, L.I.; Wu, G.; Slungaard, A.; Mortari, F.; Griffioen, A.W.; Mayo, K.H. Platelet factor 4 and interleukin-8 CXC chemokine heterodimer formation modulates function at the quaternary structural level. *J. Biol. Chem.* **2005**, *280*, 4948–4958. [CrossRef] [PubMed]

33. Ahuja, S.K.; Murphy, P.M. The CXC chemokines growth-regulated oncogene (GRO) α, GROβ, GROγ, neutrophil-activating peptide-2, and epithelial cell-derived neutrophil-activating peptide-78 are potent agonists for the type B, but not the type A, human interleukin-8 receptor. *J. Biol. Chem.* **1996**, *271*, 20545–20550. [CrossRef] [PubMed]

34. Kasper, B.; Brandt, E.; Bulfone-Paus, S.; Petersen, F. Platelet factor 4 (PF-4)-induced neutrophil adhesion is controlled by SRC-kinases, whereas PF-4-mediated exocytosis requires the additional activation of p38 map kinase and phosphatidylinositol 3-kinase. *Blood* **2004**, *103*, 1602–1610. [CrossRef] [PubMed]

35. Mayo, K.H.; Roongta, V.; Ilyina, E.; Milius, R.; Barker, S.; Quinlan, C.; La Rosa, G.; Daly, T.J. Nmr solution structure of the 32-kDa platelet factor 4 ELR-motif N-terminal chimera: A symmetric tetramer. *Biochemistry* **1995**, *34*, 11399–11409. [CrossRef] [PubMed]

36. Fairbrother, W.J.; Reilly, D.; Colby, T.J.; Hesselgesser, J.; Horuk, R. The solution structure of melanoma growth stimulating activity. *J. Mol. Biol.* **1994**, *242*, 252–270. [CrossRef] [PubMed]

37. Kim, K.S.; Clark-Lewis, I.; Sykes, B.D. Solution structure of gro/melanoma growth stimulatory activity determined by 1H NMR spectroscopy. *J. Biol. Chem.* **1994**, *269*, 32909–32915. [PubMed]

38. Clore, G.M.; Appella, E.; Yamada, M.; Matsushima, K.; Gronenborn, A.M. Three-dimensional structure of interleukin 8 in solution. *Biochemistry* **1990**, *29*, 1689–1696. [CrossRef] [PubMed]

39. Brown, A.; Sepuru, K.M.; Rajarathnam, K. Structural basis of native CXCL7 monomer binding to CXCR2 receptor N-domain and glycosaminoglycan heparin. *Int. J. Mol. Sci.* **2017**, *18*, 508. [CrossRef] [PubMed]

40. Sepuru, K.M.; Rajarathnam, K. CXCL1/MGSA is a novel glycosaminoglycan (GAG)-binding chemokine: Structural evidence for two distinct non-overlapping binding domains. *J. Biol. Chem.* **2016**, *291*, 4247–4255. [CrossRef] [PubMed]

41. Ravindran, A.; Sawant, K.V.; Sarmiento, J.; Navarro, J.; Rajarathnam, K. Chemokine CXCL1 dimer is a potent agonist for the CXCR2 receptor. *J. Biol. Chem.* **2013**, *288*, 12244–12252. [CrossRef] [PubMed]

42. Rajarathnam, K.; Prado, G.N.; Fernando, H.; Clark-Lewis, I.; Navarro, J. Probing receptor binding activity of interleukin-8 dimer using a disulfide trap. *Biochemistry* **2006**, *45*, 7882–7888. [CrossRef] [PubMed]

43. Nasser, M.W.; Raghuwanshi, S.K.; Grant, D.J.; Jala, V.R.; Rajarathnam, K.; Richardson, R.M. Differential activation and regulation of CXCR1 and CXCR2 by CXCL8 monomer and dimer. *J. Immunol.* **2009**, *183*, 3425–3432. [CrossRef] [PubMed]

44. Kuscher, K.; Danelon, G.; Paoletti, S.; Stefano, L.; Schiraldi, M.; Petkovic, V.; Locati, M.; Gerber, B.O.; Uguccioni, M. Synergy-inducing chemokines enhance CCR2 ligand activities on monocytes. *Eur. J. Immunol.* **2009**, *39*, 1118–1128. [CrossRef] [PubMed]

45. Sebastiani, S.; Danelon, G.; Gerber, B.; Uguccioni, M. CCL22-induced responses are powerfully enhanced by synergy inducing chemokines via CCR4: Evidence for the involvement of first β-strand of chemokine. *Eur. J. Immunol.* **2005**, *35*, 746–756. [CrossRef] [PubMed]

46. Vanbervliet, B.; Bendriss-Vermare, N.; Massacrier, C.; Homey, B.; de Bouteiller, O.; Brière, F.; Trinchieri, G.; Caux, C. The inducible CXCR3 ligands control plasmacytoid dendritic cell responsiveness to the constitutive chemokine stromal cell-derived factor 1 (SDF-1)/CXCL12. *J. Exp. Med.* **2003**, *198*, 823–830. [CrossRef] [PubMed]

47. Bdeir, K.; Gollomp, K.; Stasiak, M.; Mei, J.; Papiewska-Pajak, I.; Zhao, G.; Worthen, G.S.; Cines, D.B.; Poncz, M.; Kowalska, M.A. Platelet-specific chemokines contribute to the pathogenesis of acute lung injury. *Am. J. Respir. Cell Mol. Biol.* **2017**, *56*, 261–270. [CrossRef] [PubMed]

48. Zwijnenburg, P.J.; Polfliet, M.M.; Florquin, S.; van den Berg, T.K.; Dijkstra, C.D.; van Deventer, S.J.; Roord, J.J.; van der Poll, T.; van Furth, A.M. CXC-chemokines kc and macrophage inflammatory protein-2 (MIP-2) synergistically induce leukocyte recruitment to the central nervous system in rats. *Immunol. Lett.* **2003**, *85*, 1–4. [CrossRef]

49. Rzepka, J.P.; Haick, A.K.; Miura, T.A. Virus-infected alveolar epithelial cells direct neutrophil chemotaxis and inhibit their apoptosis. *Am. J. Respir. Cell Mol. Biol.* **2012**, *46*, 833–841. [CrossRef] [PubMed]

50. Crown, S.E.; Yu, Y.; Sweeney, M.D.; Leary, J.A.; Handel, T.M. Heterodimerization of CCR2 chemokines and regulation by glycosaminoglycan binding. *J. Biol. Chem.* **2006**, *281*, 25438–25446. [CrossRef] [PubMed]

51. Guan, E.; Wang, J.; Norcross, M.A. Identification of human macrophage inflammatory proteins 1α and 1β as a native secreted heterodimer. *J. Biol. Chem.* **2001**, *276*, 12404–12409. [CrossRef] [PubMed]

52. Gangavarapu, P.; Rajagopalan, L.; Kolli, D.; Guerrero-Plata, A.; Garofalo, R.P.; Rajarathnam, K. The monomer-dimer equilibrium and glycosaminoglycan interactions of chemokine CXCL8 regulate tissue-specific neutrophil recruitment. *J. Leukoc. Biol.* **2012**, *91*, 259–265. [CrossRef] [PubMed]

53. Sawant, K.V.; Poluri, K.M.; Dutta, A.K.; Sepuru, K.M.; Troshkina, A.; Garofalo, R.P.; Rajarathnam, K. Chemokine CXCL1 mediated neutrophil recruitment: Role of glycosaminoglycan interactions. *Sci. Rep.* **2016**, *6*, 33123. [CrossRef] [PubMed]

54. Schrödinger, L.L.C. *The Pymol Molecular Graphics System*, version 1.8; Schrödinger, LLC.: New York, NY, USA, 2016.

55. Duan, Y.; Wu, C.; Chowdhury, S.; Lee, M.C.; Xiong, G.; Zhang, W.; Yang, R.; Cieplak, P.; Luo, R.; Lee, T.; et al. A point-charge force field for molecular mechanics simulations of proteins based on condensed-phase quantum mechanical calculations. *J. Comput. Chem.* **2003**, *24*, 1999–2012. [CrossRef] [PubMed]

56. Case, D.A.; Darden, T.A.; Cheatham, T.E., III; Simmerling, C.L.; Wang, J.; Duke, R.E.; Luo, R.; Walker, R.C.; Zhang, W.; Merz, K.M.; et al. *Amber 12*; University of California: San Francisco, NC, USA, 2012.

57. Lee, M.C.; Deng, J.; Briggs, J.M.; Duan, Y. Large-scale conformational dynamics of the HIV-1 integrase core domain and its catalytic loop mutants. *Biophys. J.* **2005**, *88*, 3133–3146. [CrossRef] [PubMed]

58. Humphrey, W.; Dalke, A.; Schulten, K. VMD: Visual molecular dynamics. *J. Mol. Graph.* **1996**, *14*, 33–38, 27–38. [CrossRef]

59. Rajagopalan, L.; Rajarathnam, K. Ligand selectivity and affinity of chemokine receptor CXCR1. Role of N-terminal domain. *J. Biol. Chem.* **2004**, *279*, 30000–30008. [CrossRef] [PubMed]

60. Goddard, T.D.; Kneller, D.G. *Sparky 3*; University of California: San Francisco, NC, USA, 2008.

61. Ravindran, A.; Joseph, P.R.; Rajarathnam, K. Structural basis for differential binding of the interleukin-8 monomer and dimer to the CXCR1 N-domain: Role of coupled interactions and dynamics. *Biochemistry* **2009**, *48*, 8795–8805. [CrossRef] [PubMed]

62. Joseph, P.R.; Mosier, P.D.; Desai, U.R.; Rajarathnam, K. Solution NMR characterization of chemokine CXCL8/IL-8 monomer and dimer binding to glycosaminoglycans: Structural plasticity mediates differential binding interactions. *Biochem. J.* **2015**, *472*, 121–133. [CrossRef] [PubMed]

63. Dominguez, C.; Boelens, R.; Bonvin, A.M. Haddock: A protein–protein docking approach based on biochemical or biophysical information. *J. Am. Chem. Soc.* **2003**, *125*, 1731–1737. [CrossRef] [PubMed]

64. De Vries, S.J.; van Dijk, A.D.; Krzeminski, M.; van Dijk, M.; Thureau, A.; Hsu, V.; Wassenaar, T.; Bonvin, A.M. Haddock versus haddock: New features and performance of haddock2.0 on the CAPRI targets. *Proteins* **2007**, *69*, 726–733. [CrossRef] [PubMed]

65. Mulloy, B.; Forster, M.J.; Jones, C.; Davies, D.B.N.M.R. And molecular-modelling studies of the solution conformation of heparin. *Biochem. J.* **1993**, *293*, 849–858. [CrossRef] [PubMed]

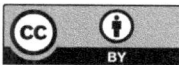

International Journal of
Molecular Sciences

MDPI

Article

Glycosaminoglycans Regulate CXCR3 Ligands at Distinct Levels: Protection against Processing by Dipeptidyl Peptidase IV/CD26 and Interference with Receptor Signaling

Mieke Metzemaekers [1], Anneleen Mortier [1], Rik Janssens [1,2], Daiane Boff [1,2], Lotte Vanbrabant [1], Nicole Lamoen [3,†], Jo Van Damme [1], Mauro M. Teixeira [2], Ingrid De Meester [3], Flávio A. Amaral [2] and Paul Proost [1,*]

[1] Laboratory of Molecular Immunology, Department of Microbiology and Immunology,
    Rega Institute for Medical Research, KU Leuven, Herestraat 49 box 1042, B-3000 Leuven, Belgium;
    mieke.metzemaekers@kuleuven.be (M.M.); anneleen_mortier@hotmail.com (A.M.);
    rik.janssens@kuleuven.be (R.J.); daianebff@gmail.com (D.B.); lotte.vanbrabant@kuleuven.be (L.V.);
    jo.vandamme@kuleuven.be (J.V.D.)
[2] Imunofarmacologia, Departamento de Bioquímica e Imunologia, Instituto de Ciências Biológicas,
    Universidade Federal de Minas Gerais, Av Antonio Carlos 6627, Pampulha, Belo Horizonte 31270-901,
    Minas Gerais, Brazil; mmtex.ufmg@gmail.com (M.M.T); dr.famaral@gmail.com (F.A.A.)
[3] Laboratory of Medical Biochemistry, Department of Pharmaceutical Sciences, University of Antwerp,
    Universiteitsplein 1 S6, B-2610 Wilrijk, Belgium; ingrid.demeester@uantwerpen.be
*   Correspondence: paul.proost@kuleuven.be; Tel.: +32-163-224-71
†   Nicole Lamoen passed away a few months ago.

Received: 7 June 2017; Accepted: 6 July 2017; Published: 13 July 2017

Abstract: CXC chemokine ligand (CXCL)9, CXCL10 and CXCL11 direct chemotaxis of mainly T cells and NK cells through activation of their common CXC chemokine receptor (CXCR)3. They are inactivated upon NH_2-terminal cleavage by dipeptidyl peptidase IV/CD26. In the present study, we found that different glycosaminoglycans (GAGs) protect the CXCR3 ligands against proteolytic processing by CD26 without directly affecting the enzymatic activity of CD26. In addition, GAGs were shown to interfere with chemokine-induced CXCR3 signaling. The observation that heparan sulfate did not, and heparin only moderately, altered CXCL10-induced T cell chemotaxis in vitro may be explained by a combination of protection against proteolytic inactivation and altered receptor interaction as observed in calcium assays. No effect of CD26 inhibition was found on CXCL10-induced chemotaxis in vitro. However, treatment of mice with the CD26 inhibitor sitagliptin resulted in an enhanced CXCL10-induced lymphocyte influx into the joint. This study reveals a dual role for GAGs in modulating the biological activity of CXCR3 ligands. GAGs protect the chemokines from proteolytic cleavage but also directly interfere with chemokine–CXCR3 signaling. These data support the hypothesis that both GAGs and CD26 affect the in vivo chemokine function.

Keywords: chemokine; glycosaminoglycan; leukocyte migration; posttranslational modification; CXCR3; dipeptidyl peptidase IV; CD26

1. Introduction

The family of chemotactic cytokines or chemokines is constituted by a group of low molecular mass proteins that direct specific leukocyte migration in a time- and site-dependent manner in health and disease [1,2]. Chemokines are not only crucial players in basal innate and adaptive immune mechanisms, but are also implicated in a broad range of additional physiological and pathophysiological processes ranging from embryonic development and angiogenesis to cancer and autoimmune diseases [3–9]. According to the localization of the conserved NH_2-terminal cysteine residues, a sub classification into CXC, CC, CX_3C and C chemokine subfamilies is respected. CXCL9, CXCL10 and CXCL11 are three CXC chemokines that lack a conserved Glu-Leu-Arg (ELR) amino acid motif and exert their chemotactic activity through interaction with their common G protein-coupled receptor (GPCR) CXCR3 [10,11]. In order of increasing potency, CXCL9, CXCL10 and CXCL11 activate CXCR3, which is strongly expressed on type-1 helper (Th1) CD4+ T cells, effector CD8+ T cells and certain innate leukocytes including natural killer (NK) cells [10–12]. In addition to their chemotactic effects, angiostatic properties have been attributed to the CXCR3 ligands [3,5,11,13]. Unique characteristics have been claimed to individual CXCR3 ligands. For example, CXCL11 is the only CXCR3 ligand that also interacts with the atypical chemokine receptor ACKR3 (also known as CXCR7) [14–16]. CXCL9 contains a unique COOH-terminal tail that consists for about 50% of basic amino acids and differs not only from the two other CXCR3 ligands, but also from almost all chemokines in general (vide infra) [1,17].

As suggested by their alternative names, being monokine induced by interferon (IFN)-γ (Mig), IFN-γ-inducible protein of 10 kDa (IP-10) and IFN-γ-inducible T cell α chemoattractant (I-TAC), for CXCL9, CXCL10 and CXCL11 respectively, these are inflammatory chemokines with IFN-γ as a major inducer. However, the specific expression of individual CXCR3 ligands is differently regulated. Induction of CXCL9 expression is truly IFN-γ dependent [18,19], whereas expression of CXCL10 is also induced by a variety of innate stimuli including IFN-α or IFN-β [18,20]. IFN-γ and IFN-β, but not IFN-α, are potent stimulators of CXCL11 expression [21]. Consequently, despite their mutual structural similarities and shared, unique signaling receptor, the CXCR3 ligands show a significant degree of redundancy only in vitro that seems less the case in vivo [10]. During the course of immune responses, the temporal and spatial expression patterns of individual CXCR3 ligands are ligand-specific, with each CXCR3 ligand being regulated by different stimuli and expressed by different cell types [10,22,23]. It is therefore believed that in vivo, CXCL9, CXCL10 and CXCL11 each play a unique role in fine-tuning the trafficking of T cells. Accordingly, in certain inflammatory in vivo models, deficiency for one specific CXCR3 ligand cannot be countervailed by the presence of the two others [24–27]. Additionally, in vivo models exist where full T cell infiltration requires cooperation between the CXCR3 ligands [28,29]. To add even more complexity to the CXCR3-chemokine loop, apparent ligand antagonism has been described between CXCR3 agonists [30]. Furthermore, one has to keep in mind that most studies in mice concern CXCL10, whereas CXCL9 and certainly CXCL11 have been studied to a lesser extend in vivo. Moreover, it has been reported that a frame shift causing the presence of a stop codon in the CXCL11 gene thus, resulting in deficiency for CXCL11 is present in one of the routinely used mouse strains, i.e., C57BL6 mice [31].

In addition to interaction with chemokine receptors, chemokine-induced leukocyte migration in vivo usually requires also interaction between chemokines and GAGs [32–39]. GAGs, e.g., heparin, heparan sulfate, chondroitin sulfate, keratan sulfate, dermatan sulfate and hyaluronic acid, are present in the extracellular matrix and at the cell surface, usually as part of proteoglycan structures (GAG chains attached to a protein core). Due to their sulfate groups, these heterogeneous polysaccharides are negatively charged and thus attractive interaction partners for the highly basic chemokines [40]. GAGs retain chemokines on endothelial surfaces and prevent washout of chemokines by the blood flow [33]. Of the three main CXCR3 agonists, CXCL9 in particular is an extremely efficient GAG interacting chemokine, due to its highly positively charged long COOH-terminal tail that consists for circa 50% of basic amino acids. To investigate the function of the COOH-terminal region of CXCL9, our lab previously synthesized several peptides, derived from the COOH-terminal region of CXCL9 [17,41]. Specifically, the longest peptide CXCL9 (74–103) was found to compete with CXCL8 for GAG-binding, thereby preventing CXCL8 from performing its neutrophil-chemotactic function in vivo [17]. CXCL8 is an ELR positive CXC chemokine that activates CXCR1 and CXCR2 and is considered the main human neutrophil-attracting chemokine [4,42,43]. In general, binding to GAGs facilitates chemokine retention and assists in generation of a chemokine gradient that directs leukocyte migration in vivo [33,44] Interaction with GAGs also mediates chemokine oligomerization [40] and is thought to play a role in either cis or trans (on endothelial cells) presentation of chemokines to their receptors [45]. In addition, GAGs were shown to serve as a protective factor that prevent the chemokines CXCL12 and CCL11 from proteolysis by specific enzymes [46,47].

Since the identification of chemokines, it has been evidenced that the biological availability and functioning of chemokines is coordinated at multiple levels. These include alternative splicing and mutual synergistic or antagonistic effects between certain chemokines, in addition to the aforementioned interactions with GAGs, specific GPCRs and atypical chemokine receptors [44] Moreover, a major role for posttranslational processing, e.g., proteolysis, citrullination, glycosylation and nitration, has been recognized in fine-tuning the exact chemokine function and receptor specificity in vitro and in vivo [44,48–51]. An enzyme that has been shown to provoke NH_2-terminal processing of various chemokines including CXCL9, CXCL10 and CXCL11 is dipeptidyl peptidase IV or CD26 [50,52,53]. In addition to its enzymatic activity as a serine protease, the multifunctional or "moonlighting" protein CD26 functions as a receptor, costimulator for T cell activation, adhesion molecule and has been associated with apoptosis [54–57]. The membrane-bound enzyme is expressed on cells of different origins, including certain immune cells, whereas soluble proteolytically active CD26 exists in several body fluids such as plasma and seminal fluid. CD26 preferentially removes the two most NH_2-terminal amino acids from substrates whose penultimate position is occupied by a (hydroxy) proline or alanine residue. Pro is present at this position in a number of chemokine sequences. The NH_2-terminal chemokine domain is responsible for GPCR binding and activation and, consequently, limited proteolysis by CD26 (but also by other enzymes) may have drastic effects on the biological functioning of a chemokine [50–52]. It turned out that the biological effect of CD26-mediated cleavage is highly complex and depends on the chemokine ligand involved. For all three CXCR3 agonists, it was previously demonstrated that processing by CD26 results in drastic loss of receptor signaling and impaired capacity to direct lymphocyte chemotaxis, while leaving the angiostatic properties of these chemokines unaffected [53]. For human CXCL10 and CXCL11, the corresponding CD26-truncated isoforms CXCL10 (3–77) and CXCL11 (3–73) were previously isolated from natural sources, including conditioned medium from MG-63-osteosarcoma cells, fibroblasts and keratinocytes [22,58–61].

In the present study, we wanted to provide new insights in the intriguing role of GAGs in the regulation of the activity of CXCR3 agonists. Specifically, we investigated the effects of GAGs on the CXCR3 chemokine dialog and on CD26-mediated processing of CXCR3 agonists. The relationship between GAGs, CD26, CXCR3 and its chemokine ligands was found to be highly complex and dual, while GAGs dose-dependently preserved CXCL9, CXCL10 and CXCL11 from cleavage by CD26, these negatively charged macromolecules also negatively affected their calcium mobilizing capacities through CXCR3.

2. Results

2.1. Soluble GAGs Protected CXCR3 Ligands against Truncation by Soluble CD26

GAGs were previously described to protect CXCL12 and CCL11 against proteolytic processing by specific enzymes, either directly or indirectly [46,47]. In the present study, we wondered whether this was also true for CD26-mediated truncation of the three most potent CXCR3 chemokine agonists and CD26 substrates CXCL9, CXCL10 and CXCL11. CXCL10, the most intensively studied CXCR3 ligand, was incubated for 2 h with 12.5 U/L natural human CD26 and final GAG concentrations up to 26.4 μg/mL. We reasoned that, following extraction of truncated and intact CXCL10 from incubation mixtures using C4 or strong cation exchange purification techniques, the percentage of CD26-mediated CXCL10-processing could be determined with mass spectrometry. However, using this protocol we failed to detect CXCL10 isoforms and we relied on automated NH_2-terminal sequencing using Edman degradation for quantification of the CD26-mediated conversion of native CXCL10 towards CXCL10(3–77). Dose response experiments were conducted with heparan sulfate and the fixed chain-length heparin variants heparin DP30 and DP8. For all GAGs tested, CXCL10 was dose-dependently protected against proteolytic processing by CD26 (Figure 1). Incubation of CXCL10 with CD26 in the absence of GAG resulted in almost complete truncation of intact CXCL10 by two amino acids towards CXCL10 (3–77). At GAG concentrations up to 2.64 µg/mL, almost all CXCL10 was processed, whereas GAG concentrations of 8.8 µg/mL offered the chemokine almost full protection against proteolytic processing by the serine protease.

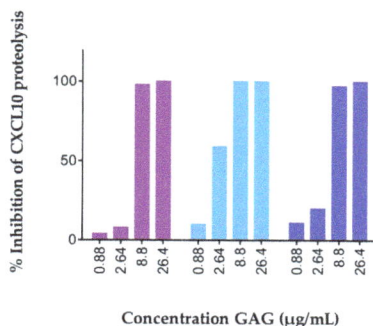

Figure 1. GAGs dose-dependently protect CXCL10 from cleavage by CD26. Recombinant human CXCL10 (20 µg/mL) was incubated with 12.5 U/L natural human CD26 and 0.88 to 26.4 µg/mL heparan sulfate (violet, ●), heparin DP30 (blue, ●), or heparin DP8 (deep blue, ●)), in 50 mM Tris buffer supplemented with 1 mM EDTA (pH 7.5). Incubation of CXCL10 with CD26 in the absence of GAG was used as a control. Reactions were terminated after 2 h by acidification to 0.08% (v/v) trifluoroacetic acid (TFA). The ratio of truncated CXCL10 (3–77) over corresponding intact chemokine was determined with automated NH$_2$-sequencing. Results are represented as percentages of GAG-mediated inhibition of proteolysis of CXCL10 by CD26.

Inspired by these drastic effects of GAGs on CD26-mediated truncation of CXCL10, we investigated the effects of GAGs on CD26-mediated processing of the two other IFN-γ-inducible CXCR3 chemokine agonists, i.e., CXCL9 and CXCL11. Accordingly, we optimized the desalting process after the CD26 incubation and found that chemokines could be detected and quantified by mass spectrometry after pre-purification on C18 pipette tips if the GAG concentrations did not exceed 8.8 µg/mL. The three main CXCR3 agonists were incubated with CD26 in the absence or presence of 8.8, 2.64 or 0.88 µg/mL heparan sulfate, heparin, chondroitin sulfate A or chondroitin sulfate C. All these GAGs had a relative molecular mass (M$_r$) of 40 kDa (data not shown). After an incubation period of 2 h, CD26 activity was stopped through acidification with TFA. Samples were desalted with C18 tips and subjected to mass spectrometry. Without GAGs, almost all CXCL10 and CXCL11 was cleaved by CD26 to CXCL10 (3–77) and CXCL11(3–73), respectively. In contrast, CXCL9 was processed by the enzyme for only about 20% (data not shown). These findings were in line with previous studies which demonstrated that CXCL10, and especially CXCL11, are highly efficient CD26 substrates, whereas the half-life of CXCL9 upon incubation with the enzyme is remarkably longer [53,62]. The presence of heparin, heparan sulfate, chondroitin sulfate A or chondroitin sulfate C in the incubation mixture protected the three IFN-induced CXCR3 ligands dose-dependently from truncation by CD26 (Figure 2, Figures S1–S3). At 8.8 µg/mL heparin, heparan sulfate, chondroitin sulfate A and C completely prevented processing of CXCL9 and CXCL10 by CD26. A comparable protective effect was obtained with heparan sulfate and chondroitin sulfate C, whereas heparin and chondroitin sulfate A were less efficient in protecting CXCL11 from proteolytic truncation by CD26. Thus, the obtained results indicated a dose-dependent, GAG-mediated chemokine protection against processing by CD26 for all GAGs tested. However, minor differences in efficiency were detected between the different GAGs although they all had a comparable molecular mass.

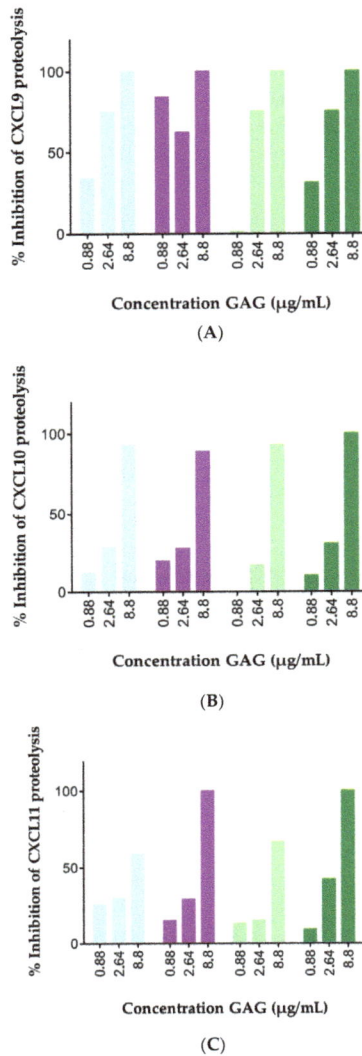

Figure 2. GAGs dose-dependently protect IFN-γ-inducible CXCR3 ligands from cleavage by CD26. Recombinant human: CXCL9 (**A**); CXCL10 (**B**) or CXCL11(**C**) (20 μg/mL) was incubated with 12.5 U/L natural human CD26 and 0.88 to 8.8 μg/mL heparan sulfate (violet, ●), heparin (light blue, ●), chondroitin sulfate A (light green, ●) or chondroitin sulfate C (green, ●) in 50 mM Tris buffer supplemented with 1 mM EDTA (pH 7,5). Reactions were terminated after 2 h by acidification to 0.08% (*v/v*) TFA. The ratio of truncated CXCL9(3–103), CXCL10(3–77) or CXCL11(3–73) over corresponding intact chemokines was determined after C18 purification and mass spectrometry. Results are represented as percentages of GAG-mediated inhibition of proteolysis of CXCL10 by CD26.

2.2. GAGs Did Not Inhibit the Enzymatic Activity of Soluble CD26 Directly

The exact enzymatic activity of the purified natural human CD26 sample was determined to be 4.6 ± 0.6 U/L (mean $\pm$ SEM, $n = 3$) using a chromogenic assay with Gly-Pro-p-nitroanilide (Gly-Pro-pNA) as the substrate. No pNA release was observed upon incubation of the substrate with the highest concentration of heparin DP30 in the absence of CD26. To investigate a direct effect of GAGs on the activity of the enzyme, the release of pNA was detected when Gly-Pro-pNA and CD26 were incubated in the absence or presence of 10 or 100 µg/mL heparin DP30. The CD26 activities in conditions with and without GAG were highly similar (Table 1). Thus, no evidence was found for GAGs to inhibit the proteolytic activity of CD26 directly, which was in line with a former study that reported that heparan sulfate did not inhibit the enzymatic activity of CD26 [46].

Table 1. Effect of heparin on the proteolytic activity of CD26.

Concentration Heparin DP30 (µg/mL)	CD26 Activity (U/L)
0	4.6
10	4.19
100	4.35

2.3. GAGs Interfered with Chemokine Signaling through CXCR3

Chemokine-induced CXCR3-signaling is associated with the release of intracellular calcium from the endoplasmic reticulum. Consequently, we reasoned that measuring the $[Ca^{2+}]_i$ after stimulation of cells with CXCL9, CXCL10 or CXCL11 with or without GAGs, would provide us with new insights on the effect of GAGs on the chemokine-induced G protein-dependent signaling through CXCR3. To this end, Chinese Hamster Ovarian (CHO) cells, stably transfected with CXCR3A and loaded with the calcium-binding fluorescent dye Fura-2, were stimulated with final concentrations of 3 ng/mL to 1 µg/mL CXCL9, CXCL10 or CXCL11. The corresponding chemokine-induced calcium responses were calculated using the Grynkiewicz equation. For CXCL10 and CXCL11, a concentration of 3 ng/mL resulted in an increase of the $[Ca^{2+}]_i$ with 106.8 nM ($n = 39$) and 304.5 nM ($n = 18$), respectively, and 3 ng/mL CXCL10 or CXCL11 was selected for further experiments in combination with GAGs. Cells were treated with CXCL10 or CXCL11 with or without 0.04 µg/mL, 2 µg/mL or 10 µg/mL GAG. Representative experiments are shown in Figure 3. The observed calcium responses were calculated as percentages of the corresponding reference values in the absence of GAGs. A dose-dependent negative correlation was found between the GAG concentration and the ability of CXCL10 and CXCL11 to evoke an intracellular calcium release through CXCR3 (Figure 4A,B). Heparin molecules with different length were tested in combination with CXCL10 and the longer heparin molecules were more potent inhibitors of the calcium response compared to the shorter DP8 form. For the less potent CXCL9, a concentration of 1 µg/mL was selected, resulting in an increase of the $[Ca^{2+}]_i$ with 598.1 nM ($n = 4$). Heparan sulfate also dose dependently inhibited the calcium response induced by this weaker CXCR3 ligand (Figure 4C). It remains to be elucidated whether the effect of GAGs on calcium signaling is due to direct binding of GAGs to chemokines, CXCR3 or both. In addition, it cannot be excluded that GAGs directly interfere with intracellular signaling. However, as expected, GAGs did not induce an increase of the $[Ca^{2+}]_i$ in the absence of chemokine (data not shown).

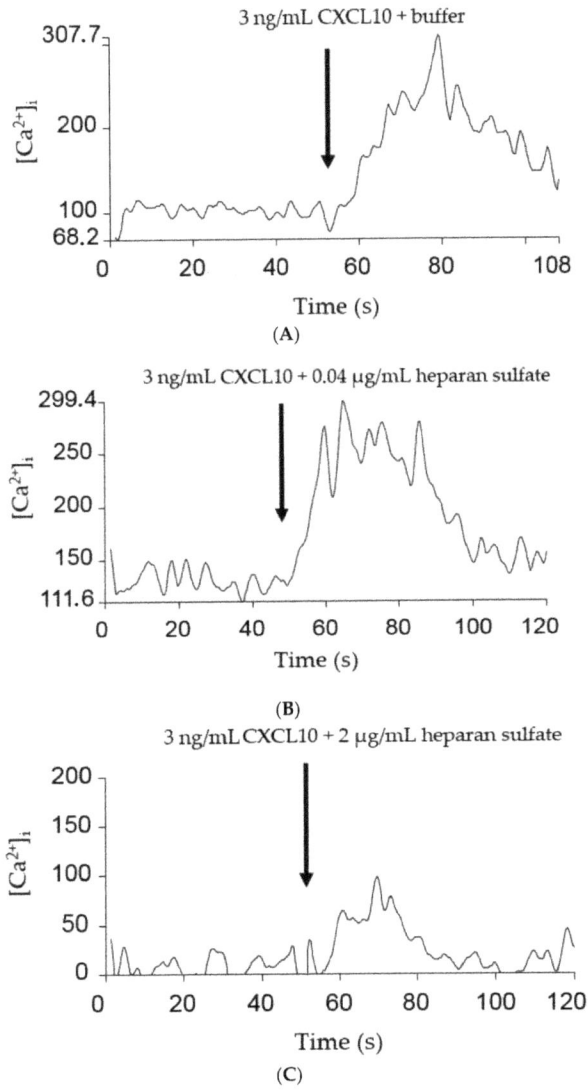

Figure 3. *Cont.*

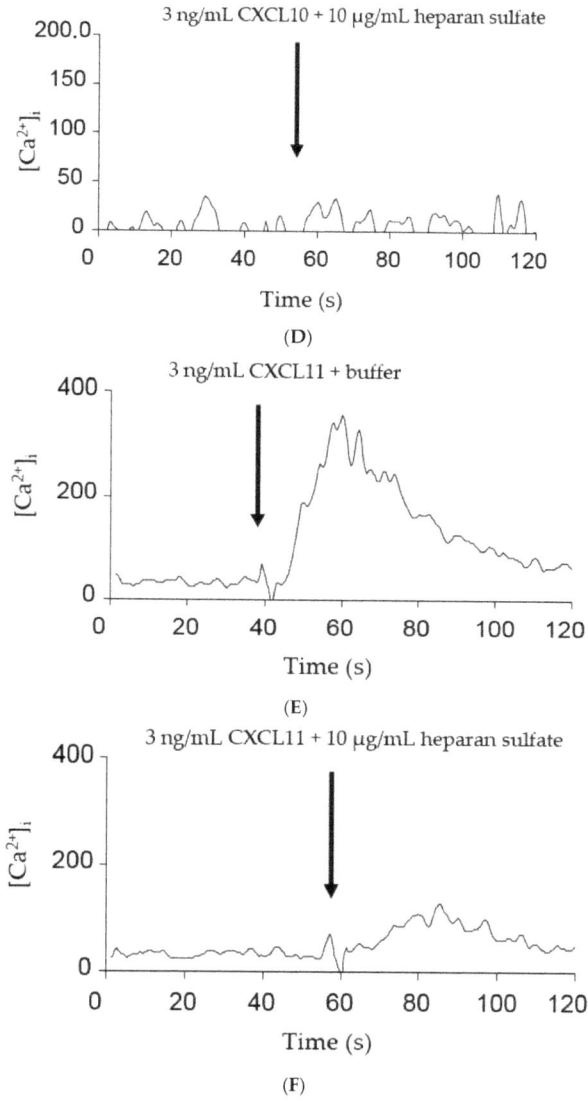

(D)

(E)

(F)

Figure 3. *Cont.*

(G)

(H)

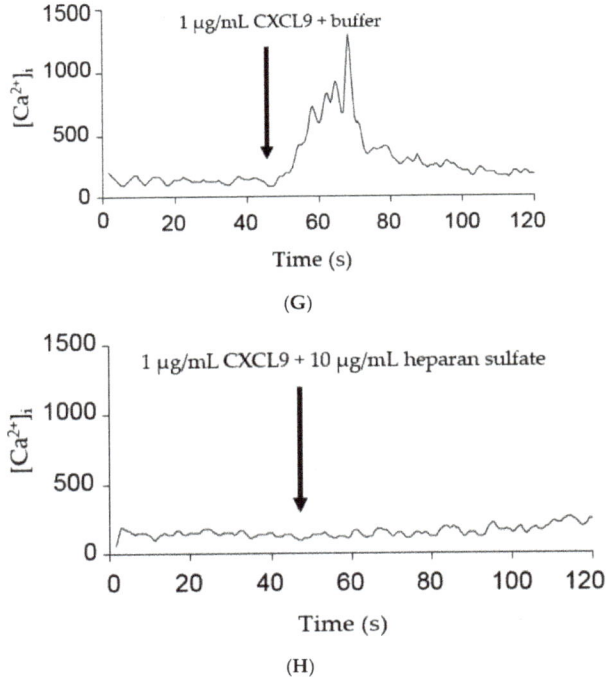

Figure 3. Effect of heparan sulfate on chemokine-induced calcium signaling through CXCR3. CHO/CXCR3A cells were stimulated with 3 ng/mL: CXCL10 (**A–D**); or CXCL11 (**E,F**); or 1 µg/mL CXCL9 (**G,H**) in the presence or absence of GAG. $[Ca^{2+}]_i$ concentrations were calculated using the equation of Grynkiewicz et al. Figures show representative experiments in which cells were simultaneously stimulated with chemokine and buffer (**A,E,G**); or 0.04 µg/mL (**B**); 2 µg/mL (**C**); or 10 µg/mL (**D,F,H**) heparan sulfate.

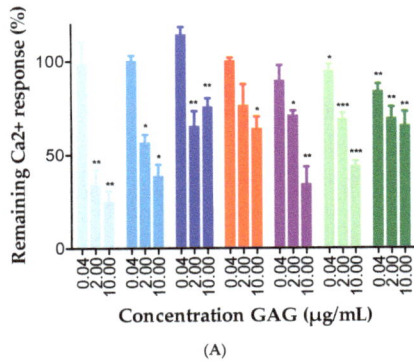

(A)

Figure 4. *Cont.*

(B)

(C)

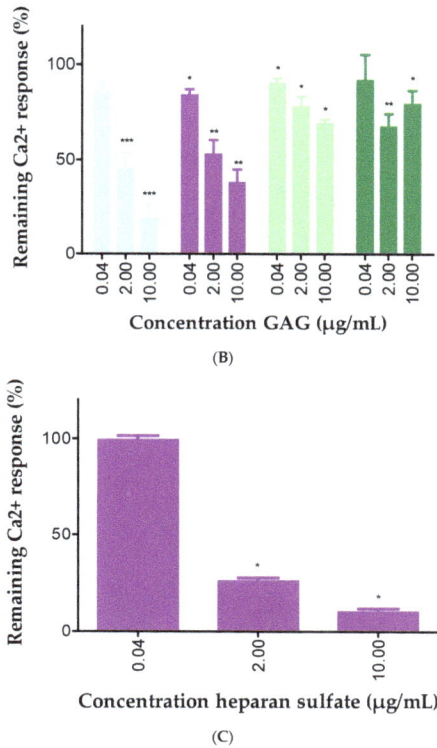

Figure 4. GAGs interfere with chemokine signaling through CXCR3. CHO/CXCR3A cells were stimulated with 3 ng/mL: CXCL10 (**A**); or CXCL11 (**B**); or 1 μg/mL CXCL9 (**C**) in the presence or absence of heparan sulfate (violet, ●), heparin (light blue,), heparin DP30 (blue, ●), heparin DP8 (deep blue, ●), dermatan sulfate (red, ●), chondroitin sulfate A (light green,) or chondroitin sulfate C (green, ●). $[Ca^{2+}]_i$ concentrations were calculated using the equation of Grynkiewicz et al. Mann–Whitney U-tests were performed to statistically compare $[Ca^{2+}]_i$ concentrations obtained after stimulation with CXCL9, CXCL10 or CXCL11 plus GAG, with $[Ca^{2+}]_i$ concentrations that resulted from stimulation with, respectively, CXCL9, CXCL10 or CXCL11 only (* = $p < 0.05$; ** = $p < 0.01$; *** = $p < 0.001$). Results are represented as mean percentages (±SEM) compared to conditions in which cells were stimulated with CXCL9, CXCL10 or CXCL11 without GAG. Percentages are means of 3–8 independent experiments.

2.4. Effect of Soluble GAGs on CXCL10-Mediated CD26-Positive T Cell Chemotaxis In Vitro

Activated T cells express membrane-bound CD26. Thus, we wondered whether the observed GAG-mediated protection of CXCL10 against inactivation by CD26 was reflected in an increased CXCL10-induced T cell chemotaxis. To this end, we first confirmed CD26 expression and activity on cultured T cells. Flow cytometry was performed and revealed that, as expected, the majority of cultured cells expressed CD26 in addition to CD3 and CXCR3 (data not shown). Different cell concentrations were incubated with the CD26 substrate Gly-Pro-pNA and the enzymatic activity was determined. As expected, an increased enzymatic activity was found with increasing concentrations of T cells (data not shown). Purified soluble natural seminal fluid-derived CD26 was used as a positive control.

Subsequently, in vitro Boyden chamber assays were conducted to evaluate the effects of GAGs on CXCL10-mediated chemotaxis of T cells. We investigated the migratory response of T cells towards 3 to 300 ng/mL CXCL10 with or without 0.04 or 4 µg/mL soluble heparin or heparan sulfate (Figure 5). Chemotactic indices were calculated by dividing the number of migrated cells to chemokine by the number of cells that migrated in response to buffer. As expected, a dose-dependent CXCL10-mediated T cell chemotaxis was observed with 10 ng/mL to 300 ng/mL CXCL10. In contrast to our expectations, presence of soluble heparan sulfate did not significantly affect CXCL10-induced T cell chemotaxis in vitro (Figure 5A). Heparin (4 µg/mL) significantly inhibited T cell chemotaxis to 300 ng/mL CXCL10 and a trend towards reduced chemotaxis was found for other CXCL10 concentrations (Figure 5B). It remains to be determined whether the lack of inhibition with heparan sulfate was due to in vitro counteraction between the two observed GAG-mediated phenomena, i.e. heparan sulfate-mediated protection of CXCL10 against processing by CD26 on the one hand, and the negative effect of heparan sulfate on the CXCR3-CXCL10 dialog on the other hand.

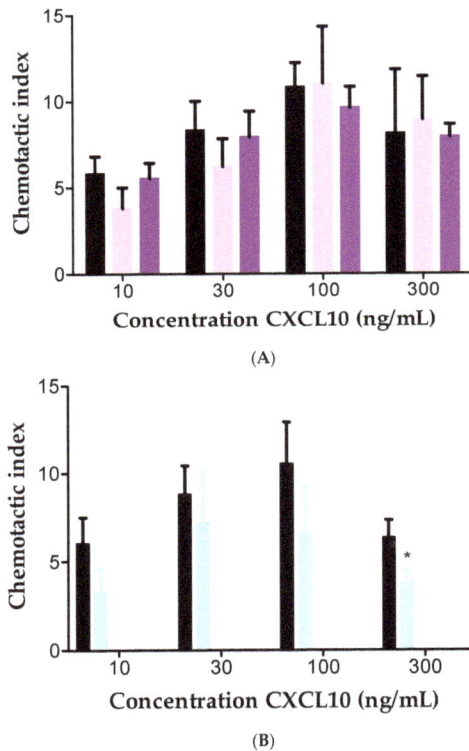

(A)

(B)

Figure 5. Effect of GAGs on CXCL10-induced T cell chemotaxis in vitro. The effects of: 0.04 µg/mL (light violet, ●), or 4 µg/mL (violet, ●) soluble heparan sulfate (**A**); or 4 µg/mL (light blue, ●) heparin (**B**) on the in vitro migratory response of PHA-activated T cells towards10–300 ng/mL CXCL10 was investigated using the 48 well Boyden chamber chemotaxis assay. Values represent the mean chemotactic index (±SEM) ($n = 7$). Statistical analysis was performed using the Mann-Whitney U test. * = $p < 0.05$; compared to stimulation with CXCL10 without GAG (black, ●).

2.5. Inhibition of Membrane-Bound CD26 Did Not Affect CXCL10-Mediated T Cell Chemotaxis In Vitro

To directly investigate the effects of specific inhibition of CD26-mediated cleavage of CXCL10 on CXCL10-directed T cell migration, chemotaxis assays were performed in the presence of the specific CD26 inhibitor sitagliptin. We first conducted a CD26 activity test with T cells that were treated with 0 to 2 mM sitagliptin and demonstrated that sitagliptin dose-dependently decreased the CD26 activity of cultured T cells (Figure 6). A concentration of 200 μM was selected for use in in vitro chemotaxis experiments. No significantly increased CXCL10-mediated T cell chemotaxis was observed when cells were treated with sitagliptin, which was in contrast with our expectations and with former in vivo studies [52,63] (Figure 7). However, in vivo, soluble CD26 is present on capillary endothelial cells and in body fluids including plasma, whereas, in our in vitro chemotaxis experiments, CXCL10 was only confronted with membrane-bound CD26 on the T cells. Therefore, it could be speculated that CXCL10 in in vitro assays was already bound to CXCR3 prior to potential truncation by CD26. Additionally, it cannot be excluded that, under the usedin vitro conditions, the amount of membrane-bound CD26 was too low to be able to detect a significant influence of its inhibition by sitagliptin.

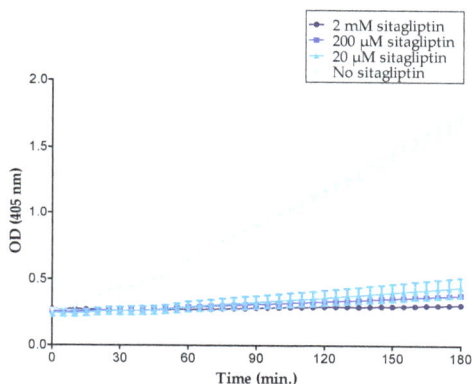

Figure 6. Sitagliptin inhibits CD26 proteolytic activity on T cells. In total, 3×10^6 cells per mL were incubated with 500 μM Gly-Pro-pNA with or without 20 μM to 2 mM sitagliptin in 75 mM Tris-HCl buffer (pH 8.3). OD values were measured at 405 nm and plotted in function of time to construct CD26 activity curves. The figure shows mean values (±SEM) of a representative experiment.

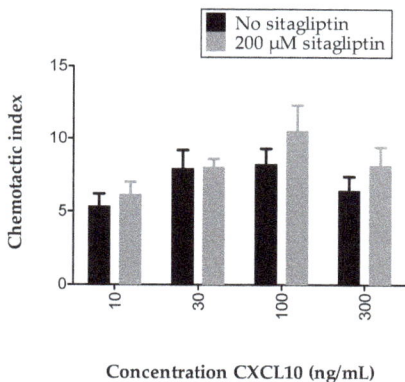

Figure 7. Sitagliptin did not affect CXCL10-induced T cell chemotaxis in vitro. The effects of treatment with 200 μM sitagliptin on the in vitro migratory response of PHA-activated T cells towards 10–300 ng/mL CXCL10 was investigated using the 48 well Boyden chamber chemotaxis assay. Values represent the mean chemotactic index (±SEM) ($n = 6$). Statistical analysis was performed using the Mann-Whitney U test.

2.6. Inhibition of CD26 Significantly Increased CXCL10-Induced Lymphocyte Influx into the Joint In Vivo

Chemokine injection into the tibiofemoral articulation was used as an experimental model to study the effect of specific CD26 inhibition in vivo, since this model has the advantage of very low basal leukocyte counts upon vehicle injection (Figure 8). Moreover, CXCL10 is typically a chemokine found in high concentrations in synovial fluids from inflammatory joints of patients with septic, rheumatoid or psoriatic arthritis [22,23]. To investigate the in vivo effect of CD26 inhibition on CXCL10-induced lymphocyte recruitment into the joint, CXCL10 was injected into the tibiofemoral articulation of sitagliptin-treated and untreated mice.

No lymphocyte infiltration was seen in mice that did receive vehicle injection in the joint. Injection of CXCL10 resulted in a lymphocyte recruitment in both untreated and sitagliptin treated mice (Figure 8). However, the number of lymphocytes in joints of mice that had received sitagliptin was significantly higher than the lymphocyte counts in mice that were not treated with the CD26 inhibitor These results provide direct in vivo evidence that CD26 inhibition protects CXCL10 against cleavage, which is reflected into an enhanced lymphocyte extravasation into the joint. Moreover, these findings are in line with previous studies that reported that sitagliptin treatment in mice is translated into increased CXCL10-mediated lymphocyte infiltration into tumor tissue [63] and increased lymphocyte recruitment to intraperitoneally injected CXCL10 [52].

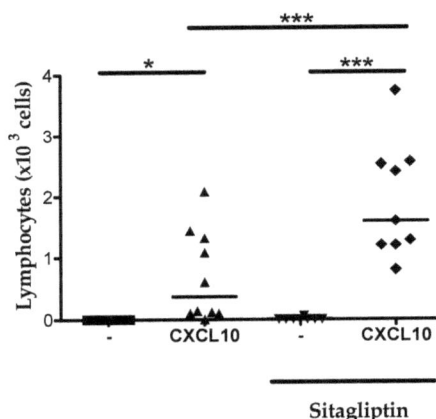

Figure 8. Sitagliptin-treatment of mice enhances CXCL10-mediated lymphocyte extravasation into the joint. The effect of CD26 inhibition on CXCL10-induced lymphocyte extravasation was determined in vivo. Vehicle or CXCL10 were injected into the tibiofemoral articulation of sitagliptin-treated C57BL/6 mice. Total leukocyte numbers migrated into the joint were determined 3 h post injection. Percentages of lymphocytes were differentially counted on May–Grünwald–Giemsa stained cytospins and were used to calculate total lymphocyte numbers. Each symbol represents an individual mouse ($n \geq 8$). Horizontal lines indicate the median number of lymphocytes for each treatment group. Statistical analysis was performed using the Mann-Whitney U test. * $p < 0.05$, *** $p < 0.001$.

3. Discussion

Binding of chemokines to GAGs is essential to generate chemotactic gradients in vivo [32–39]. Moreover, it has been evidenced that the impact of the interaction with GAGs extends beyond the mere facilitation of chemokine retention on the endothelium, thereby locally concentrating chemokines on the cell surface [44]. Interaction with GAGs was found to mediate chemokine oligomerization and to provoke protection against proteolysis by specific enzymes. For example, CXCL12 was protected by heparan sulfate and heparin oligosaccharides against cleavage by CD26 [46]. CXCL12 or stromal derived factor 1 (SDF-1) is an ELR negative CXC chemokine that induces chemotaxis of lymphocytes and CD34 positive progenitor cells through activation of CXCR4. Via interaction with the same receptor, CXCL12 holds anti-HIV properties [64–67]. The chemotactic, CXCR4 dependent signaling and antiviral effects of CXCL12 are lost upon truncation by CD26 [68,69]. In the present study, we demonstrated that GAGs also protect CXCL9, CXCL10 and CXCL11 against proteolytic processing by CD26. Of note, the study by Sadir et al. [46] relied on colon carcinoma cells as source of CD26 activity whereas in our experiments, natural soluble CD26, isolated from human seminal fluid and purified to homogeneity, was used.

Another study reported that murine CCL11, also named eotaxin, is no longer processed by plasmin, elastase and cathepsin G upon interaction with immobilized heparin [47]. Here, the authors found that heparin directly inhibits the enzymatic activity of elastase and cathepsin G but not plasmin. In the present study, no evidence was found for GAGs to directly block the enzymatic activity of CD26. These results are in line with the aforementioned CXCL12 study were the investigators showed that the enzymatic activity of CD26 was not blocked by heparan sulfate [46]. We therefore suppose that the observed role for GAGs in offering the CXCR3 ligands protection against processing by CD26 is rooted at the level of chemokine–GAG interactions, thereby providing steric hindrance at the level of the NH_2-terminal domain of the chemokine. For CXCL12 it was shown that the protection of the NH_2-terminus depends on GAG-induced oligomerization of the chemokine rather than straight interaction with the NH_2-terminal Lys residue [70]. It remains to be elucidated whether the protective effect of GAG interaction on CXCR3 ligands is a result of GAG-mediated chemokine oligomerization or direct steric hindrance at their NH_2-terminus. Nota bene, GAG-mediated chemokine oligomerization seems an intriguing mechanism on its own, but the molecular details remain largely unknown. Indeed, although chemokine monomers seem responsible for GPCR activation, GAG-mediated induction or stabilization of chemokine oligomers is a prerequisite for the in vivo activity of certain chemokines including CXCL10 [33,36,71]. In return, oligomerization may enhance chemokine affinity for GAGs, which is also dependent on specific GAG density [72]. Oligomeric forms were described for CXCL9 and CXCL10 at physiological concentrations, whereas the oligomeric state of CXCL11 is less understood [36,73–75]. However, a key role for oligomerization of several chemokines including CXCL11 was recently demonstrated in facilitating reorganization and bridging of GAG chains, thereby conferring another level of complexity to the chemokine–GAG dialog [72].

The CXCR3 agonists, specifically CXCL9, CXCL10 and CXCL11, all contain a proline residue in the penultimate NH_2-terminal sequence and are biologically relevant CD26 substrates. Upon incubation of 5 μM chemokine with a normal plasma concentration of 25 U/L CD26, the half-lives of CXCL10 and CXCL11 were previously demonstrated to be, respectively, not more than 4 and 2 min, whereas CD26-mediated cleavage of CXCL9 was found to occur less efficiently (half-life of 24 min under the same experimental conditions) [62]. Following cleavage by CD26, the three CXCR3 agonists are biologically inactive in chemotaxis and CXCR3-dependent signaling assays and show a decreased effect on T cells. Moreover, CXCL10(3–77) and CXCL11(3–73) act as CXCR3 antagonists [53]. The CD26-truncated isoform CXCL10(3–77) was originally isolated from natural sources including conditioned medium from MG-63 osteosarcoma cells and fibroblasts [22,58]. Studies with CXCL10$^{-/-}$ mice established a crucial role for CXCL10 in the generation of effector T cells and in T cell trafficking in general [76]. This important physiological role of CXCL10, but also CXCL9 and CXCL11, combined with the fact that CXCL9(3–103), CXCL10(3–77) and CXCL11(3–73) are inactive, supports the idea that CD26-mediated proteolysis of the CXCR3 agonists may have major biological consequences. Results of multiple studies provided evidence in favor of this hypothesis. In mice, truncation of CXCL10 by CD26 reduces the infiltration of T cells into tumor tissue [63] and towards intraperitoneally injected CXCL10 [52] and consequently impairs the natural antitumor immunity Administration of the CD26 inhibitor sitagliptin significantly improved the natural antitumor immunity of these mice and their response to existing immunotherapies. In human, the biologically inactive isoform CXCL10(3–77) was found in plasma from patients that suffer from chronical hepatitis C viral infections [77]. Moreover, two prospective studies recently confirmed the CD26-mediated processing of human CXCL10 in vivo, and provided direct evidence in favor of CD26 inhibition to preserve intact CXCL10 [78]. Although human CXCL11 activates CXCR3 with higher potency and is even more efficiently processed by CD26 than CXCL10, the CD26—CXCL11 axis has been studied to a lesser extend in an in vivo context. It is likely to assume that this can be at least partially explained by the fact that murine CXCL11, in contrast to its human counterpart, contains a methionine residue in its penultimate position and is therefore no substrate for CD26. Interestingly, natural human CXCL11(3–73) was previously isolated from IFN-γ stimulated keratinocytes [59–61]. In addition, murine CXCL9 is no CD26 substrate due to the leucine residue that occupies the penultimate position in its NH_2-terminal amino acid sequence. However, in view of the efficient cleavage of all three human CXCR3 agonists, our observed GAG-mediated protection may be highly significant depending on the local conditions in specific human tissues. Indeed injection of CXCL10 in joints still induces limited lymphocyte migration (Figure 8), whereas injection of CXCL10 in the peritoneum did not attract lymphocytes [52].

In the present study, we found that soluble GAGs significantly reduce the calcium mobilizing capacities of CXCL9, CXCL10 and CXCL11 through CXCR3. Given the general idea that the NH_2-terminal chemokine domain facilitates receptor interaction whereas the COOH-region is considered the major GAG-binding domain, this observation may seem somewhat unexpected. However, it was previously suggested that both interaction domains are not necessarily restricted to, respectively, the NH_2- and COOH-terminus. The relevance of this hypothesis for CXCL10 for example, is supported by the fact that mutation of amino acids 20 to 24, 46 and 47 impairs both the heparin affinity of the chemokine and its binding and signalization through CXCR3 [79]. Furthermore, citrullination of the most NH_2-terminal arginine in CXCL10 or CXCL11 reduced their interaction with heparin [80]. At this point it remains to be elucidated whether the negative effect of GAGs on the potency of CXCR3 agonists to induce intracellular calcium release results from competition between chemokines and GAGs for CXCR3 binding or is rooted at the level of signal transduction, where GAGs potentially exert an inhibitory effect either directly or indirectly. Noteworthy, former studies reported that soluble GAGs also significantly reduce the CXCL8, CCL2, CCL3 and CCL5 mediated intracellular calcium mobilization [81]. Specifically, the authors showed that GAGs, in a competitive fashion, bind to chemokine receptors CXCR1, CXCR2 and CCR1. To our notice, no calcium mobilization studies with GAGs, CXCR3 and its chemokine ligands have been conducted before, but we speculate that GAGs may also interact with CXCR3.

Membrane-bound CD26 is a lymphocyte surface marker that is expressed by activated T cells [82]. In our study, we confirmed that cultured T cells were indeed characterized by CD26 expression and we demonstrated that the expressed enzyme was enzymatically active. Combined with the fact that CXCL10(3–77) is biologically inactive and our observation that GAGs protect CXCL10 against cleavage by CD26, we reasoned that in the presence of GAGs, intact CXCL10 would be preserved, thus resulting in enhanced CXCL10-mediated T cell chemotaxis compared to a condition without GAG. However, we found no significant differences in CXCL10-mediated T cell chemotaxis in vitro in the presence of heparan sulfate and a moderately reduced migration in the presence of heparin. Possibly, this could be explained by the negative effect of GAGs on the CXCL10-CXCR3 dialog. Indeed, it appears that the reduced CXCL10(3–77)-CXCR3 interaction overwrites the inhibitory effect of GAGs on CD26-mediated truncation of intact CXCL10 towards inactive CXCL10(3–77). To investigate the effect of specific inhibition of CD26-mediated cleavage on CXCL10-induced T cell chemotaxis in vitro, we evaluated the effect of administration of the CD26 inhibitor sitagliptin. In contrast to our expectations, no significant increase in CXCL10-directed T cell migration was found in vitro when cells were treated with sitagliptin. However, it was previously demonstrated that sitagliptin treatment in mice resulted in enhanced infiltration of T cells into the peritoneum or in tumor tissue in vivo [52,63]. Moreover, in the present study, we showed that intra articular injection of CXCL10 in sitagliptin-treated mice significantly enhances lymphocyte recruitment to the joint compared to mice that did not receive the CD26 inhibitor. These observations are in line with the idea that specific CD26 inhibition protects CXCL10 from inactivation in vivo. Indeed, in contrast to what is the case in our in vitro experiments, soluble CD26 and membrane-bound CD26 on non-lymphoid cells such as certain endothelial cells, fibroblasts and epithelial cells is present in vivo in addition to T cell-associated membrane-bound CD26 [83]. Therefore, in in vitro chemotaxis experiments, CXCL10 was not hindered by soluble CD26, but could only be inactivated by CD26 when it directly contacted the membrane-bound enzyme. A possible explanation for the lack of a significant effect of sitagliptin-mediated CD26 inhibition on CXCL10-induced chemotaxis in vitro, consequently, could be that CXCL10 was already bound to its receptor prior to interaction with membrane-bound CD26 on T cells. Furthermore, the amount of T cells in our experiments was fixed whereas during inflammation in vivo, for example, the number of activated T cells and consequently the availability of membrane-bound CD26, may drastically increase. Additionally, although we confirmed the CD26 expression and activity on cultured T cells, the CD26 activity on these cells was rather low. Thus, one could speculate that the amount of cell-bound CD26 activity in our in vitro tests was too low.

4. Materials and Methods

4.1. Cells and Reagents

4.1.1. Chemokines and CD26

Full length recombinant human chemokines CXCL9, CXCL10 and CXCL11 were purchased from PeproTech (Rocky Hill, NJ, USA). An Activo-P11 automated solid phase peptide synthesizer (Activotec, Cambridge, UK) was used to chemically synthesize CXCL10, based on *N*-(9-fluorenyl) methoxycarbonyl (Fmoc) chemistry as described previously [84]. To avoid synthesis problems due to its COOH-terminal proline, a H-Pro-2Cl-Trityl resin (Activotec) was used for synthesis of CXCL10. The synthesized chemokine was purified to homogeneity with reverse phase–high performance liquid chromatography using a Source 5-RPC column (4.6 × 150 mm; GE Healthcare, Uppsala, Sweden). An acetonitrile gradient in 0.1% (*v/v*) TFA was used for elution of the synthesized protein and 0.7% of the effluent was directly injected into an electrospray–ion trap mass spectrometer (Bruker AmaZon SL mass spectrometer; Bruker Daltonics, Bremen, Germany). Fractions containing homogenous CXCL10 were selected, pooled, evaporated and dissolved in ultrapure water. Following folding of purified CXCL10 according to the protocol described by Loos et al. [84], the identity of the chemokine was confirmed by ion trap mass spectrometry and automated NH_2-terminal sequencing based on the principle of Edman degradation (Procise 491 cLC sequencer, Applied Biosystems, Foster City, CA, USA). In addition, SDS-PAGE and bicinchoninic acid (BCA) protein assays (Pierce, Woodland Hills, CA, USA) were used to determine protein concentrations and purity.

Natural human soluble CD26 was isolated from human seminal fluid and purified to homogeneity by anion exchange and affinity chromatography as described [85].

4.1.2. Cells

Chinese hamster ovary cells, stably transfected with CXCR3A (CHO/CXCR3A cells), were a gift from M. Parmentier (Université Libre de Bruxelles, Brussels, Belgium) and were cultured in Ham's F12 medium (Lonza, Basel, Switzerland) enriched with 1 mM sodium pyruvate, 400 µg/mL geneticin and 10% (*v/v*) fetal calf serum (FCS; Gibco, Paisley, UK). Peripheral blood mononuclear cells (PBMCs) were isolated from buffy coats or from fresh blood after centrifugation (10 min., 20 °C, 218 g) in a density gradient (Pancoll human, 1,077 g/mL; PAN Biotech GmbH, Aidenbach, Germany). Isolated PBMCs were washed with phosphate buffered saline (PBS) and cultivated in "Roswell Park Memorial Institute" 1640 (RPMI1640) medium (Cambrex Corporation, East Rutherford, NJ, USA) complemented with 10% (*v/v*) FCS, 0.1% (*w/v*) $NaHCO_3$ (Gibco) and 0.05% (*w/v*) gentamycin (Gibco). T cells were activated with 0.002% (*w/v*) phytoheamagglutinin L (PHA; Sigma-Aldrich, St. Louis, MO, USA) at 37 °C during 2–5 days. Activated T cells were stimulated with recombinant human IL-2 (Peprotech) in fresh medium every 2–3 days, and were used in experiments 10–20 days after PHA activation and 2 days after IL-2 stimulation.

4.2. Proteolytic Processing of Chemokines by CD26 In Vitro

The chemokines CXCL9, CXCL10 or CXCL11 (20 µg/mL) were incubated with 12.5 units per liter (U/L) natural human CD26, with or without 0.88 to 26.4 µg/mL heparin, heparin DP8, heparin DP30, heparan sulfate, dermatan sulfate (Iduron, Chechire, U.K.), chondroitin sulfate A or chondroitin sulfate C (Sigma-Aldrich) in 50 mM EDTA; 1 mM Tris buffer (pH 7.5) in a total volume of 25 µL in low-binding tubes (Eppendorf LoBind Tube 1,5 mL, Eppendorf AG, Hamburg, Germany). An overview of the GAGs used in experiments is provided in Table 2. Nota bene, "DP" refers to the number of disaccharides. After 2 h of incubation, enzymatic reactions were terminated by acidification up to 0.08% (*v/v*) TFA. Chemokines were extracted and desalted from total samples on C18 ZipTip pipet tips (Millipore Corporation), eluted with 50% (*v/v*) acetonitrile in 0.1% (*v/v*) TFA, and analyzed by mass spectrometry.

Table 2. Specifications of GAGs used in experiments.

GAG	Source	Company	Composition	Relative Molecular Mass M_r
Heparin	Porcine mucosa	Iduron	ΔHexA,2S–GlcNS,6S–(IdoUA,2S–GlcNS,6S)n	±40 kDa [a]
Heparin DP30	Porcine mucosa	Iduron	ΔHexA,2S–GlcNS,6S–(IdoUA,2S–GlcNS,6S)$_{30}$	>9 kDa [b]
Heparin DP8	Porcine mucosa	Iduron	ΔHexA,2S–GlcNS,6S–(IdoUA,2S–GlcNS,6S)$_8$	±2.4 kDa [b]
Heparan sulfate	Porcine mucosa	Iduron	GlcA-GlcNAc and IdoA/Glc-GlcNS (variable O-sulfation); contains both low and high sulfated heparan sulfates	±40 kDa [a]
Dermatan sulfate	Porcine mucosa	Iduron	HexA-GalNAc,4S (88%); HexA-GalNAc (5%); HexA,2S-GalNAc,4S (7%)	±41 kDa [b]
Chondroitin sulfate A	Bovine trachea	Sigma-Aldrich	Alternating Copoly β-glucuronic acid-(1→3)-N-acetyl-β-galactosamine-4-sulfate-(1→4)	±40 kDa [a]
Chondroitin sulfate C	Shark cartilage	Sigma-Aldrich	Poly[β-glucuronic acid-(1→3)-N-acetyl-β-galactosamine-6-sulfate-(1→4)] alternating	±40 kDa [a]

[a] as experimentally determined by mass spectrometry; [b] according to the data sheet of the company.

4.3. CD26 Activity Assays

In a flat bottom 96 well plate, (Greiner Bio-One, Kremsmünster, Austria), 5 U/L purified natural human CD26 was incubated with 500 µM of the substrate Gly-Pro-*p*-nitroanilide (Gly-Pro-pNA; Sigma-Aldrich), with or without GAG, in 0.22 µm-filtered 75 mM Tris-HCl buffer (pH 8.3). Evolution of the optic density (OD) at 405 nm was followed using a spectrophotometer (BioTek PowerWave XS, Winooski, VT, USA) and represented the kinetics of CD26-mediated enzymatic conversion of colorless Gly-Pro-pNA into yellowish pNA. OD measurements were performed at 37 °C every 5 min for 3 h. CD26 activity curves were constructed by plotting OD values against time. Slopes of activity curves reflected the number of converted substrate molecules per min and were used to calculate enzymatic activities in U/L using the Lambert-Beer law. CD26 activity assays were also used to investigate the CD26 activity of PHA-activated T cells. Briefly, 10^4 to 3×10^6 T cells per mL in 75 mM Tris-HCl buffer (pH 8.3), with or without 20 µM to 2 mM sitagliptin (Merck Sharpe & Dohme (MSD) Whitehouse Station, NJ, USA), were incubated with 500 µM Gly-Pro pNA and the same protocol was followed.

4.4. Calcium-Mobilization Assays

CHO/CXCR3A cells (10×10^6 per mL) in Ham's F12 medium (Lonza) containing 10% (*v/v*) FCS were treated with 2.5 µM of the fluorescent dye Fura-2AM (Invitrogen, Carlsbad, CA, USA), 0.01% (*w/v*) Pluronic-F127 (Sigma) and 125 µM Probenecid solution (ICN Biomedicals Inc., Aurora, OH, USA) for 30 min at room temperature. Cells were washed with Ham's F12 medium containing 10% (*v/v*) FCS, centrifuged (10 min, 4 °C, 177 g) and suspended in pH 7.0 Ca^{2+} buffer ("Hanks Balanced Salt Solution" (HBSS; Invitrogen) containing Ca^{2+} and Mg^{2+} and complemented with 10 mM HEPES (Gibco) and 0.1% (v/v) FCS) enriched with 125 μM Probenecid. Cells were kept on ice, centrifuged (10 min, 4 °C, 177 g), and suspended in Ca^{2+} buffer with Probenecid at final concentrations of 10^6 cells per mL. An LS50 B luminescence spectrometer (Perkin Elmer, Waltham, MA, USA) was used to measure fluorescence and intracellular Ca^{2+} concentrations ([Ca^{2+}]$_i$) were calculated using the Grynkiewicz equation [86]. For each individual test condition, 1.8 × 10^6 cells were preheated for 10 min at 30 °C, followed by stimulation with 3 to 1000 ng/mL CXCL9, CXCL10 or CXCL11, with or without 0.04 μg/mL, 2 μg/mL or 10 μg/mL GAG. R$_{max}$ and R$_{min}$ values were determined via treatment of cells with 50 μM digitonin and 10 mM EGTA (Sigma-Aldrich) in 20 mM Tris (pH 8.5; Merck, Darmstadt, Germany), respectively. Results were analyzed with WinLab32 software (Perkin Elmer). Fluorescence intensities of unloaded cells (not treated with Fura-2AM) were used to correct results for auto-fluorescence intrinsic to CHO/CXCR3A cells.

4.5. In Vitro Chemotaxis Assays

In vitro, 48-well Boyden chamber cell migration assays were used to determine chemotaxis of PHA-activated T cells in response to CXCL10 with or without GAG [87]. Briefly, CXCL10 and T cells were diluted in HBSS buffer enriched with 0.5% (v/v) human serum albumin (HSA; Red Cross Blood transfusion center, Leuven, Belgium). Wells in the lower part of the chamber were filled with 10–300 ng/mL CXCL10 with or without 0.04 or 4 μg/mL GAG in a total volume of 30 μL per well. Buffer without chemokine or GAG was used as a negative control. The lower chamber was covered with a 5 μm polycarbonate membrane (Nuclepore Track-Etch Membrane, Whatman, Little Chalfont, UK) that was treated with 20 μg/mL fibronectin (Gibco) in PBS overnight. The upper part of the chamber was filled with 2 × 10^6 T cells per mL in buffer (50 μL per well), with or without 200 μM sitagliptin. Following 3 h of incubation at 37 °C, membranes were fixed and stained (Hemacolor Solution I–III, Merck). For each individual test condition, numbers of migrated T cells were counted microscopically in 10 separate fields. Chemotactic indices were determined by dividing total numbers of T cells that migrated to the sample through the total number of cells that migrated in response to buffer alone.

4.6. In Vivo Cell Migration Assay

The effect of CD26 inhibition on lymphocyte attraction was determined after intra-articular (i.a.) injection of human CXCL10 as described by Janssens et al. [88]. Briefly, the drinking water of 8-week-old C57BL/6 mice was complemented with 1.7 mg/mL sitagliptin from 3 days prior to i.a. injection of 1 μg synthetic full length CXCL10 diluted in 0.9% (w/v) NaCl. A *Limulus* amoebocyte lysate assay (Cambrex) demonstrated that endotoxin levels in injected samples were lower than 0.125 pg LPS per μg chemokine. During injection of 10 μL of the CXCL10 dilution, mice were anaesthetized using 3.75% (w/v) ketamine plus 0.25% (w/v) xylazine in PBS. Mice were sacrificed after 3 h of incubation, and articular cavities were washed with 3% (w/v) BSA in PBS. Total leukocyte numbers were calculated after staining with Turk's solution in a Neubauer chamber, followed by differential counting of samples on cytospins that were stained with May–Grünwald–Giemsa. All in vivo experiments were conducted in the animal research facility of the University of Minas Gerais after approval by the Animal Ethical Committee.

4.7. Flow Cytometry

Flow cytometry was used to confirm the CXCR3 and CD26 expression of cultivated T cells. Tubes were filled with 3 × 10^5 cells and centrifuged (5 min, 4 °C, 315 g). Supernatant was removed and cells were suspended in PBS containing Fc block (MACS Miltenyi Biotec, Bergisch Gladbach, Germany) and Aqua Zombie-BV510 (Biolegend, San Diego, CA, USA), according to the recommendations of the companies. Following 15 min of incubation at 20 °C, cells were centrifuged (5 min, 4 °C,

315 g) and pellets were suspended in flow cytometry buffer (PBS containing 2% (*v*/*v*) FCS and 2 mM EDTA). Samples were centrifuged (5 min, 4 °C, 315 g) and cells were diluted in fresh buffer. For each sample, recommended amounts of BV421-labeled anti-human CXCR3, PE-labeled anti-human CD3, PerCP-Cy5.5-labeled anti-human CD14, FITC-labeled anti-human CD26 (BD Pharmingen, San Diego, CA, USA) or APC-labeled anti-human CD14 (Biolegend), were added. Combined stainings were conducted with anti-CD3-PE, anti-CXCR3-BV421, anti-CD26-FITC and anti-CD14-PerCP-Cy5.5; anti-CD3-PE, anti-CXCR3-BV421 and anti-CD26-FITC; anti-CD3, anti-CD3-PE, anti-CXCR3-BV421 and anti-CD14-PerCP-Cy5.5 and finally with anti-CD3-PE, anti-CXCR3-BV421 and anti-CD14-APC. Isotype controls were performed to exclude non-specific binding. Untreated cells were used as negative controls. One sample of unstained cells was heated at 56 °C for 10–15 min to kill part of the cells, and served as a positive control for the Aqua Zombie staining. Antibody-treated cells were kept at 4 °C for 30 min, and were, respectively, suspended in flow cytometry buffer, centrifuged (5 min, 4 °C, 315 g) and decanted 3 times in a row. Resulting pellets were diluted in fixation buffer (flow cytometry buffer plus 0.04% (*w*/*v*) paraformaldehyde) and fluorescence intensities were determined with a BD LSRFORTESSA X-20 flow cytometer (BD Biosciences, Franklin Lakes, NJ, USA) equipped with 5 lasers. Results were analyzed with FlowJo software.

4.8. Statistics

Mann–Whitney U tests were performed to evaluate whether results of unpaired groups were significantly different or not. A *p* value of 0.05 or less was considered significant.

Supplementary Materials: Supplementary materials can be found at www.mdpi.com/1422-0067/18/7/1513/s1.

Acknowledgments: This research was financially supported by the Interuniversity Attraction Poles Programme initiated by the Belgian Science Policy Office (I.A.P. Project 7/40), the Fund for Scientific Research of Flanders, the Brazilian National Council for Scientific and Technological Development (CNPq) and the Concerted Research Actions of the Regional Government of Flanders (GOA/12/017) and C1 funding from KU Leuven. The Hercules foundation of the Flemish government funded the purchase of LC-MS/MS equipment (Contract AKUL/11/31). AM obtained a postdoctoral research scholarship of the FWO-Vlaanderen

Author Contributions: Mieke Metzemaekers, Anneleen Mortier, Rik Janssens, Daiane Boff, Lotte Vanbrabant, Flávio A. Amaral and Paul Proost performed experiments; Nicole Lamoen purified natural CD26 enzyme; Mieke Metzemaekers, Anneleen Mortier and Paul Proost wrote the manuscript; Mieke Metzemaekers, Anneleen Mortier, Jo Van Damme, Mauro M. Teixeira, Ingrid De Meester, Flávio A. Amaral and Paul Proost designed the study and were responsible for data interpretation and manuscript correction. All authors approved the final version of the manuscript.

Conflicts of Interest: The authors declare no conflict of interest.

Abbreviations

$[Ca^{2+}]_i$	Intracellular calcium concentration
GAG	glycosaminoglycan
GPCR	G protein-coupled receptor
M_r	Relative molecular mass

References

1. Zlotnik, A.; Yoshie, O. The chemokine superfamily revisited. *Immunity* **2012**, *36*, 705–716. [CrossRef] [PubMed]
2. Blanchet, X.; Langer, M.; Weber, C.; Koenen, R.R.; von Hundelshausen, P. Touch of chemokines. *Front. Immunol.* **2012**, *3*, 175. [CrossRef] [PubMed]
3. Romagnani, P.; Lasagni, L.; Annunziato, F.; Serio, M.; Romagnani, S. CXC chemokines: The regulatory link between inflammation and angiogenesis. *Trends Immunol.* **2004**, *25*, 201–209. [CrossRef] [PubMed]
4. Russo, R.C.; Garcia, C.C.; Teixeira, M.M.; Amaral, F.A. The CXCL8/IL-8 chemokine family and its receptors in inflammatory diseases. *Expert. Rev. Clin. Immunol.* **2014**, *10*, 593–619. [CrossRef] [PubMed]

5.   Keeley, E.C.; Mehrad, B.; Strieter, R.M. Chemokines as mediators of tumor angiogenesis and neovascularization. *Exp. Cell Res.* **2011**, *317*, 685–690. [CrossRef] [PubMed]

6.   Bachelerie, F.; Ben-Baruch, A.; Burkhardt, A.M.; Combadiere, C.; Farber, J.M.; Graham, G.J.; Horuk, R.; Sparre-Ulrich, A.H.; Locati, M.; Luster, A.D.; et al. International union of basic and clinical pharmacology. LXXXIX. Update on the extended family of chemokine receptors and introducing a new nomenclature for atypical chemokine receptors. *Pharmacol. Rev.* **2014**, *66*, 1–79. [CrossRef] [PubMed]

7.   Corsiero, E.; Nerviani, A.; Bombardieri, M.; Pitzalis, C. Ectopic lymphoid structures: Powerhouse of autoimmunity. *Front. Immunol.* **2016**, *7*, 430. [CrossRef] [PubMed]

8.   Opdenakker, G.; Proost, P.; Van Damme, J. Microbiomic and posttranslational modifications as preludes to autoimmune diseases. *Trends Mol. Med.* **2016**, *22*, 746–757. [CrossRef] [PubMed]

9.   Rot, A.; von Andrian, U.H. Chemokines in innate and adaptive host defense: Basic chemokinese grammar for immune cells. *Annu. Rev. Immunol.* **2004**, *22*, 891–928. [CrossRef] [PubMed]

10. Groom, J.R.; Luster, A.D. CXCR3 ligands: Redundant, collaborative and antagonistic functions. *Immunol. Cell Biol.* **2011**, *89*, 207–215. [CrossRef] [PubMed]

11. Van Raemdonck, K.; Van den Steen, P.E.; Liekens, S.; Van Damme, J.; Struyf, S. CXCR3 ligands in disease and therapy. *Cytokine Growth Factor Rev.* **2015**, *26*, 311–327. [CrossRef] [PubMed]

12. Groom, J.R.; Luster, A.D. CXCR3 in T cell function. *Exp. Cell Res.* **2011**, *317*, 620–631. [CrossRef] [PubMed]

13. Lasagni, L.; Francalanci, M.; Annunziato, F.; Lazzeri, E.; Giannini, S.; Cosmi, L.; Sagrinati, C.; Mazzinghi, B.; Orlando, C.; Maggi, E.; et al. An alternatively spliced variant of CXCR3 mediates the inhibition of endothelial cell growth induced by IP-10, Mig, and I-TAC, and acts as functional receptor for platelet factor 4. *J. Exp. Med.* **2003**, *197*, 1537–1549. [CrossRef] [PubMed]

14. Naumann, U.; Cameroni, E.; Pruenster, M.; Mahabaleshwar, H.; Raz, E.; Zerwes, H.G.; Rot, A.; Thelen, M. CXCR7 functions as a scavenger for CXCL12 and CXCL11. *PLoS ONE* **2010**, *5*, e9175. [CrossRef] [PubMed]

15. Girard, M.; Rhainds, D.; St-Onge, G. Mutational analysis of atypical chemokine receptor 3 (ACKR3/CXCR7) interaction with its chemokine ligands CXCL11 and CXCL12. *J. Biol. Chem.* **2017**, *292*, 31–42.

16. Burns, J.M.; Summers, B.C.; Wang, Y.; Melikian, A.; Berahovich, R.; Miao, Z.; Penfold, M.E.; Sunshine, M.J.; Littman, D.R.; Kuo, C.J.; et al. A novel chemokine receptor for SDF-1 and I-TAC involved in cell survival, cell adhesion, and tumor development. *J. Exp. Med.* **2006**, *203*, 2201–2213. [CrossRef] [PubMed]

17. Vanheule, V.; Janssens, R.; Boff, D.; Kitic, N.; Berghmans, N.; Ronsse, I.; Kungl, A.J.; Amaral, F.A.; Teixeira, M.M.; Van Damme, J.; et al. The Positively charged COOH-terminal glycosaminoglycan-binding CXCL9(74–103) peptide inhibits CXCL8-induced neutrophil extravasation and monosodium urate crystal-induced gout in mice. *J. Biol. Chem.* **2015**, *290*, 21292–21304. [CrossRef] [PubMed]

18. Farber, J.M. Mig and IP-10: CXC chemokines that target lymphocytes. *J. Leukoc. Biol.* **1997**, *61*, 246–257. [PubMed]

19. Ohmori, Y.; Schreiber, R.D.; Hamilton, T.A. Synergy between interferon-gamma and tumor necrosis factor-α in transcriptional activation is mediated by cooperation between signal transducer and activator of transcription 1 and nuclear factor κB. *J. Biol. Chem.* **1997**, *272*, 14899–14907. [CrossRef] [PubMed]

20. Ohmori, Y.; Wyner, L.; Narumi, S.; Armstrong, D.; Stoler, M.; Hamilton, T.A. Tumor necrosis factoralpha induces cell type and tissue-specific expression of chemoattractant cytokines in vivo. *Am. J. Pathol.* **1993**, *142*, 861–870. [PubMed]

21. Rani, M.R.; Foster, G.R.; Leung, S.; Leaman, D.; Stark, G.R.; Ransohoff, R.M. Characterization of β-R1, a gene that is selectively induced by interferon β (IFN-β) compared with IFN-α. *J. Biol. Chem.* **1996**, *271*, 22878–22884. [CrossRef] [PubMed]

22. Proost, P.; Struyf, S.; Loos, T.; Gouwy, M.; Schutyser, E.; Conings, R.; Ronsse, I.; Parmentier, M.; Grillet, B.; Opdenakker, G.; et al. Coexpression and interaction of CXCL10 and CD26 in mesenchymal cells by synergising inflammatory cytokines: CXCL8 and CXCL10 are discriminative markers for autoimmune arthropathies. *Arthritis Res. Ther.* **2006**, *8*, R107. [CrossRef] [PubMed]

23. Proost, P.; Vynckier, A.K.; Mahieu, F.; Put, W.; Grillet, B.; Struyf, S.; Wuyts, A.; Opdenakker, G.; Van Damme, J. Microbial Toll-like receptor ligands differentially regulate CXCL10/IP-10 expression in fibroblasts and mononuclear leukocytes in synergy with IFN-γ and provide a mechanism for enhanced synovial chemokine levels in septic arthritis. *Eur. J. Immunol.* **2003**, *33*, 3146–3153. [CrossRef] [PubMed]

24. Hsieh, M.F.; Lai, S.L.; Chen, J.P.; Sung, J.M.; Lin, Y.L.; Wu-Hsieh, B.A.; Gerard, C.; Luster, A.; Liao, F. Both CXCR3 and CXCL10/IFN-inducible protein 10 are required for resistance to primary infection by dengue virus. *J. Immunol.* **2006**, *177*, 1855–1863. [CrossRef] [PubMed]

25. Christen, U.; McGavern, D.B.; Luster, A.D.; von Herrath, M.G.; Oldstone, M.B. Among CXCR3 chemokines, IFN-γ-inducible protein of 10 kDa (CXC chemokine ligand (CXCL) 10) but not monokine induced by IFN-γ (CXCL9) imprints a pattern for the subsequent development of autoimmune disease. *J. Immunol.* **2003**, *171*, 6838–6845. [CrossRef] [PubMed]

26. Li, B.; Xu, W.; Xu, L.; Jiang, Z.; Wen, Z.; Li, K.; Xiong, S. I-TAC is a dominant chemokine in controlling skin intragraft inflammation via recruiting CXCR3+ cells into the graft. *Cell. Immunol.* **2010**, *260*, 83–91. [CrossRef] [PubMed]

27. Klein, R.S.; Lin, E.; Zhang, B.; Luster, A.D.; Tollett, J.; Samuel, M.A.; Engle, M.; Diamond, M.S. Neuronal CXCL10 directs CD8+ T-cell recruitment and control of West Nile virus encephalitis. *J. Virol.* **2005**, *79*, 11457–11466. [CrossRef] [PubMed]

28. Campanella, G.S.; Tager, A.M.; El Khoury, J.K.; Thomas, S.Y.; Abrazinski, T.A.; Manice, L.A.; Colvin, R.A.; Luster, A.D. Chemokine receptor CXCR3 and its ligands CXCL9 and CXCL10 are required for the development of murine cerebral malaria. *Proc. Natl. Acad. Sci. USA* **2008**, *105*, 4814–4819. [CrossRef] [PubMed]

29. Thapa, M.; Welner, R.S.; Pelayo, R.; Carr, D.J. CXCL9 and CXCL10 expression are critical for control of genital herpes simplex virus type 2 infection through mobilization of HSV-specific CTL and NK cells to the nervous system. *J. Immunol.* **2008**, *180*, 1098–1106. [CrossRef] [PubMed]

30. Rosenblum, J.M.; Shimoda, N.; Schenk, A.D.; Zhang, H.; Kish, D.D.; Keslar, K.; Farber, J.M.; Fairchild, R.L. CXC chemokine ligand (CXCL) 9 and CXCL10 are antagonistic costimulation molecules during the priming of alloreactive T cell effectors. *J. Immunol.* **2010**, *184*, 3450–3460. [CrossRef] [PubMed]

31. Sierro, F.; Biben, C.; Martínez-Muñoz, L.; Mellado, M.; Ransohoff, R.M.; Li, M.; Woehl, B.; Leung, H.; Groom, J.; Batten, M.; et al. Disrupted cardiac development but normal hematopoiesis in mice deficient in the second CXCL12/SDF-1 receptor, CXCR7. *Proc. Natl. Acad. Sci. USA* **2007**, *104*, 14759–14764. [CrossRef] [PubMed]

32. Sarris, M.; Masson, J.B.; Maurin, D.; Van der Aa, L.M.; Boudinot, P.; Lortat-Jacob, H.; Herbomel, P. Inflammatory chemokines direct and restrict leukocyte migration within live tissues as glycan-bound gradients. *Curr. Biol.* **2012**, *22*, 2375–2382. [CrossRef] [PubMed]

33. Proudfoot, A.E.; Handel, T.M.; Johnson, Z.; Lau, E.K.; LiWang, P.; Clark-Lewis, I.; Borlat, F.; Wells, T.N.; Kosco-Vilbois, M.H. Glycosaminoglycan binding and oligomerization are essential for the in vivo activity of certain chemokines. *Proc. Natl. Acad. Sci. USA* **2003**, *100*, 1885–1890. [CrossRef] [PubMed]

34. Wang, L.; Fuster, M.; Sriramarao, P.; Esko, J.D. Endothelial heparan sulfate deficiency impairs L-selectin- and chemokine-mediated neutrophil trafficking during inflammatory responses. *Nat. Immunol.* **2005**, *6*, 902–910. [CrossRef] [PubMed]

35. Severin, I.C.; Gaudry, J.P.; Johnson, Z.; Kungl, A.; Jansma, A.; Gesslbauer, B.; Mulloy, B.; Power, C.; Proudfoot, A.E.; Handel, T. Characterization of the chemokine CXCL11-heparin interaction suggests two different affinities for glycosaminoglycans. *J. Biol. Chem.* **2010**, *285*, 17713–17724. [CrossRef] [PubMed]

36. Campanella, G.S.; Grimm, J.; Manice, L.A.; Colvin, R.A.; Medoff, B.D.; Wojtkiewicz, G.R.; Weissleder, R.; Luster, A.D. Oligomerization of CXCL10 is necessary for endothelial cell presentation and in vivo activity. *J. Immunol.* **2006**, *177*, 6991–6998. [CrossRef] [PubMed]

37. Massena, S.; Christoffersson, G.; Hjertström, E.; Zcharia, E.; Vlodavsky, I.; Ausmees, N.; Rolny, C.; Li, J.P.; Phillipson, M. A chemotactic gradient sequestered on endothelial heparan sulfate induces directional intraluminal crawling of neutrophils. *Blood* **2010**, *116*, 1924–1931. [CrossRef] [PubMed]

38. Bao, X.; Moseman, E.A.; Saito, H.; Petryanik, B.; Thiriot, A.; Hatakeyama, S.; Ito, Y.; Kawashima, H.; Yamaguchi, Y.; Lowe, J.B.; et al. Endothelial heparan sulfate controls chemokine presentation in recruitment of lymphocytes and dendritic cells to lymph nodes. *Immunity* **2010**, *33*, 817–829. [CrossRef] [PubMed]

39. Kumar, A.V.; Katakam, S.K.; Urbanowitz, A.K.; Gotte, M. Heparan sulfate as a regulator of leukocyte recruitment in inflammation. *Curr. Protein Pept. Sci.* **2015**, *16*, 77–86. [CrossRef] [PubMed]

40. Xu, D.; Esko, J.D. Demystifying heparan sulfate-protein interactions. *Annu. Rev. Biochem.* **2014**, *83*, 129–157. [CrossRef] [PubMed]

41. Vanheule, V.; Vervaeke, P.; Mortier, A.; Noppen, S.; Gouwy, M.; Snoeck, R.; Andrei, G.; Van Damme, J.; Liekens, S.; Proost, P. Basic chemokine-derived glycosaminoglycan binding peptides exert antiviral properties against dengue virus serotype 2, herpes simplex virus-1 and respiratory syncytial virus. *Biochem. Pharmacol.* **2016**, *100*, 73–85. [CrossRef] [PubMed]

42. Baggiolini, M. CXCL8—The First Chemokine. *Front. Immunol.* **2015**, *6*, 285. [CrossRef] [PubMed]

43. Van Damme, J.; Van Beeumen, J.; Conings, R.; Decock, B.; Billiau, A. Purification of granulocyte chemotactic peptide/interleukin-8 reveals N-terminal sequence heterogeneity similar to that of beta-thromboglobulin. *Eur. J. Biochem.* **1989**, *181*, 337–344. [CrossRef] [PubMed]

44. Mortier, A.; Van Damme, J.; Proost, P. Overview of the mechanisms regulating chemokine activity and availability. *Immunol. Lett.* **2012**, *145*, 2–9. [CrossRef] [PubMed]

45. Krohn, S.C.; Bonvin, P.; Proudfoot, A.E. CCL18 exhibits a regulatory role through inhibition of receptor and glycosaminoglycan binding. *PLoS ONE* **2013**, *8*, e72321. [CrossRef] [PubMed]

46. Sadir, R.; Imberty, A.; Baleux, F.; Lortat-Jacob, H. Heparan sulfate/heparin oligosaccharides protect stromal cell-derived factor-1 (SDF-1)/CXCL12 against proteolysis induced by CD26/dipeptidyl peptidase IV. *J. Biol. Chem.* **2004**, *279*, 43854–43860. [CrossRef] [PubMed]

47. Ellyard, J.I.; Simson, L.; Bezos, A.; Johnston, K.; Freeman, C.; Parish, C.R. Eotaxin selectively binds heparin. An interaction that protects eotaxin from proteolysis and potentiates chemotactic activity in vivo. *J. Biol. Chem.* **2007**, *282*, 15238–15247. [CrossRef] [PubMed]

48. Mortier, A.; Gouwy, M.; Van Damme, J.; Proost, P. Effect of posttranslational processing on the in vitro and in vivo activity of chemokines. *Exp. Cell Res.* **2011**, *317*, 642–654. [CrossRef] [PubMed]

49. Moelants, E.A.; Mortier, A.; Van Damme, J.; Proost, P. In vivo regulation of chemokine activity by post-translational modification. *Immunol. Cell Biol.* **2013**, *91*, 402–407. [CrossRef] [PubMed]

50. Metzemaekers, M.; Van Damme, J.; Mortier, A.; Proost, P. Regulation of chemokine activity—A focus on the role of dipeptidyl peptidase IV/CD26. *Front. Immunol.* **2016**, *7*, 483. [CrossRef] [PubMed]

51. Janssens, R.; Mortier, A.; Boff, D.; Ruytinx, P.; Gouwy, M.; Vantilt, B.; Larsen, O.; Daugvilaite, V.; Rosenkilde, M.M.; Parmentier, M.; et al. Truncation of CXCL12 by CD26 reduces its CXC chemokine receptor 4- and atypical chemokine receptor 3-dependent activity on endothelial cells and lymphocytes. *Biochem. Pharmacol.* **2017**, *132*, 92–101. [CrossRef] [PubMed]

52. Mortier, A.; Gouwy, M.; Van Damme, J.; Proost, P.; Struyf, S. CD26/dipeptidylpeptidase IV-chemokine interactions: Double-edged regulation of inflammation and tumor biology. *J. Leukoc. Biol.* **2016**, *99*, 955–969. [CrossRef] [PubMed]

53. Proost, P.; Schutyser, E.; Menten, P.; Struyf, S.; Wuyts, A.; Opdenakker, G.; Detheux, M.; Parmentier, M.; Durinx, C.; Lambeir, A.M.; et al. Amino-terminal truncation of CXCR3 agonists impairs receptor signaling and lymphocyte chemotaxis, while preserving antiangiogenic properties. *Blood* **2001**, *98*, 3554–3561. [CrossRef] [PubMed]

54. Lambeir, A.M.; Durinx, C.; Scharpé, S.; De Meester, I. Dipeptidyl-peptidase IV from bench to bedside: An update on structural properties, functions, and clinical aspects of the enzyme DPP IV. *Crit. Rev. Clin. Lab. Sci.* **2003**, *40*, 209–294. [CrossRef] [PubMed]

55. Klemann, C.; Wagner, L.; Stephan, M.; von Hörsten, S. Cut to the chase: A review of CD26/dipeptidyl peptidase-4's (DPP4) entanglement in the immune system. *Clin. Exp. Immunol.* **2016**, *185*, 1–21. [CrossRef] [PubMed]

56. Wagner, L.; Klemann, C.; Stephan, M.; von Hörsten, S. Unravelling the immunological roles of dipeptidyl peptidase 4 (DPP4) activity and/or structure homologue (DASH) proteins. *Clin. Exp. Immunol.* **2016**, *184*, 265–283. [CrossRef] [PubMed]

57. Boonacker, E.; Van Noorden, C.J. The multifunctional or moonlighting protein CD26/DPPIV. *Eur. J. Cell Biol.* **2003**, *82*, 53–73. [CrossRef] [PubMed]

58. Proost, P.; De Wolf-Peeters, C.; Conings, R.; Opdenakker, G.; Billiau, A.; Van Damme, J. Identification of a novel granulocyte chemotactic protein (GCP-2) from human tumor cells. In vitro and in vivo comparison with natural forms of GRO, IP-10, and IL-8., IP-10, and IL-8. *J. Immunol.* **1993**, *150*, 1000–1010. [PubMed]

59. Ludwig, A.; Schiemann, F.; Mentlein, R.; Lindner, B.; Brandt, E. Dipeptidyl peptidase IV (CD26) on T cells cleaves the CXC chemokine CXCL11 (I-TAC) and abolishes the stimulating but not the desensitizing potential of the chemokine. *J. Leukoc. Biol.* **2002**, *72*, 183–191. [PubMed]

60. Proost, P.; Mortier, A.; Loos, T.; Vandercappellen, J.; Gouwy, M.; Ronsse, I.; Schutyser, E.; Put, W.; Parmentier, M.; Struyf, S.; et al. Proteolytic processing of CXCL11 by CD13/aminopeptidase N impairs CXCR3 and CXCR7 binding and signaling and reduces lymphocyte and endothelial cell migration. *Blood* **2007**, *110*, 37–44. [CrossRef] [PubMed]

61. Hensbergen, P.J.; van der Raaij-Helmer, E.M.; Dijkman, R.; van der Schors, R.C.; Werner-Felmayer, G.; Boorsma, D.M.; Scheper, R.J.; Willemze, R.; Tensen, C.P. Processing of natural and recombinant CXCR3-targeting chemokines and implications for biological activity. *Eur. J. Biochem.* **2001**, *268*, 4992–4999. [CrossRef] [PubMed]

62. Lambeir, A.M.; Proost, P.; Durinx, C.; Bal, G.; Senten, K.; Augustyns, K.; Scharpé, S.; Van Damme, J.; De Meester, I. Kinetic investigation of chemokine truncation by CD26/dipeptidyl peptidase IV reveals a striking selectivity within the chemokine family. *J. Biol. Chem.* **2001**, *276*, 29839–29845. [CrossRef] [PubMed]

63. Barreira da Silva, R.; Laird, M.E.; Yatim, N.; Fiette, L.; Ingersoll, M.A.; Albert, M.L. Dipeptidylpeptidase 4 inhibition enhances lymphocyte trafficking, improving both naturally occurring tumor immunity and immunotherapy. *Nat. Immunol.* **2015**, *16*, 850–858. [CrossRef] [PubMed]

64. Bleul, C.C.; Fuhlbrigge, R.C.; Casasnovas, J.M.; Aiuti, A.; Springer, T.A. A highly efficacious lymphocyte chemoattractant, stromal cell-derived factor 1 (SDF-1). *J. Exp. Med.* **1996**, *184*, 1101–1109. [CrossRef] [PubMed]

65. Lim, K.; Hyun, Y.M.; Lambert-Emo, K.; Capece, T.; Bae, S.; Miller, R.; Topham, D.J.; Kim, M. Neutrophil trails guide influenza-specific CD8(+) T cells in the airways. *Science* **2015**, *349*, aaa4352. [CrossRef] [PubMed]

66. Möhle, R.; Bautz, F.; Rafii, S.; Moore, M.A.; Brugger, W.; Kanz, L. The chemokine receptor CXCR-4 is expressed on CD34+ hematopoietic progenitors and leukemic cells and mediates transendothelial migration induced by stromal cell-derived factor-1. *Blood* **1998**, *91*, 4523–4530. [PubMed]

67. Aiuti, A.; Webb, I.J.; Bleul, C.C.; Springer, T.; Gutierrez-Ramos, J.C. The chemokine SDF-1 is a chemoattractant for human CD34+ hematopoietic progenitor cells and provides a new mechanism to explain the mobilization of CD34+ progenitors to peripheral blood. *J. Exp. Med.* **1997**, *185*, 111–120. [CrossRef] [PubMed]

68. Shioda, T.; Kato, H.; Ohnishi, Y.; Tashiro, K.; Ikegawa, M.; Nakayama, E.E.; Hu, H.; Kato, A.; Sakai, Y.; Liu, H.; et al. Anti-HIV-1 and chemotactic activities of human stromal cell-derived factor 1alpha (SDF-1α) and SDF-1β are abolished by CD26/dipeptidyl peptidase IV-mediated cleavage. *Proc. Natl. Acad. Sci. USA* **1998**, *95*, 6331–6336. [CrossRef] [PubMed]

69. Proost, P.; Struyf, S.; Schols, D.; Durinx, C.; Wuyts, A.; Lenaerts, J.P.; De Clercq, E.; De Meester, I.; Van Damme, J. Processing by CD26/dipeptidyl-peptidase IV reduces the chemotactic and anti-HIV-1 activity of stromal-cell-derived factor-1α. *FEBS Lett.* **1998**, *432*, 73–76. [CrossRef]

70. Ziarek, J.J.; Veldkamp, C.T.; Zhang, F.; Murray, N.J.; Kartz, G.A.; Liang, X.; Su, J.; Baker, J.E.; Linhardt, R.J.; Volkman, B.F. Heparin oligosaccharides inhibit chemokine (CXC motif) ligand 12 (CXCL12) cardioprotection by binding orthogonal to the dimerization interface, promoting oligomerization, and competing with the chemokine (CXC motif) receptor 4 (CXCR4) N terminus. *J. Biol. Chem.* **2013**, *288*, 737–746. [CrossRef] [PubMed]

71. Gangavarapu, P.; Rajagopalan, L.; Kolli, D.; Guerrero-Plata, A.; Garofalo, R.P.; Rajarathnam, K. The monomer-dimer equilibrium and glycosaminoglycan interactions of chemokine CXCL8 regulate tissue-specific neutrophil recruitment. *J. Leukoc. Biol.* **2012**, *91*, 259–265. [CrossRef] [PubMed]

72. Dyer, D.P.; Migliorini, E.; Salanga, C.L.; Thakar, D.; Handel, T.M.; Richter, R.P. Differential structural remodelling of heparan sulfate by chemokines: The role of chemokine oligomerization. *Open Biol.* **2017**, *7*, 160286. [CrossRef] [PubMed]

73. Dyer, D.P.; Salanga, C.L.; Volkman, B.F.; Kawamura, T.; Handel, T.M. The dependence of chemokine-glycosaminoglycan interactions on chemokine oligomerization. *Glycobiology.* **2016**, *26*, 312–326. [CrossRef] [PubMed]

74. Egesten, A.; Eliasson, M.; Johansson, H.M.; Olin, A.I.; Morgelin, M.; Mueller, A.; Pease, J.E.; Frick, I.M.; Bjorck, L. The CXC chemokine MIG/CXCL9 is important in innate immunity against Streptococcus pyogenes. *J. Infect. Dis.* **2007**, *195*, 684–693. [CrossRef] [PubMed]

75. Swaminathan, G.J.; Holloway, D.E.; Colvin, R.A.; Campanella, G.K.; Papageorgiou, A.C.; Luster, A.D.; Acharya, K.R. Crystal structures of oligomeric forms of the IP-10/CXCL10 chemokine. *Structure* **2003**, *11*, 521–532. [CrossRef]

76. Dufour, J.H.; Dziejman, M.; Liu, M.T.; Leung, J.H.; Lane, T.E.; Luster, A.D. IFN-γ-inducible protein 10 (IP-10; CXCL10)-deficient mice reveal a role for IP-10 in effector T cell generation and trafficking. *J. Immunol.* **2002**, *168*, 3195–3204. [CrossRef] [PubMed]

77. Casrouge, A.; Decalf, J.; Ahloulay, M.; Lababidi, C.; Mansour, H.; Vallet-Pichard, A.; Mallet, V.; Mottez, E.; Mapes, J.; Fontanet, A.; et al. Evidence for an antagonist form of the chemokine CXCL10 in patients chronically infected with HCV. *J. Clin. Investig.* **2011**, *121*, 308–317. [CrossRef] [PubMed]

78. Decalf, J.; Tarbell, K.V.; Casrouge, A.; Price, J.D.; Linder, G.; Mottez, E.; Sultanik, P.; Mallet, V.; Pol, S.; Duffy, D.; et al. Inhibition of DPP4 activity in humans establishes its in vivo role in CXCL10 post-translational modification: Prospective placebo-controlled clinical studies. *EMBO Mol. Med.* **2016**, *8*, 679–683. [CrossRef] [PubMed]

79. Campanella, G.S.; Lee, E.M.; Sun, J.; Luster, A.D. CXCR3 and heparin binding sites of the chemokine IP-10 (CXCL10). *J. Biol. Chem.* **2003**, *278*, 17066–17074. [CrossRef] [PubMed]

80. Loos, T.; Mortier, A.; Gouwy, M.; Ronsse, I.; Put, W.; Lenaerts, J.P.; Van Damme, J.; Proost, P. Citrullination of CXCL10 and CXCL11 by peptidylarginine deiminase: A naturally occurring posttranslational modification of chemokines and new dimension of immunoregulation. *Blood* **2008**, *112*, 2648–2656. [CrossRef] [PubMed]

81. Kuschert, G.S.; Coulin, F.; Power, C.A.; Proudfoot, A.E.; Hubbard, R.E.; Hoogewerf, A.J.; Wells, T.N. Glycosaminoglycans interact selectively with chemokines and modulate receptor binding and cellular responses. *Biochemistry* **1999**, *38*, 12959–12968. [CrossRef] [PubMed]

82. Gorrell, M.D.; Gysbers, V.; McCaughan, G.W. CD26: A multifunctional integral membrane and secreted protein of activated lymphocytes. *Scand. J. Immunol.* **2001**, *54*, 249–264. [CrossRef] [PubMed]

83. Waumans, Y.; Baerts, L.; Kehoe, K.; Lambeir, A.M.; De Meester, I. The Dipeptidyl Peptidase Family, Prolyl Oligopeptidase, and Prolyl Carboxypeptidase in the Immune System and Inflammatory Disease, Including Atherosclerosis. *Front. Immunol.* **2015**, *6*, 387. [CrossRef] [PubMed]

84. Loos, T.; Mortier, A.; Proost, P. Chapter 1. Isolation, identification, and production of posttranslationally modified chemokines. *Methods Enzymol.* **2009**, *461*, 3–29. [PubMed]

85. De Meester, I.; Vanhoof, G.; Lambeir, A.M.; Scharpé, S. Use of immobilized adenosine deaminase for the rapid purification of native human CD26/dipeptidyl peptidase IV. *J. Immunol. Methods* **1996**, *189*, 99–105. [CrossRef]

86. Grynkiewicz, G.; Poenie, M.; Tsien, R.Y. A new generation of Ca^{2+} indicators with greatly improved fluorescence properties. *J. Biol. Chem.* **1985**, *260*, 3440–3450. [PubMed]

87. Boyden, S. The chemotactic effect of mixtures of antibody and antigen on polymorphonuclear leucocytes. *J. Exp. Med.* **1962**, *115*, 453–466. [CrossRef] [PubMed]

88. Janssens, R.; Mortier, A.; Boff, D.; Vanheule, V.; Gouwy, M.; Franck, C.; Larsen, O.; Rosenkilde, M.M.; Van Damme, J.; Amaral, F.A.; et al. Natural nitration of CXCL12 reduces its signaling capacity and chemotactic activity in vitro and abrogates intra-articular lymphocyte recruitment in vivo. *Oncotarget* **2016**, *7*, 62439–62459. [CrossRef] [PubMed]

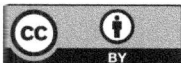

International Journal of
Molecular Sciences

MDPI

Article

The Effect of N-Terminal Cyclization on the Function of the HIV Entry Inhibitor 5P12-RANTES

Anna F. Nguyen, Megan S. Schill, Mike Jian and Patricia J. LiWang *

Molecular Cell Biology and the Health Sciences Research Institute, University of California Merced,
5200 North Lake Rd., Merced, CA 95343, USA; aankirskaia@ucmerced.edu (A.F.N.);
mschill@caltech.edu (M.S.S.); jian.mike2@gmail.com (M.J.)
* Correspondence: pliwang@ucmerced.edu; Tel.: +1-209-228-4568

Received: 1 July 2017; Accepted: 14 July 2017; Published: 20 July 2017

Abstract: Despite effective treatment for those living with Human Immunodeficiency Virus (HIV), there are still two million new infections each year. Protein-based HIV entry inhibitors, being highly effective and specific, could be used to protect people from initial infection. One of the most promising of these for clinical use is 5P12-RANTES, a variant of the chemokine RANTES/CCL5. The N-terminal amino acid of 5P12-RANTES is glutamine (Gln; called Q0), a residue that is prone to spontaneous cyclization when at the N-terminus of a protein. It is not known how this cyclization affects the potency of the inhibitor or whether cyclization is necessary for the function of the protein, although the N-terminal region of RANTES has been shown to be critical for receptor interactions, with even small changes having a large effect. We have studied the kinetics of cyclization of 5P12-RANTES as well as N-terminal variations of the protein that either produce an identical cyclized terminus (Glu0) or that cannot similarly cyclize (Asn0, Phe0, Ile0, and Leu0). We find that the half life for N-terminal cyclization of Gln is roughly 20 h at pH 7.3 at 37 °C. However, our results show that cyclization is not necessary for the potency of this protein and that several replacement terminal amino acids produce nearly-equally potent HIV inhibitors while remaining CC chemokine receptor 5 (CCR5) antagonists. This work has ramifications for the production of active 5P12-RANTES for use in the clinic, while also opening the possibility of developing other inhibitors by varying the N-terminus of the protein.

Keywords: 5P12-RANTES; Chemokine (C-C Motif) Ligand 5 (CCL5); HIV entry inhibition; N-terminal cyclization; chemokine

1. Introduction

HIV, the virus that causes acquired immune deficiency syndrome (AIDS), infects about 2 million people each year, mostly throughout the developing world [1]. While effective treatments are available, particularly in economically advanced countries, there is no cure, and prevention remains a critical issue. A major strategy to prevent HIV infection is the development of microbicides, substances that could be used topically to prevent the sexual spread of HIV. Ideally, a microbicide would be active and remain functional in both the vaginal compartment (pH 4.0–4.5) [2] and the rectal compartment (pH 7) [3].

One of the most promising proteins under consideration for use as a microbicide is 5P12-RANTES. This protein was developed using random mutagenesis at the N-terminus of the chemokine RANTES (also called Chemokine (C-C Motif) Ligand 5 (CCL5)) [4], itself a weak HIV inhibitor. 5P12-RANTES binds tightly to the chemokine receptor CCR5 (CC chemokine receptor 5), which is the major co-receptor used by HIV to gain entry to the cell during initial infection [5,6]. 5P12-RANTES has also been shown to be stable at biological temperatures and in the presence of relevant bodily fluids [7], and it was fully protective as a topical microbicide when tested in macaques [8]. More recently, it has been reported as being under clinical development [9].

The N-terminal region of chemokines are known to be critical for function, with slight alterations or truncations known to cause significant differences in their interaction with their respective receptors [10–13]. For example, the simple addition of an N-terminal methionine caused RANTES/CCL5 to act as a CCR5 antagonist rather than an agonist [10], and truncation of the N-terminal residues of chemokines likewise led to proteins with the ability to bind but not activate CCR5 [12,14]. In developing chemokines as HIV inhibitors, chemically modifying the N-terminus of RANTES was found to be particularly effective. For example, one potent analog was AOP-RANTES, in which an organic extension replaced the first residue of RANTES [15]. This modified protein was not only a potent HIV inhibitor, but it also prevented chemotaxis of human monocytes; this is a valuable property because it is important to avoid bringing immune cells to a site where they could potentially be infected with HIV [16]. Researchers then used this design as a scaffold and tested various synthetic modifications to the N-terminus, resulting in the discovery of the even more potent PSC-RANTES; both AOP-RANTES and PSC-RANTES induce internalization of the CCR5 receptor [17,18]. However, neither of these variants could be produced recombinantly. To circumvent this issue, Hartley et al. developed a random mutagenesis/phage display technique with changes to the N-terminal resides of RANTES that led first to the production of P2-RANTES [13] and then to the discovery of 5P12-RANTES [4]. The mutations that produced 5P12-RANTES were focused on just the first ten amino acids in RANTES and showed over two orders of magnitude variation in inhibitory potency [4].

Interestingly, 5P12-RANTES as well as the other resultant inhibitors carried forward from the study, such as 5P14-RANTES and 6P4-RANTES, have a glutamine as the first amino acid (termed "Q0" because this is an additional amino acid added to the wild type RANTES sequence). N-terminal glutamines are able to chemically cyclize [19–21] (Figure 1), leading to possible heterogeneity in the protein product with two forms (cyclized and uncyclized) that are significantly different in charge and other chemical properties. This has also been a topic of significance in the development of antibodies as therapeutics, where N-terminal Gln and Glu are both common [19,22–24]. The increasing use of antibodies as therapeutics has led to several reports about the importance of cyclization of both Gln and Glu at the N-terminus of these and other clinically-relevant proteins [20,23–25].

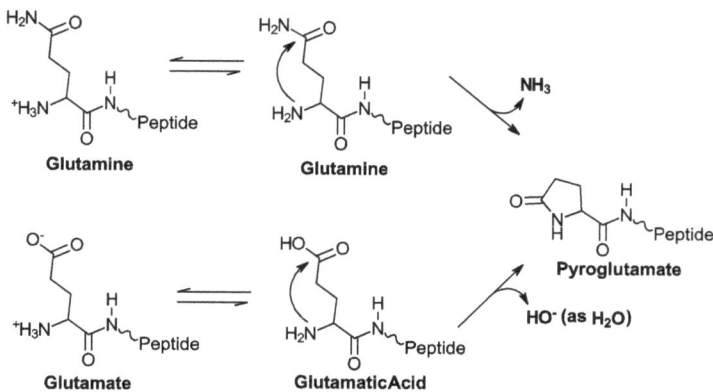

Figure 1. Cyclization reactions of N-terminal glutamine and glutamate residues in a polypeptide chain. Conditions such as pH are important factors in the rate of cyclization; low pH leads to a higher proportion of a good leaving group, while high pH leads to better nucleophilicity in the attacking amino group [22,26].

While it has been recognized that 5P12-RANTES is likely to undergo N-terminal cyclization, the functional impact of this modification at such a critical region of the protein, as well as the details of the kinetics of cyclization, have not yet been reported [4,9,27]. Such information is critical both from the standpoint of understanding the mechanism of HIV inhibition and from the standpoint of identifying all forms of a molecule that may enter the clinic.

Here, we report a study on the N-terminal cyclization of 5P12-RANTES, including the effect of cyclization on CCR5 receptor function and HIV inhibition in two representative strains, as well as the rate of cyclization under various conditions. We also show the effect of mutating the N-terminal "QC" to other amino acids, such as the residue glutamate, which cyclizes to form an identical molecule to "wild type" cyclized 5P12-RANTES.

2. Results

2.1. 5P12-RANTES N-Terminal Cyclization

^{15}N labeled 5P12-RANTES was produced from *E. coli* with an N-terminal fusion partner to disallow N-terminal cyclization of Q0 for most of the purification process. Cleavage of the fusion tag by enterokinase was carried out at pH 7.4 at 4 °C followed by reversed-phase chromatography and lyophilization of the pure protein so that it could be stored as dry powder to inhibit cyclization. The purified 5P12-RANTES was solubilized at pH 2.8 for Nuclear Magnetic Resonance (NMR) spectroscopy, where it was observed that less than 5% of the protein had undergone N-terminal cyclization during the purification process (Figure 2).

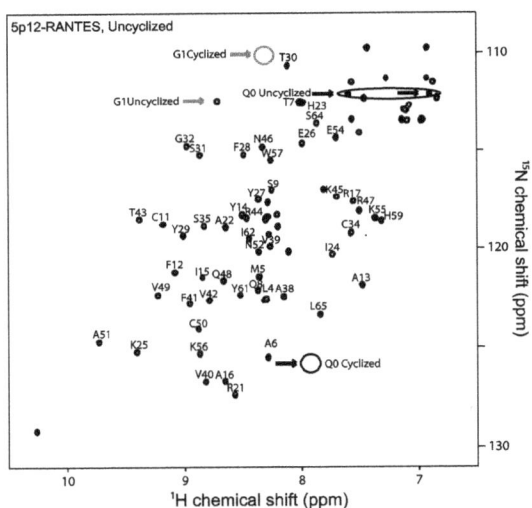

Figure 2. Heteronuclear single quantum coherence (HSQC) nuclear magnetic resonance (NMR) spectrum of ^{15}N-labeled 5P12-RANTES directly after dissolution in pH 2.8 20 mM sodium phosphate buffer at 25 °C. Little or no cyclization is observed at this time. Cyclization of Q0 results in a shift of the G1 peak (labeled, grey arrows; cyclized position circled) which can be used to quantify the amount of cyclized 5P12-RANTES in solution. Cyclization also results in loss of Q0 side chain amide peaks (black arrows, circled) and appearance of cyclized Q0 lactam peak (black arrow, circle). Chemical shift assignments from Wiktor et al. [28]; no assignments are shown for region near E66, where these authors used a variant. Also not shown are side chain assignments for W57 and Asn/Gln (except for the relevant N-terminal side chain amide). Percent cyclization was determined by peak height at lower contour level than shown.

The cyclization rate of the N-terminal Gln of 5P12-RANTES at 37 °C was monitored by NMR at pH 7.3 and at pH 2.8 as shown in Figure 3B. A clear indication of cyclization at the N-terminal "Q0" position is the peak position of the backbone amide of glycine 1. This peak shows a clear shift from 8.7 ppm (^{1}H) and 112.5 ppm (^{15}N) to 8.4 ppm (^{1}H) and 109.5 ppm (^{15}N) as its neighboring side chain cyclizes [9] (Figures 2 and 3A). Concomitantly, the lactam peak of the cyclized pyroglutamate (derived from Q0) is observed to grow in at 7.9 ppm (^{1}H) and 125.5 ppm (^{15}N) upon cyclization. At pH 7.3 these peaks are not discernable in an HSQC spectrum, likely due to faster amide exchange. Therefore NMR analysis for the pH 7.3 incubation was carried out at pH 2.8.

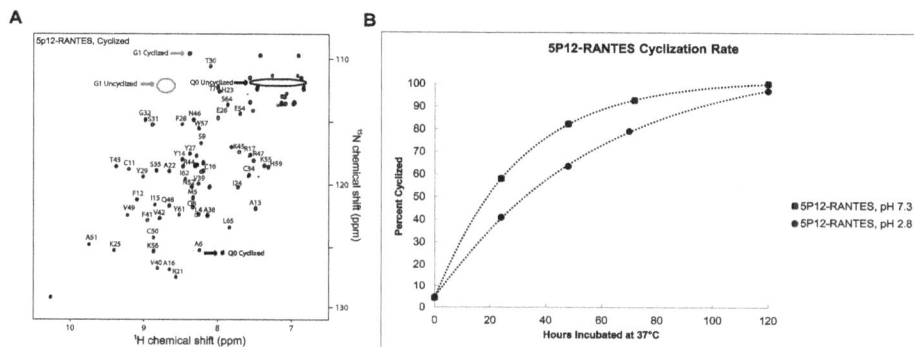

Figure 3. 5P12-RANTES cyclization. (**A**) HSQC spectrum of cyclized ^{15}N-labeled 5P12-RANTES after being incubated at 37 °C for 5 days at pH 2.8. NMR was performed in 20 mM sodium phosphate at pH 2.8, 25 °C. Cyclization results in a shift of the G1 residue (grey arrows; G1 resonances denoted by gray arrows and circles), as well as an appearance of the N-terminal pyroglutamate residue (black arrow; Q0 resonances denoted with black circles and arrows) as well as loss of Q0 amide side chain peaks (black arrow, circled). Assignments are not shown for certain areas as described in Figure 2. (**B**) Cyclization over time of 5P12-RANTES at pH = 7.3 and pH = 2.8, incubated at 37 °C. Amount of cyclization was determined by obtaining peak heights of the amide of G1 when the N-terminus of the protein (Gln0) was cyclized and uncyclized using NMRPipe, and dividing the cyclized peak height by the total of all G1 (cyclized and uncyclized) peak heights.

In order to monitor cyclization at pH 7.3, lyophilized powder of 5P12-RANTES was dissolved at pH 7.3, incubated at 37 °C, and aliquots were removed at various time intervals. These aliquots were lyophilized to halt further cyclization. Then immediately prior to measurement by NMR, each dry aliquot was dissolved in pH = 2.8 buffer. In this way, incubation occurred at neutral pH, but spectroscopy occurred at low pH where key peaks were visible in the spectrum, chemokine solubility is optimal, and on a time scale that would not allow significant further cyclization.

As shown in Figure 3B, Q0 cyclization of 5P12-RANTES at pH 7.3 (37 °C) exhibits a half life of about 20 h. When cyclization is measured with constant incubation at pH 2.8 (37 °C), the half life is about 33 h, with cyclization essentially complete at 120 h.

2.2. 5P12-Q0E Also Cyclizes to Produce Mature 5P12-RANTES

To further investigate the properties of the N-terminus of 5P12-RANTES, we produced 5P12-RANTES-Q0E, in which the Gln is replaced by the amino acid Glutamate, which is also capable of cyclizing when placed at the amino terminus of a protein. While the cyclization is expected to be slower due to the poor leaving group on the Glu side chain, the product of cyclization should be identical to cyclized Q0. This variant allows further study of cyclization and also provides an alternate route to the presumed mature product i.e., fully cyclized 5P12-RANTES containing a pyroglutamate at the N-terminus.

Isotopically labeled [15]N 5P12-RANTES-Q0E was produced with an N-terminal fusion protein to disallow cyclization until cleavage near the end of purification, in a similar manner as with 5P12-RANTES. Initial solubilization of purified, lyophilized protein followed by NMR revealed that less than 4% of this protein was cyclized during purification (Figure 4A). Incubation of [15]N 5P12-RANTES-Q0E was carried out at pH 7.3 and pH 2.8 and monitored by NMR as described above. As shown in Figure 4B, the reaction to produce N-terminal pyroglutamate takes many days, with a half-life of greater than 150 days at pH 7.3 and a half-life of about 60 days at pH 2.8. This faster cyclization at low pH is expected due to improvement of the leaving group upon protonation. When cyclization is complete, the spectrum is identical to cyclized "wild type" 5P12-RANTES as expected (Figure S1).

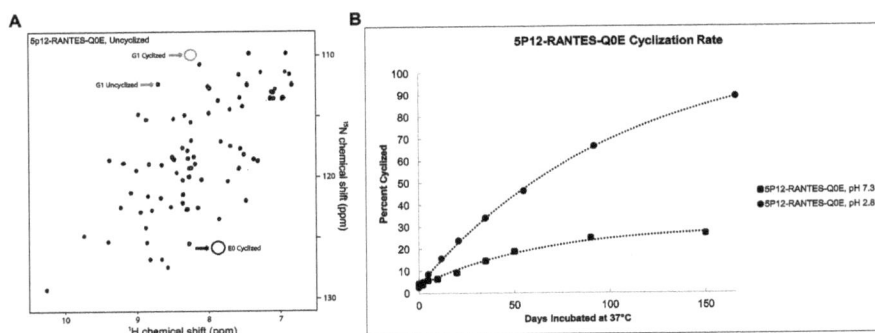

Figure 4. 5P12-RANTES-Q0E. (**A**) HSQC spectrum of ^{15}N-labeled 5P12-RANTES-Q0E. The spectrum is identical to that of 5P12-RANTES except for a slight G1 shift (grey arrows) and a loss of two side chain amide peaks corresponding to the Gln-0 NH_2 group and no cyclized peak (black arrow, circled, lower right). Cyclization results in a shift of the G1 residue (labeled) which can be used to quantify the amount of cyclized 5P12-RANTES-Q0E in solution. Spectrum was measured in 20 mM sodium phosphate, pH 2.8, 25 °C. Percent cyclization was measured by peak height at lower contour levels than shown. (**B**) Cyclization over time of 5P12-RANTES-Q0E in pH = 7.3 and pH = 2.8, incubated at 37 °C. Spectrum at the 150 day time point shows folded protein, with some degradation (Figure S2).

2.3. High Potency HIV Inhibition Does Not Require N-terminal Cyclization or N-Terminal Glutamine

To determine the relative importance of N-terminal cyclization on the anti-HIV potency of 5P12-RANTES, single round viral assays were carried out using two representative strains of HIV. Since these assays necessarily use mammalian cells, conditions are constrained to physiological pH (pH 7.3). In these assays, cells are aliquoted into 96 well plates and allowed to divide overnight. Various dilutions of inhibitor (freshly made from lyophilized powder and minimally cyclized) were incubated with the cells for 30 min. Virus was then added and the cells incubated overnight. Medium containing virus and inhibitor were removed the following day as medium was changed and cells were allowed to grow an additional two days with fresh medium. Infection was monitored with a standard β-galactosidase readout as described in Methods. The total time the inhibitor is in solution and able to cyclize is 20 h at pH 7.3 in this assay.

As shown in Table 1, "immature" 5P12-RANTES that was essentially uncyclized at the start of the assay gave an IC_{50} of 1.51 ± 0.10 nM for strain PVO.4 and 1.61 ± 0.12 nM for strain ZM53. Given the length of the assay, it is estimated that roughly 50% of the immature 5P12-RANTES did cyclize during the course of the assay. However, virus entry has been demonstrated to take place over the course of minutes [29], so a significant amount of virus-cell interaction could be expected before the inhibitor was significantly cyclized. "Matured" 5P12-RANTES (that was incubated for 36 h, pH 2.8 at 50 °C to allow full cyclization prior to use in the HIV assay) showed essentially equal potency, with an IC_{50} of 1.27 ± 0.10 nM for PVO.4 and 1.46 ± 0.15 nM for ZM53.

Table 1. IC_{50} values of 5P12-RANTES variants (in nM) against a Clade B HIV viral strain (PVO.4) or Clade C viral strain (ZM53) in single-round pseudoviral infection assays. Assays were performed in triplicate and repeated three times.

IC_{50} Values of 5P12 Variants		
5P12 Variant	**PVO.4 (nM)**	**ZM53 (nM)**
5P12-RANTES Uncyclized	1.51 ± 0.10	1.61 ± 0.12
5P12-RANTES Cyclized	1.27 ± 0.10	1.46 ± 0.15
5P12-RANTES-Q0E Uncyclized	6.30 ± 0.14	4.04 ± 0.29
5P12-RANTES-Q0E Cyclized	1.09 ± 0.06	1.23 ± 0.09
5P12-RANTES-Q0N	2.20 ± 0.33	1.31 ± 0.19
5P12-RANTES-Q0I	1.21 ± 0.24	1.43 ± 0.11
5P12-RANTES-Q0F	1.26 ± 0.19	1.84 ± 0.12
5P12-RANTES-Q0L	1.31 ± 0.12	1.45 ± 0.15

The mutant 5P12-Q0E showed somewhat poorer inhibition in its immature, uncyclized form, with an IC_{50} of 6.30 ± 0.14 nM for PVO.4. This variant has a negatively charged glutamate at position 0, a part of the protein that is presumed to interact with the receptor CCR5 in or near the hydrophobic membrane of the cell [30]. Given the half-life of cyclization described above, it is expected that during the assay, under 5% of this protein would be cyclized. When the matured, cyclized 5P12-Q0E (prepared as described in Methods) was used in these inhibition assays, its potency was essentially identical to wild type, cyclized 5P12-RANTES (Table 1), as expected for these two now-identical proteins.

As a control for uncyclized Q0 ("wild type") 5P12-RANTES, we produced and purified 5P12-Q0N, in which the Gln is replaced by Asn. This amino acid is identical to Gln but has a shorter side chain so cannot similarly cyclize. As expected, the NMR spectrum of ^{15}N 5P12-Q0N shows no indication of a cyclized N-terminus (Figure S3A). In HIV inhibition assays, this protein shows high potency, with an IC_{50} of 2.20 ± 0.33 nM against PVO.4 and 1.31 ± 0.19 against ZM53, essentially the same as for the wild type (Q0) protein, indicating that the presence of a cyclized pyroglutamate is not necessary for the anti-HIV activity of 5P12-RANTES.

Since both uncyclized and cyclized 5P12 variants were shown to be potent inhibitors of HIV, we made other mutations at the Q0 position of the protein to determine the effect of changes at this position on HIV inhibitory ability. For these experiments the Gln0 was changed to Phe, Ile, and Leu. Each of these variants was expressed and shown to be folded by NMR (Figure S3B–D); none of these side chains are expected to undergo significant chemical transformation upon incubation. As shown in Table 1, each variant was highly potent and very similar in activity to 5P12-RANTES, with IC_{50} values ranging from 1.21 ± 0.24 nM to 1.31 ± 0.13 nM (PVO.4) and 1.43 ± 0.11 nM to 1.84 ± 0.12 nM (ZM53).

2.4. The Effect of the N-Terminal Amino Acid and Its State of Cyclization on Activation of CC Chemokine Receptor 5 (CCR5)

5P12-RANTES has been reported to be an antagonist of CCR5, not inducing calcium mobilization; lack of calcium mobilization is a property that is favorable (and likely necessary) in the context of therapeutic HIV inhibition. To determine whether the cyclization of Q0 or the placement of other amino acids at the N-terminus affect activation of CCR5, calcium flux assays were carried out on Chinese Hamster Ovary (CHO) cells expressing CCR5, $G_{\alpha 16}$, and apo-aequorin, a calcium-responsive protein. As shown in Figure 5, neither N-terminally cyclized nor N-terminally uncyclized 5P12-RANTES (i.e., having Q0) caused a calcium flux until concentrations reached 500 nM, while wild type RANTES/CCL5 showed calcium release at low nM concentrations as expected. Further, the N-terminal variants of 5P12-RANTES (-Q0E cyclized and uncyclized, -Q0N, -Q0I, -Q0F, -Q0L) also exhibited no ability to cause the release of calcium until reaching 500 nM concentration (Figure 5). These results were further confirmed with a fluorescence assay using human HeLa-P5L cells, which showed similar results (Table S1).

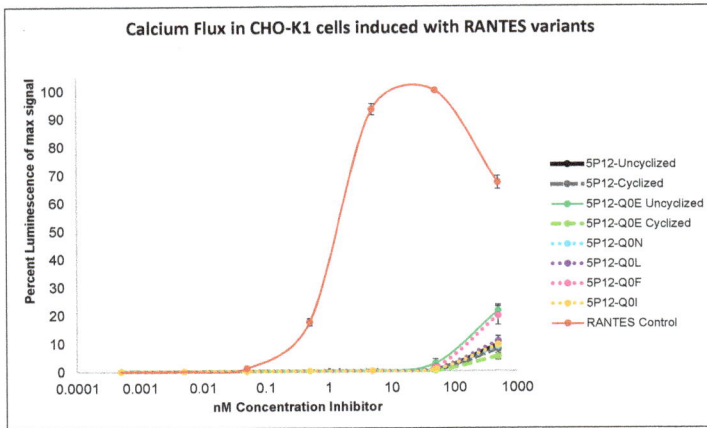

Figure 5. Calcium Flux Assay. CHO-K1 cells expressing CCR5 on their surface were incubated with various concentration of chemokine (either wild type RANTES/CCL5 or a 5P12-RANTES variant) and monitored for luminescence of aequorin upon calcium release. At very high "supraoptimal" concentrations, RANTES/CCL5 exhibits aggregation with alternate effects on receptor activation [31].

3. Discussion

There are at least four highly potent classes of protein HIV entry inhibitors, each with great potential for clinical use in preventing viral infection. The first of these is broadly neutralizing antibodies [32], which bind gp120 or gp41 and show great promise, particularly when used in combination [33], but are generally produced in eukaryotic cells. [34,35] A second class of entry inhibitors includes lectins, which bind to glycosylation sites on HIV env and include the highly studied Griffithsin and Cyanovirin-N, both of which are being evaluated for potential clinical trials [36,37]. A third group are variations of peptides that are derived from HIV gp41, called fusion inhibitors [38], that are particularly effective in combination with other inhibitors [39,40].

Finally, in the fourth group, certain chemokine variants have been shown to inhibit entry of HIV due to their ability to bind the chemokine receptors that act as co-receptors for HIV. The most effective chemokine variants have been derived from the chemokine RANTES (Figure S4), originally by using synthetic modification at the N-terminus to produce PSC-RANTES, for example, which was shown to be effective in protecting macaques from infection [8,18]. Structural studies have shown that the N-terminus of the chemokine is likely to interact with the receptor at or near the cell membrane [41], and work on synthetic RANTES variants supported these results, showing that hydrophobic groups at the N-terminus were more effective at interacting with the CCR5 receptor than similar variants with hydrophilic modifications [18].

More recently, random mutagenesis/phage display was employed to select for RANTES N-terminal variants with enhanced ability to inhibit HIV. This work first led to P2-RANTES [13], which was used as a starting point for later selection of a series of even more highly potent, fully-recombinant RANTES variants [4]. This latter set of inhibitors included 5P12-RANTES, 5P14-RANTES, and 6P4-RANTES, each of which has slight differences in its 10 N-terminal amino acids, leading to differing ability to activate and/or internalize the CCR5 receptor, and again, providing evidence that the N-terminal region of the chemokine is critical in interacting with the receptor and affecting its conformational changes in the membrane. The most clinically promising of these inhibitors is generally considered to be 5P12-RANTES, due to its combination of high potency and inability to induce downstream signaling or internalization of the CCR5 receptor. Therefore, this inhibitor can inhibit HIV without activating the immune system or mediating an influx of immune cells (and by virtue of being a CCR5 antagonist, may actually reduce immune activity).

5P12-RANTES has been shown to have many properties necessary for use as a topical microbicide, including stability at elevated temperatures, a range of pH conditions, and within environments containing bodily fluids [7,42]. This inhibitor demonstrated the ability to prevent infection in macaques [8] and has shown effectiveness against many strains of HIV with little or no indication that HIV is able to mutate to lose sensitivity to it [43]. Therefore, this protein is a top candidate for a clinical HIV microbicide.

A critical issue for any protein moving to the clinic is a clear understanding of its function, as well as characterization of any variation in its chemical or structural composition. For instance, antibodies often have Glu or Gln as N-terminal residues, and the growing importance of antibodies as therapeutics has led to the study of these residues' propensity to cyclize [19,22–24]. 5P12-RANTES has an N-terminal Gln (referred to as Q0), an amino acid that is known to cyclize when at this position in a protein [19,44], leading to an extra cyclization step during clinical-grade production [27]. However, a detailed study of the rate and functional effect of this cyclization in 5P12-RANTES has not been reported.

Wiktor et al. have provided NMR chemical shift assignments and the structure of a non-aggregating variant of 5P12-RANTES [9,28]. This group estimated a half-life for Q0 cyclization as approximately two days at pH 3.8, although the sample was refrigerated during part of this time, since the primary goal of the work was not to study N-terminal cyclization but rather to investigate the overall structure of the protein and its interactions with detergents.

We have shown here that the N-terminus of 5P12-RANTES cyclizes to form pyroglutamate with a half-life of roughly 20 h at pH 7.3 and 33 h at pH 2.8 (37 °C). This indicates that the protein, if purified without regard to cyclization, would still cyclize on the time scale of a typical HIV assay (20 h at pH 7.3), leaving inconclusive whether high potency is reserved for only the cyclized form. However, when Q0 is replaced with N, such cyclization is not observed, and this variant (5P12-Q0N) shows essentially identical HIV-inhibitory ability as 5P12-RANTES, indicating that a cyclized N-terminus is not important for the function of this inhibitor. Other hydrophobic N-terminal variants, -Q0I, -Q0F, -Q0L, also show very high potency, nearly equivalent to 5P12-RANTES (Table 1).

To further investigate the importance of the cyclized form of 5P12-RANTES, we made 5P12-Q0E, in which glutamate replaces glutamine at the N-terminus of the protein. Glutamate can also be expected to cyclize and form the same pyroglutamate as is formed by glutamine (Figure 1), although a poorer leaving group is expected to cause this reaction to be slower. Upon cyclization, this variant will yield a product that is identical to cyclized 5P12-RANTES.

It was observed that at 37 °C, 5P12-Q0E cyclization occurs with a half-life of well over 150 days at pH 7.3 (with still only 25% cyclization observed at 150 days) and roughly 60 days at pH 2.8. The fully cyclized version of the variant (prepared by prolonged incubation at higher temperatures) was tested against two strains of HIV and shown to be essentially identical in function to cyclized 5P12-RANTES containing the original Q0. Interestingly, the uncyclized 5P12-Q0E also showed good inhibitory properties despite the timescale of the assay not allowing significant cyclization and therefore leaving a negatively charged Glu at the terminus of the protein throughout the assay (Table 1).

These results clarify the conditions necessary to cyclize 5P12-RANTES if it were to be used clinically in a homogeneous form. They further show that not only is cyclization not necessary for anti-HIV activity, but also that a variety of amino acids at the N-terminus would be expected to provide protection against HIV infection. This allows a greater range of amino acid sequences as potential inhibitors, which could lead to flexibility in determining which sequence most easily results in production of the large amounts of protein required for clinical use.

In conclusion, 5P12-RANTES is a highly potent HIV inhibitor that could be used as a microbicide to prevent HIV infection. However, chemical cyclization of its N-terminal glutamine causes this protein to exist as a heterogeneous mixture when expressed recombinantly. We show that the protein is still a highly effective inhibitor of HIV in both its cyclized and uncyclized forms and have determined the rate of cyclization under various conditions, with relevance both for the manufacture and clinical use of this protein. We also show that several amino acids are suitable replacements for the N-terminal glutamine if changes in the sequence are necessary or desirable.

4. Materials and Methods

4.1. Protein Purification

In brief, the following method was used (with the exception of wild type RANTES/CCL5, which required some differences as noted): Plasmids were transformed into *Escherichia coli* BL21 (DE3) (Novagen) competent cells and expressed in minimal media with $^{15}NH_4Cl$ as the sole nitrogen source. Protein production was induced with the addition of isopropyl β-d-1-thiogalactopyranoside (IPTG) and incubated with shaking at 22 °C for 20 h (wild type RANTES/CCL5 was induced with IPTG followed by shaking at 37 °C for 6 h). The cell pellet was resuspended in 6 M guanidine hydrochloride, 200 mM NaCl, 10 mM benzamidine, and 50 mM Tris (pH 8.0) and was then disrupted by French press and then centrifuged at $27,000 \times g$ for 1 h. The soluble portion was loaded onto a nickel chelating column (Qiagen, Hilden, Germany) equilibrated with the resuspension buffer. Proteins were eluted from the column using a pH gradient with 6 M guanidine hydrochloride, 200 mM NaCl, and 60 mM NaOAc (pH 4) followed by addition of 10 mM β-mercaptoethanol with stirring for one hour at room temperature. The proteins were then refolded by dropwise addition to $10\times$ volume of refolding buffer (550 mM L-Arginine Hydrochloride, 200 mM NaCl, 1 mM EDTA, 1 mM reduced glutathione (GSH), 0.1 mM oxidized glutathione (GSSG), 50 mM Tris, pH 8), and then allowed to stir overnight at 4 °C. The solution was dialyzed twice into 4 liters 200 mM NaCl, 2 mM $CaCl_2$, 20 m Tris, pH 7.4 buffer at 4 °C (into 4 L of 200 mM NaCl, 20 mM Tris pH 8 for wild type RANTES).

To cleave fusion tags from the purified protein, the samples were incubated for 24 h with 650 nM of the protease enterokinase (5P12-RANTES-Q0E required 3 days at a 2 µM; 100 nM ULP-1/SUMC protease was used to cleave wild type RANTES/CCL5; protease purification described below) The protein solution was then centrifuged to remove precipitated material and added onto a second nickel chelating column (Qiagen, Hilden, Germany), with unbound eluate (containing the cleaved 5P12-RANTES or its variants) being collected. (This second nickel column is not necessary for wild type RANTES/CCL5 purification). The samples were then dialyzed and purified on a C_4 reversed-phase chromatography column (Vydac, Hesperia, CA, USA), using an acetonitrile gradient. Wild type RANTES/CCL5 was also purified with the C_4 column, allowing separation from the SUMO tag. Overall, samples were near neutral pH for about a day during proteolytic cleavage (3 days for 5P12-Q0E due to slow cleavage) and a day for dialysis to prepare conditions for the C4 column, during which time N-terminal cyclization was possible. However, dialysis was carried out at 4 °C to minimize this reaction, and as noted in Results, little cyclization was observed after this point. The fractions were analyzed on an SDS-PAGE gel to confirm purity and then lyophilized in a Labconco freeze-dry system

N-terminally cyclized proteins used for functional assays (below) were prepared as follows: purified and lyophilized 5P12-RANTES was incubated for 36 h at 50 °C in 20 mM sodium phosphate buffer pH 2.8 to ensure 100% cyclization. 5P12-RANTES-Q0E was incubated for 50 days at 50 °C in 20 mM sodium phosphate buffer pH 2.8 to fully cyclize. Both samples were tested by NMR to confirm structural integrity and full cyclization (Figure S1).

The proteases used in these purifications were produced and purified in our laboratory as briefly described: Ubl-specific protease 1 or enterokinase protease were proteins were expressed in Luria Broth (LB) medium using a pET-28b vector and the cells were collected and French pressed. The ULP1 protease from the supernatant was purified using a nickel chelating column [45]. The enterokinase was found in the inclusion body and resuspended in 6 M guanidinium chloride buffer before being purified using a nickel chelating column. Enterokinase was then dialyzed in buffer to allow for refolding and tested for activity through self-cleavage of the fusion tag (manuscript in preparation).

4.2. Obtaining Rates of 5P12-RANTES and 5P12-RANTES-Q0E Cyclization

Samples incubated at pH 2.8 were prepared by adding ^{15}N-labeled lyophilized protein (5P12-RANTES or 5P12-RANTES-Q0E) to 20 mM sodium phosphate buffer with 10% D_2O and 5 µM DSS, resulting in a final pH = 2.8. Samples were placed into Shigemi NMR tubes (Shigemi, Inc., Allison Park, PA, USA) and incubated at 37 °C. NMR spectra were periodically measured at 37 °C for these samples (see below).

Samples at pH = 7.3 (the same pH as the pseudoviral assay medium) were prepared by adding ^{15}N-labeled lyophilized protein (5P12-RANTES or 5P12-RANTES-Q0E) to 5 mM Sodium Phosphate buffer with 0.02% sodium azide with a final pH of pH 7.3. Proteins were incubated at 37 °C, and samples were removed at selected time points, flash-frozen using liquid nitrogen, and lyophilized. Samples were then dissolved in 20 mM Phosphate buffer, 5% D_2O, and 5 µM DSS with a final pH = 2.8, and then measured by NMR at 25 °C (see below). All measurements for the pH of protein samples were taken with a micro electrode (Thermo Scientific/Orion).

4.3. NMR Spectroscopy

^{15}N-labeled lyophilized proteins were added into 20 mM Sodium Phosphate buffer with 10% D_2O and 5 µM 2,2-dimethyl-2-silapentane-5-sulfonic acid (DSS), with a final pH = 2.8 for all samples. Concentration of protein ranged from 30 uM to 80 uM. Sample preparation for cyclization time points are further described above. All NMR data were acquired on a four-channel 600 MHz Bruker Avance III spectrometer equipped with a GRASP II gradient accessory and a TCI cryoprobe with an actively shielded Z-gradient coil. Spectra were measured at 25 °C and 37 °C. The chemical shift was referenced relative to internal DSS [46]. The data were processed using NmrPipe [47] and analyzed using PIPP [48]. For HSQC spectra, sweep width = 8474.576 (^{1}H) and 1766.784 Hz (^{15}N), with 1280 points in ^{1}H and 128 * (256 total) points in ^{15}N.

4.4. Quantifying N-Terminal Cyclization

N-terminal cyclization of 5P12-RANTES or 5P12-RANTES-Q0E results in the appearance of an N-terminal lactam peak "Gln0" (Figures 1 and 2), as well as a shift in the Gly1 backbone amide peak. [9,28] (Figures 2 and 3A). Peak height comparison of the Gly1 amide when the N-terminus of the protein is cyclized versus uncyclized was used to estimate the percent of the protein cyclized in the sample as follows. NmrPipe was used to obtain peak heights for the Gly1 amide. The percent cyclization was obtained by dividing the height of the Gly1 peak when the N-term was cyclized by the sum of the heights of both cyclized and uncyclized Gly1 peaks in a spectrum. Similar values were obtained when using the peak height of the cyclized Q0 peak to measure the cyclized amount. Using peak volumes rather than height did not appreciably change the result.

4.5. Cell Lines and Viruses

HeLa-TZM-bl cells were obtained through the AIDS Research and Reference Reagent Program, Division of AIDS, National Institute of Allergy and Infectious Diseases (NIAID), National Institutes of Health; the HeLa-TZM-bl cell line was from John C. Kappes, Xiaoyun Wu, and Tranzyme Inc. 293FT cells were originally obtained from Invitrogen; CHO-K1 cells stably expressing CCR5, $G_{\alpha16}$, and apo-aequorin were a kind gift from Marc Parmentier from the Institute of Interdisciplinary Research of the Free University of Brussels (ULB) Medical School, Brussels, Belgium. HeLa-P5L Cells (a cell line stably expressing human receptor CD4 and CCR5) was a kind gift from M. Alizon (Cochin Institute, Paris, France) [49].

Viral plasmids used to create pseudovirus, including HIV-1 PVO clone 4 (SVPB11), ZM53M.PB12 (SVPC11), and pSG3$^{\Delta env}$, were obtained from the AIDS Research and Reference Reagent Program, Division of AIDS, NIAID, National Institutes of Health; PVO, clone 4 (SVPB11) was from David

Montefiori and Feng Gao [50]; ZM53M.PB12, SVPC11 was from Cynthia A. Derdeyn and Eric Hunter [51]; plasmid pSG3$^{\Delta env}$ was obtained from John C. Kappes and Xiaoyun Wu [51–53].

4.6. Single Round Pseudovirus Production

293FT cells were co-transfected with the pSG3$^{\Delta env}$ plasmid and an envelope plasmid using the XTreme Gene Transfection Reagent (Roche/Sigma-Aldrich, St. Louis, MO, USA). 48 h post-transfection, the supernatant was collected, centrifuged, and filtered with a 0.45-µm syringe filter. The viral stocks were then stored at −80 °C.

4.7. Single-Round Pseudoviral Assay

HeLa-TZM-bl cells were grown in culture media (10% Fetal Bovine Serum (FBS), penicillin/streptomycin, 25 mM HEPES in Dulbecco's Modified Eagle's Medium (DMEM)). 10^4 cells per well were seeded into a 96-well plate and allowed to incubate at 37 °C overnight. Media was then aspirated and replaced with 50 µL fresh media and allowed to incubate for 2 h. For preparation of inhibitor, a deep-well dish was made with varying concentrations of inhibitor diluted into phosphate-buffered saline (PBS) and mixed thoroughly. 20 µL of inhibitor from these dilutions (or 20 µL PBS for controls) were added to the TZM cell-containing wells, and the plate was rotated for 1 min to mix, before incubating for 30 min at 37 °C. 30 µL of single-round virus (described above) in media was then added (with non-viral media to the negative control) for a final volume of 100 µL/well and the plate was rotated for 1 min to mix. This "layering" method differs from other similar pseudoviral assays, where the inhibitor is mixed in-well. In our hands, mixing in-well leads to lower IC$_{50}$ (apparent better inhibition), but current experiments use "layering" addition to more closely mimic conditions under which a topical microbicide may be used. After 20 h, media was aspirated and replaced with 100 µL/well of fresh media. After 48 more hours, the media was aspirated and the cells were lysed using 30 µL/well of 0.5% NP-40 in PBS. Lysed cells were incubated at room temperature for 25 min. Substrate was added (30 µL/well; 8 mM chlorophenol red-β-D-galactopyranoside, 10 mM β mercaptoethanol, 20 mM KCl in PBS). The absorbance signals at wavelengths 570 and 630 nm were measured, and the 570:630 ratio for each well was calculated. All inhibitors were tested in triplicate repeated three times. The data were plotted using Microsoft Excel, and the IC$_{50}$ value was determined using a linear equation fitted between two data points surrounding 50% inhibition.

4.8. CCR5 Functional Assays in CHO-K1 Cells

The functional response of CCR5-expressing cells to RANTES and its variants was analyzed by measuring the luminescence of aequorin in response to release of Ca^{2+} as described previously [54]. Briefly, CHO-K1 cells were cultured in Ham's F12 medium (Corning, Cellgro, Manassas, VA, USA) supplemented with 10% FBS (Life Technologies, Carlsbad, CA, USA), 100 units/mL penicillin, 100 µg/mL streptomycin, and 400 µg/mL G418 (Life technologies, Carlsbad, CA, USA), then removed from plates by incubating at 37 °C with versene (Gibco, Gaithersburg, MD, USA), and then adding 3× volume Ca^{2+}- and Mg^{2+}-free DMEM (GE Healthcare, Little Chalfont, UK) to gently resuspend. The cells were gently pelleted for 4 min at 600× g and then resuspended at a density of 5 × 10^6 cells/mL using Ham's F12 Medium supplemented with 10% FBS, penicillin/streptomycin, 25 mM HEPES. Cells were then incubated in the dark at room temperature, for 1 h with 5 µM coelenterazine H (Promega, Madison, WI, USA). Cells were then diluted five-fold using Ham's F-12 medium, and 50 µL (50,000 cells) were added per well in a 96-well plate. 50 µL of each inhibitor diluted in Ham's F-12 medium were added to each well at varying concentrations. Luminescence was measured in 30 s increments using an Orion II microplate luminometer (Berthold Techniques, Bad Wildbad , Germany).

4.9. CCR5 Activity in HeLa-P5L

The functional response of CCR5-expressing cells HeLa-P5L to RANTES and its variants was analyzed by measuring the fluorescence using Fluo-4 dye (Thermo Scientific, Waltham, MA, USA) according to the manufacturer's suggested protocol. Briefly, HeLa-P5L cells were cultured in RPMI-1640 (Invitrogen, Carlsbad, CA, USA) supplemented with 10% FBS, and 100 units of penicillin and 0.1 mg/mL streptomycin. The expression of CCR5 was selectively expressed by adding zeocin (Invitrogen, Carlsbad, CA, USA) at 0.5 mg/mL. Cells were then removed from plates by incubating at 37 °C with versene solution (Gibco, Gaithersburg, MD, USA) and then gently resuspended with culture media. The cells were gently pelleted for 4 min at $600 \times g$ and then resuspended at a density of 1×10^6 cells/mL and 100 µL was plated onto 96 well plates with black polystyrene wells and a flat, micro-clear bottom (Greiner CELLSTAR). After a 15 h incubation at 37 °C, wells were washed three times with sterile Hank's buffered salt solution (HBSS), 137 mM NaCl, 5.4 mM KCl, 0.25 mM Na_2HPO_4, 0.44 mM KH_2PO_4, 1.3 mM $CaCl_2$, 1.0 mM $MgSO_4$, 1.0 mM $MgCl_2$, 10 mM glucose, 10 mM HEPES, with pH adjusted to 7.4 using 1N NaOH. 50 µL of 2 µM Fluo-4-AM Ester (Invitrogen, Carlsbad, CA, USA) in HBSS was added. The plate was incubated in the dark at room temperature for 30 min, then washed three times with HBSS supplemented with 2 mM Probenecid (Tocris, Bristol, UK), then left to incubate with 80 µL/well of HBSS with 2 mM Probenecid for 30 min at 37 °C. Fluorescence was measured after addition of 20 µL of chemokine variants in HBSS for a final chemokine concentration of 300 nM/well. Fluorescence reading was done on a Cytation 5 Cell Imaging Multi-Mode Reader (Biotek, Winooski, VT, USA) with an absorption/emission at 494/516 nm at 35 s, with wild type RANTES/CCL5 as a positive control and HBSS containing no inhibitor as a negative control.

Supplementary Materials: Supplementary materials can be found at www.mdpi.com/1422-0067/18/7/1575/s1.

Acknowledgments: The authors are grateful for the assistance of Li Zhang and Kathryn Fischer (University of California Merced). Funding was provided by NIH R01AI112011.

Author Contributions: Anna F. Nguyen and Patricia J. LiWang conceived and designed experiments and wrote the paper. Megan S. Schill and Mike Jian aided in DNA work and protein purification. All other experiments were performed by Anna F. Nguyen.

Conflicts of Interest: The authors declare no conflict of interest.

Abbreviations

HIV	Human Immunodeficiency Virus
AIDS	Acquired Immune Deficiency Syndrome
CCL5	Chemokine (C-C Motif) Ligand 5; also called RANTES
RANTES	Regulated on Activation, Normal T-cell Expressed and Secreted; also called CCL5
Gln/Q	Glutamine
Glu/E	Glutamate
Asn/N	Asparagine
Phe/F	Phenylalanine
Ile/I	Isoleucine
DMEM	Dulbecco's Modified Eagle's Medium
NMR	Nuclear Magnetic Resonance
HBSS	Hank's Buffered Salt Solution
FBS	Fetal Bovine Serum
HSQC	Heteronuclear Single Quantum Coherence
CHO	Chinese Hamster Ovary
IPTG	Isopropyl β-D-1-thiogalactopyranoside
TFA	Trifluoroacetic Acid

References

1. Global Report: Unaids UNAIDS Report on the Global AIDS Epidemic 2013. Available online: http://www.unaids.org/sites/default/files/media_asset/UNAIDS_Global_Report_2013_en_1.pdf (accessed on 17 July 2017).

2. Boskey, E.R.; Telsch, K.M.; Whaley, K.J.; Moench, T.R.; Cone, R.A. Acid production by vaginal flora in vitro is consistent with the rate and extent of vaginal acidification. *Infect. Immun.* **1999**, *67*, 5170–5175. [PubMed]
3. Evans, D.F.; Pye, G.; Bramley, R.; Clark, A.G.; Dyson, T.J.; Hardcastle, J.D. Measurement of gastrointestinal pH profiles in normal ambulant human subjects. *Gut* **1988**, *29*, 1035–1041. [CrossRef] [PubMed]
4. Gaertner, H.; Cerini, F.; Escola, J.-M.; Kuenzi, G.; Melotti, A.; Offord, R.; Ne Rossitto-Borlat, I.; Nedellec, R.; Salkowitz, J.; Gorochov, G.; et al. Highly potent, fully recombinant anti-HIV chemokines: Reengineering a low-cost microbicide. *Proc. Natl. Acad. Sci. USA* **2008**, *105*, 17706–17711. [CrossRef] [PubMed]
5. Suresh, P.; Wanchu, A. Chemokines and chemokine receptors in HIV infection: Role in pathogenesis and therapeutics. *J. Postgrad. Med.* **2006**, *52*, 210–217. [PubMed]
6. Dragic, T.; Litwin, V.; Allaway, G.P.; Martin, S.R.; Huang, Y.; Nagashima, K.A.; Cayanan, C.; Maddon, P.J.; Koup, R.A.; Moore, J.P.; et al. HIV-1 entry into CD4+ cells is mediated by the chemokine receptor CC-CKR-5. *Nature* **1996**, *381*, 667–673. [CrossRef] [PubMed]
7. Cerini, F.; Landay, A.; Gichinga, C.; Lederman, M.M.; Flyckt, R.; Starks, D.; Offord, R.E.; Xois, F.; Gal, L.; Hartley, O. Chemokine Analogues Show Suitable Stability for Development as Microbicides. *J. Acquir. Immune Defic. Syndr.* **2008**, *49*, 472–476. [CrossRef] [PubMed]
8. Veazey, R.S.; Ling, B.; Green, L.C.; Ribka, E.P.; Lifson, J.D.; Piatak, M.; Lederman, M.M.; Mosier, D.; Offord, R.; Hartley, O. Topically Applied Recombinant Chemokine Analogues Fully Protect Macaques from Vaginal Simian-Human Immunodeficiency Virus Challenge. *J. Infect. Dis.* **2009**, *199*, 1525–1527. [CrossRef] [PubMed]
9. Wiktor, M.; Hartley, O.; Grzesiek, S. Characterization of structure, dynamics, and detergent interactions of the anti-HIV chemokine variant 5P12-RANTES. *Biophys. J.* **2013**. [CrossRef] [PubMed]
10. Proudfoot, A.E.I.; Power, C.A.; Hoogewerf, A.J.; Montjovent, M.O.; Borlat, F.; Offord, R.E.; Wells, T.N.C. Extension of recombinant human RANTES by the retention of the initiating methionine produces a potent antagonist. *J. Biol. Chem.* **1996**, *271*, 2599–2603. [CrossRef] [PubMed]
11. Laurence, J.S.; Blanpain, C.; De Leener, A.; Parmentier, M.; LiWang, P.J. Importance of basic residues and quaternary structure in the function of MIP-1β: CCR5 binding and cell surface sugar interactions. *Biochemistry* **2001**, *40*, 4990–4999. [CrossRef] [PubMed]
12. Laurence, J.S.; LiWang, A.C.; LiWang, P.J. Effect of N-terminal truncation and solution conditions on chemokine dimer stability: Nuclear magnetic resonance structural analysis of macrophage inflammatory protein 1β mutants. *Biochemistry* **1998**, *37*, 9346–9354. [CrossRef] [PubMed]
13. Hartley, O.; Dorgham, K.; Perez-Bercoff, D.; Cerini, F.; Heimann, A.; Gaertner, H.; Offord, R.E.; Pancino, G.; Debré, P.; Gorochov, G. Human Immunodeficiency Virus Type 1 Entry Inhibitors Selected on Living Cells from a Library of Phage Chemokines. *J. Virol.* **2003**, *77*, 6637–6644. [CrossRef] [PubMed]
14. Arenzana-Seisdedos, F.; Virelizier, J.-L.; Rousset, D.; Clark-Lewis, I.; Loetscher, P.; Moser, B.; Baggiolini, M. HIV blocked by chemokine antagonist. *Nature* **1996**, *383*, 400. [CrossRef] [PubMed]
15. Simmons, G.; Clapham, P.R.; Picard, L.; Offord, R.E.; Rosenkilde, M.M.; Schwartz, T.W.; Buser, R.; Wells, T.N.; Proudfoot, A.E.; Cocchi, F.; et al. Potent inhibition of HIV-1 infectivity in macrophages and lymphocytes by a novel CCR5 antagonist. *Science* **1997**, *276*, 276–279. [CrossRef] [PubMed]
16. White, G.E.; Iqbal, A.J.; Greaves, D.R. CC chemokine receptors and chronic inflammation—therapeutic opportunities and pharmacological challenges. *Pharmacol. Rev.* **2013**, *65*, 47–89. [CrossRef] [PubMed]
17. Pastore, C.; Picchio, G.R.; Galimi, F.; Fish, R.; Hartley, O.; Offord, R.E.; Mosier, D.E. Two mechanisms for human immunodeficiency virus type 1 inhibition by N-terminal modifications of RANTES. *Antimicrob. Agents Chemother.* **2003**, *47*, 509–517. [CrossRef] [PubMed]
18. Hartley, O.; Gaertner, H.; Wilken, J.; Thompson, D.; Fish, R.; Ramos, A.; Pastore, C.; Dufour, B.; Cerini, F.; Melotti, A.; et al. Medicinal chemistry applied to a synthetic protein: Development of highly potent HIV entry inhibitors. *Proc. Natl. Acad. Sci. USA* **2004**, *101*, 16460–16465. [CrossRef] [PubMed]
19. Kumar, M.; Chatterjee, A.; Khedkar, A.P.; Kusumanchi, M.; Adhikary, L. Mass spectrometric distinction of in-source and in-solution pyroglutamate and succinimide in proteins: A case study on rhG-CSF. *J. Am. Soc. Mass Spectrom.* **2013**, *24*, 202–212. [CrossRef] [PubMed]
20. Liu, Y.D.; Goetze, A.M.; Bass, R.B.; Flynn, G.C. N-terminal glutamate to pyroglutamate conversion in vivo for human IgG2 antibodies. *J. Biol. Chem.* **2011**, *286*, 11211–11217. [CrossRef] [PubMed]
21. Tritsch, G.L.; Moore, G.E. Spontaneous decomposition of glutamine in cell culture media. *Exp. Cell Res.* **1962**, *28*, 360–364. [CrossRef]

22. Yu, L.; Vizel, A.; Huff, M.B.; Young, M.; Remmele, R.L.; He, B. Investigation of N-terminal glutamate cyclization of recombinant monoclonal antibody in formulation development. *J. Pharm. Biomed. Anal.* **2006**, *42*, 455–463. [CrossRef] [PubMed]

23. Chelius, D.; Jing, K.; Lueras, A.; Rehder, D.S.; Dillon, T.M.; Vizel, A.; Rajan, R.S.; Li, T.; Treuheit, M.J.; Bondarenko, P.V. Formation of pyroglutamic acid from N-terminal glutamic acid in immunoglobulin gamma antibodies. *Anal. Chem.* **2006**, *78*, 2370–2376. [CrossRef] [PubMed]

24. Yan, B.; Valliere-Douglass, J.; Brady, L.; Steen, S.; Han, M.; Pace, D.; Elliott, S.; Yates, Z.; Han, Y.; Balland, A.; et al. Analysis of post-translational modifications in recombinant monoclonal antibody IgG1 by reversed-phase liquid chromatography/mass spectrometry. *J. Chromatogr. A* **2007**, *1164*, 153–161. [CrossRef] [PubMed]

25. Kumar, A.; Bachhawat, A.K. Pyroglutamic acid: Throwing light on a lightly studied metabolite. *Curr. Sci.* **2012**, *102*, 288–297.

26. Dick, L.W.; Kim, C.; Qiu, D.; Cheng, K.-C. Determination of the origin of the N-terminal pyro-glutamate variation in monoclonal antibodies using model peptides. *Biotechnol. Bioeng.* **2007**, *97*, 544–553. [CrossRef] [PubMed]

27. Cerini, F.; Gaertner, H.; Madden, K.; Tolstorukov, I.; Brown, S.; Laukens, B.; Callewaert, N.; Harner, J.C.; Oommen, A.M.; Harms, J.T.; et al. A scalable low-cost cGMP process for clinical grade production of the HIV inhibitor 5P12-RANTES in Pichia pastoris. *Protein Expr. Purif.* **2016**. [CrossRef] [PubMed]

28. Towards NMR Analysis of the HIV-1 Coreceptor CCR5 and Its Interaction with RANTES. Available online: http://edoc.unibas.ch/30282/ (accessed on 17 July 2017).

29. Grewe, C.; Beck, A.; Gelderblom, H.R. HIV: Early virus-cell interactions. *J. Acquir. Immune Defic. Syndr.* **1990**, *3*, 965–974. [PubMed]

30. Allen, S.J.; Crown, S.E.; Handel, T.M. Chemokine:Receptor Structure, Interactions, and Antagonism. *Annu. Rev. Immunol.* **2007**, *25*, 787–820. [CrossRef] [PubMed]

31. Appay, V.; Brown, A.; Cribbes, S.; Randle, E.; Czaplewski, L.G. Aggregation of RANTES Is Responsible for Its Inflammatory Properties: Characterization of Nonaggregating, Noninflammatory RANTES Mutants. *J. Biol. Chem.* **1999**, *274*, 27505–27512. [CrossRef] [PubMed]

32. Burton, D.R.; Hangartner, L. Broadly Neutralizing Antibodies to HIV and Their Role in Vaccine Design. *Annu. Rev. Immunol.* **2016**, *34*, 635–659. [CrossRef] [PubMed]

33. Klein, F.; Halper-Stromberg, A.; Horwitz, J.A.; Gruell, H.; Scheid, J.F.; Bournazos, S.; Mouquet, H.; Spatz, L.A.; Diskin, R.; Abadir, A.; et al. HIV therapy by a combination of broadly neutralizing antibodies in humanized mice. *Nature* **2012**, *492*, 118–122. [CrossRef] [PubMed]

34. Clark, A.J.; Gindin, T.; Zhang, B.; Wang, L.; Abel, R.; Murret, C.S.; Xu, F.; Bao, A.; Lu, N.J.; Zhou, T.; et al. Free Energy Perturbation Calculation of Relative Binding Free Energy between Broadly Neutralizing Antibodies and the gp120 Glycoprotein of HIV-1. *J. Mol. Biol.* **2016**, *429*, 930–947. [CrossRef] [PubMed]

35. Pancera, M.; Shahzad-ul-Hussan, S.; Doria-Rose, N.A.; McLellan, J.S.; Bailer, R.T.; Dai, K.; Loesgen, S.; Louder, M.K.; Staupe, R.P.; Yang, Y.; et al. Structural basis for diverse N-glycan recognition by HIV-1–neutralizing V1–V2–directed antibody PG16. *Nat. Struct. Mol. Biol.* **2013**. [CrossRef] [PubMed]

36. Alexandre, K.B.; Gray, E.S.; Lambson, B.E.; Moore, P.L.; Choge, I.A.; Mlisana, K.; Karim, S.S.A.; McMahon, J.; O'Keefe, B.; Chikwamba, R.; et al. Mannose-rich glycosylation patterns on HIV-1 subtype C gp120 and sensitivity to the lectins, Griffithsin, Cyanovirin-N and Scytovirin. *Virology* **2010**, *402*, 187–196. [CrossRef] [PubMed]

37. Akkouh, O.; Ng, T.B.; Singh, S.S.; Yin, C.; Dan, X.; Chan, Y.S.; Pan, W.; Cheung, R.C.F. Lectins with anti-HIV activity: A review. *Molecules* **2015**, *20*, 648–668. [CrossRef] [PubMed]

38. Pang, W.; Tam, S.-C.; Zheng, Y.-T. Current peptide HIV type-1 fusion inhibitors. *Antivir. Chem. Chemother.* **2009**, *20*, 1–18. [CrossRef] [PubMed]

39. Zhao, B.; Mankowski, M.K.; Snyder, B.A.; Ptak, R.G.; Liwang, P.J. Highly potent chimeric inhibitors targeting two steps of HIV cell entry. *J. Biol. Chem.* **2011**, *286*, 28370–28381. [CrossRef] [PubMed]

40. Kagiampakis, I.; Gharibi, A.; Mankowski, M.K.; Snyder, B.A.; Ptak, R.G.; Alatas, K.; LiWang, P.J. Potent Strategy To Inhibit HIV-1 by Binding both gp120 and gp41. *Antimicrob. Agents Chemother.* **2011**, *55*, 264–275. [CrossRef] [PubMed]

41. Qin, L.; Kufareva, I.; Holden, L.G.; Wang, C.; Zheng, Y.; Zhao, C.; Fenalti, G.; Wu, H.; Han, G.W.; Cherezov, V.; et al. Crystal structure of the chemokine receptor CXCR4 in complex with a viral chemokine. *Science* **2015**, *347*, 1117–1122. [CrossRef] [PubMed]

42. Zhang, L.; Herrera, C.; Coburn, J.; Olejniczak, N.; Ziprin, P.; Kaplan, D.L.; LiWang, P.J. Stabilization and sustained release of HIV inhibitors by encapsulation in silk fibroin disks. *ACS Biomater. Sci. Eng.* **2017**. [CrossRef]

43. Nedellec, R.; Coetzer, M.; Lederman, M.M.; Offord, R.E.; Hartley, O.; Mosier, D.E. Resistance to the CCR5 inhibitor 5P12-RANTES requires a difficult evolution from CCR5 to CXCR4 Coreceptor use. *PLoS ONE* **2011**, *6*, e22020. [CrossRef] [PubMed]

44. Paul, D.; Boyer, E.G.; Krebs, D.S.S. *The Enzymes*, 3rd ed.; Academic Press: New York, NY, USA, 1970; pp. 127–130.

45. Chang, Y.-G.; Kuo, N.-W.; Tseng, R.; LiWang, A. Flexibility of the C-terminal, or CII, ring of KaiC governs the rhythm of the circadian clock of cyanobacteria. *Proc. Natl. Acad. Sci. USA* **2011**, *108*, 14431–14436. [CrossRef] [PubMed]

46. Wishart, D.S.; Bigam, C.G.; Yao, J.; Abildgaard, F.; Dyson, H.J.; Oldfield, E.; Markley, J.L.; Sykes, B.D. 1 H, 13 C and 15 N chemical shift referencing in biomolecular NMR. *J. Biomol. NMR* **1995**, *6*, 135–140. [CrossRef] [PubMed]

47. Delaglio, F.; Grzesiek, S.; Vuister, G.W.; Zhu, G.; Pfeifer, J.; Bax, A. NMRPipe: A multidimensional spectral processing system based on UNIX pipes. *J. Biomol. NMR* **1995**, *6*, 277–293. [CrossRef] [PubMed]

48. Garrett, D.S.; Powers, R.; Gronenborn, A.M.; Clore, G.M. A common sense approach to peak picking in two-, three-, and four-dimensional spectra using automatic computer analysis of contour diagrams. *J. Magn. Reson.* **1991**, *95*, 214–220. [CrossRef]

49. Laurence, J.S.; Blanpain, C.; Burgner, J.W.; Parmentier, M.; LiWang, P.J. CC chemokine MIP-1β can function as a monomer and depends on Phe13 for receptor binding. *Biochemistry* **2000**, *39*, 3401–3409. [CrossRef] [PubMed]

50. Li, M.; Gao, F.; Mascola, J.R.; Stamatatos, L.; Polonis, V.R.; Koutsoukos, M.; Voss, G.; Goepfert, P.; Gilbert, P.; Greene, K.M.; et al. Human Immunodeficiency Virus Type 1 env Clones from Acute and Early Subtype B Infections for Standardized Assessments of Vaccine-Elicited Neutralizing Antibodies. *J. Virol.* **2005**, *79*, 10108–10125. [CrossRef] [PubMed]

51. Derdeyn, C.A.; Decker, J.M.; Bibollet-Ruche, F.; Mokili, J.L.; Muldoon, M.; Denham, S.A.; Heil, M.L.; Kasolo, F.; Musonda, R.; Hahn, B.H.; et al. Envelope-constrained neutralization-sensitive HIV-1 after heterosexual transmission. *Science* **2004**, *303*, 2019–2022. [CrossRef] [PubMed]

52. Wei, X.; Decker, J.M.; Liu, H.; Zhang, Z.; Arani, R.B.; Kilby, J.M.; Saag, M.S.; Shaw, G.M.; Kappes, J.C.; Wu, X. Emergence of Resistant Human Immunodeficiency Virus Type 1 in Patients Receiving Fusion Inhibitor (T-20) Monotherapy Emergence of Resistant Human Immunodeficiency Virus Type 1 in Patients Receiving Fusion Inhibitor (T-20) Monotherapy. *Antimicrob. Agents Chemother.* **2002**, *46*, 1896–1905. [CrossRef] [PubMed]

53. Wei, X.; Decker, J.M.; Wang, S.; Hui, H.; Kappes, J.C.; Wu, X.; Salazar-Gonzalez, J.F.; Salazar, M.G.; Kilby, J.M.; Saag, M.S.; et al. Antibody neutralization and escape by HIV-1. *Nature* **2003**, *422*, 307–312. [CrossRef] [PubMed]

54. Jin, H.; Shen, X.; Baggett, B.R.; Kong, X.; LiWang, P.J. The human CC chemokine MIP-1β dimer is not competent to bind to the CCR5 receptor. *J. Biol. Chem.* **2007**, *282*, 27976–27983. [CrossRef] [PubMed]

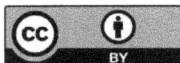

International Journal of
Molecular Sciences

MDPI

Article

Differences in Sulfotyrosine Binding amongst CXCR1 and CXCR2 Chemokine Ligands

Natasha A. Moussouras [1], Anthony E. Getschman [2], Emily R. Lackner [3],
Christopher T. Veldkamp [3], Michael B. Dwinell [1,*] and Brian F. Volkman [2,*]

[1] Department of Microbiology and Immunology, Medical College of Wisconsin, Milwaukee, WI 53226,
    USA; nmoussouras@mcw.edu
[2] Department of Biochemistry, Medical College of Wisconsin, Milwaukee, WI 53226, USA;
    agetschman@mcw.edu
[3] Department of Chemistry, University of Wisconsin-Whitewater, Whitewater, WI 53190, USA;
    LacknerER29@uww.edu (E.R.L.); veldkamc@uww.edu (C.T.V.)
*   Correspondence: mdwinell@mcw.edu (M.B.D.); bvolkman@mcw.edu (B.F.V.);
    Tel.: +1-414-955-7427 (M.B.D.); +1-414-955-8400 (B.F.V.)

Received: 2 August 2017; Accepted: 1 September 2017; Published: 3 September 2017

Abstract: Tyrosine sulfation, a post-translational modification found on many chemokine receptors, typically increases receptor affinity for the chemokine ligand. A previous bioinformatics analysis suggested that a sulfotyrosine (sY)-binding site on the surface of the chemokine CXCL12 may be conserved throughout the chemokine family. However, the extent to which receptor tyrosine sulfation contributes to chemokine binding has been examined in only a few instances. Computational solvent mapping correctly identified the conserved sulfotyrosine-binding sites on CXCL12 and CCL21 detected by nuclear magnetic resonance (NMR) spectroscopy, demonstrating its utility for hot spot analysis in the chemokine family. In this study, we analyzed five chemokines that bind to CXCR2, a subset of which also bind to CXCR1, to identify hot spots that could participate in receptor binding. A cleft containing the predicted sulfotyrosine-binding pocket was identified as a principal hot spot for ligand binding on the structures of CXCL1, CXCL2, CXCL7, and CXCL8, but not CXCL5. Sulfotyrosine titrations monitored via NMR spectroscopy showed specific binding to CXCL8, but not to CXCL5, which is consistent with the predictions from the computational solvent mapping. The lack of CXCL5–sulfotyrosine interaction and the presence of CXCL8–sulfotyrosine binding suggests a role for receptor post-translational modifications regulating ligand selectivity.

Keywords: CXCL5; CXCL8; CXCR1; CXCR2; sulfotyrosine; post-translational modification; chemokines; NMR

1. Introduction

Chemokines comprise a family of approximately 50 small globular proteins that coordinate the migration of immune cells along an increasing chemokine concentration gradient by activating specific G protein-coupled receptors (GPCRs) expressed on the surface of responding cells. The two main classes of chemokines and their receptors, CC and CXC, exhibit varying degrees of promiscuity, with some receptors binding multiple ligands, and certain ligands binding multiple receptors [1–3]. Chemokines adopt a highly conserved tertiary fold comprised of a three-stranded antiparallel β-sheet and a C-terminal α-helix stabilized by one or two disulfide bonds. Receptor binding and activation is described by a two-site, two-step model, whereby the N-terminus of the receptor binds the N-loop and chemokine core (site 1), followed by the insertion of the flexible N-terminus of the chemokine into the orthosteric pocket of the GPCR (site 2), leading to receptor activation [4].

For some chemokine receptors, tyrosine residues in the N-terminal domain (site 1) are post-translationally modified by tyrosyl protein sulfotransferases [5–7], and for the large majority that have been characterized, tyrosine sulfation enhances chemokine–receptor recognition [8–14]. NMR studies of CXCL12 bound to the N-terminal extracellular domain of its receptor CXCR4 provided the first structural details of sulfotyrosine (sY) recognition by a chemokine [12,13]. Of the three tyrosines in the CXCR4 N-terminal domain (Y7, Y12, and Y21) that are potential sites of sulfation, Y21 is the most important for CXCL12 binding [15]. Y21 makes specific contacts with the N-loop and β3 strand, which may represent a conserved "hot spot" for receptor binding in the chemokine family (Figure 1A) [16]. More recently, the NMR structure of a CCR3-chemokine complex demonstrated that a pair of adjacent sulfotyrosines occupied the same N-loop/β3 cleft of CCL11 [17]. In the case of CCR3, different patterns of sulfation for its two N-terminal tyrosines enhanced the site 1 binding affinity for its ligands CCL11, CCL24, and CCL26 to varying degrees [11]. Thus, tyrosine sulfation can increase the selectivity of a promiscuous receptor by promoting interactions with a subset of its cognate chemokine ligands [11].

A subset of CXC chemokines positive for the ELR (Glu-Leu-Arg) motif are potent neutrophil chemoattractants that activate the CXCR1 and/or CXCR2 receptor [18,19] and play critical roles in inflammatory responses, particularly in response to bacterial infections and autoimmune diseases [18,20,21]. Specifically, CXCL5, which binds both CXCR1 and CXCR2 [22], has been implicated in mediating pain in rheumatoid arthritis and UVB irradiation, and insulin resistance in obesity [23–25]. CXCR2, the most promiscuous of the six known CXC chemokine receptors, binds to CXCL1, CXCL2, CXCL3, CXCL5, CXCL6, CXCL7, and CXCL8 [1]. In contrast, CXCR1 predominantly binds CXCL8 and CXCL6, though CXCL5 is reported as a ~10-fold less potent ligand [22,26]. The CXCR2 N-terminal domain contains two tyrosines, neither of which is a likely candidate for sulfation based on local sequence analysis by Sulfinator [27] and Sulfosite [28], while the position-specific scoring matrix (PSSM) developed by Liu et al. [29] gives an intermediate sulfation likelihood score. In contrast, the Sulfosite algorithm predicts that the single tyrosine, Y27, of CXCR1 will be modified with a 92% probability, and similarly, the PSSM also predicts Y27 sulfation with high scoring. While tyrosine sulfation has not been experimentally verified for CXCR1, we speculated that the potencies of CXCL5 and CXCL8 as CXCR1 agonists might correlate with the relative importance of sulfotyrosine recognition for each chemokine ligand.

We have previously validated the modified amino acid sulfotyrosine as a chemical probe in 2D NMR studies [16]. Sulfotyrosine binding to CXCL12 induced chemical shifts in a subset of the residues that were also perturbed upon the binding of CXCR4-derived sulfopeptides [15]. Based on their location in the N-loop/β3 cleft, we concluded that the amino acid probe bound at or near the location of sulfotyrosine 21 in the structure of a CXCR4 sulfopeptide bound to CXCL12 [12]. So far, each chemokine tested (CXCL12, XCL1, CCL5, CX3CL1, and CCL21 [16,30]) bound the sulfotyrosine probe in at least one common pocket, which is consistent with our hypothesis that sulfotyrosine recognition is a conserved feature of the chemokine–receptor site 1 interface (Figure 1). Computational solvent mapping analysis confirmed this hypothesis by clustering organic solvent probe molecules in and around the conserved sulfotyrosine binding sites on the surfaces of CXCL12 [31] and CCL21 [30]. In the present study, computational solvent mapping consistently identified a similar binding pocket on all CXCR2 ligands with available structures, with the exception of CXCL5. Consistent with the computational hot spot analysis, we observed specific binding of sulfotyrosine to CXCL8, but not CXCL5, as monitored by 2D NMR. These findings suggest that receptor recognition by CXCL5 may differ from the other CXCR1/2 chemokine ligands, and that sulfotyrosine may help CXCR1 discriminate between CXCL5 and CXCL8.

2. Results

2.1. Sulfotyrosine Recognition Sites Correspond to Predicted Chemokine Hot Spots

Previous computational solvent mapping of CXCL12 and CCL21 using FTMap identified sulfotyrosine recognition sites as hot spots for ligand binding [30,31]. The FTMap algorithm surveys the protein surface with 16 small organic molecule probes, then clusters and ranks these probes based on positions with the lowest Boltzmann averaged energies, the highest ranking having the lowest energy [32,33]. We began by using the FTMap server (ftmap.bu.edu) to validate the analysis by testing CXCL12 and CCL21, for which there are both FTMap and sulfotyrosine/sulfopeptide-binding data available (Figure 1). Indeed, the top-ranking FTMap clusters localized to the sulfotyrosine-binding pocket of both of these representative CXC and CC chemokines, which indicated that the lowest energy-binding hot spot was likely to be the sulfotyrosine-binding pocket.

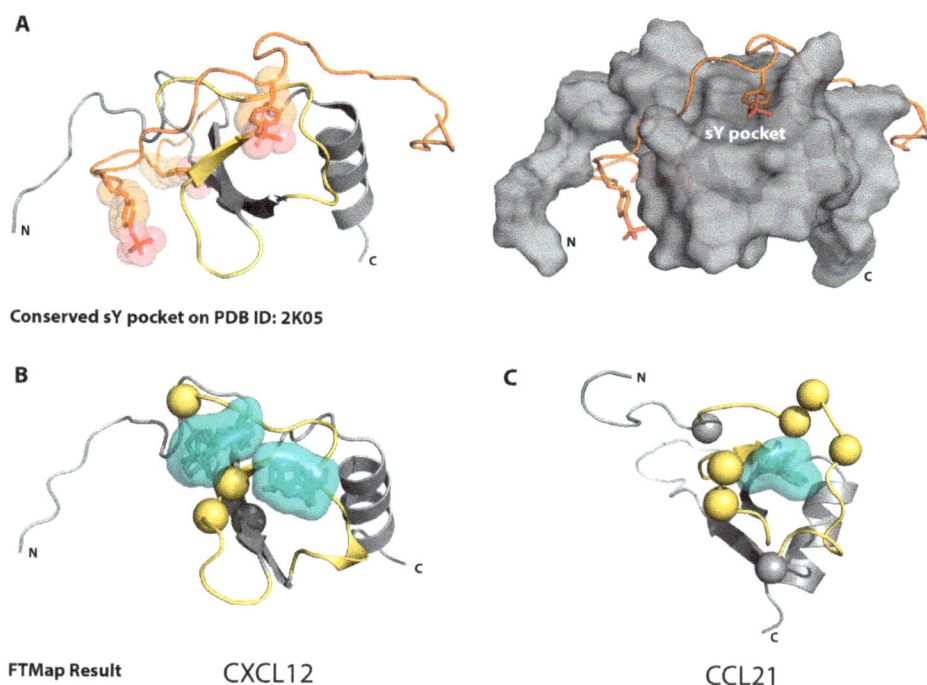

Figure 1. FTMap correctly identifies the NMR-verified sulfotyrosine-binding pocket on CXCL12 and CCL21. (**A**) The solved solution structure of CXCL12 bound to the CXCR4 N-terminal peptide (residues 1-38, sY7, sY12, sY21; Protein Data Bank (PDB) ID: 2K05), left. The CXCR4 N-terminal peptide and surface view of CXCL12 with the sY-binding pocket labeled are shown in the right panel. The tyrosine side chains of the CXCR4 peptide are displayed, the sulfate group is highlighted in red, the canonical sY-binding pocket highlighted in yellow; (**B**) First and fourth top-ranking FTMap clusters (shown in teal) map to the CXCL12 (PDB ID: 2K05) sY-binding pocket (backbone highlighted in yellow) identified by NMR sulfopeptide studies. Spheres reflect specific residues identified by NMR sY titrations [16]; (**C**) Third top-ranking FTMap cluster maps to the CCL21 sY-binding pocket (backbone highlighted in yellow), identified by NMR sY titrations (specific residues highlighted with spheres [30]) (PDB ID: 2L4N).

We next analyzed each of the CXCR2 chemokine ligands for which a solved 3D structure was available, including all members of the NMR ensemble where applicable. As shown in Figure 2A, the top-ranking clusters identified by FTMap for CXCL1, CXCL2, CXCL7, and CXCL8 were consistently located between the N-loop and β3-strand near the conserved sulfotyrosine-binding site. While a solved structure of sulfated CXCR1 or CXCR2 (or the sulfopeptide region of the receptor) with any of their ligands has not been solved, the solved NMR structure of CXCL8 with an N-terminal CXCR1 peptide [34] shows the tyrosine near the proposed sulfotyrosine-binding pocket, at the same location of many of the FTMap clusters (Figure 2A). These clusters include those of CXCL1, which lie slightly behind the N-loop, but are still within range that might encounter a CXCR2 peptide. This tyrosine of CXCR1 does not rest in the same position on CXCL8 as the tyrosine 21 of CXCR4 (PDB ID: 2K04) [12], which may account for the different positioning of the clusters relative to those in the CXCL12 analysis. For CXCL5 (Figure 2B), however, only the last, or second to last-ranking cluster identified the pocket, which suggested that for CXCL5, it is a less favorable binding pocket. Furthermore, clusters only found the pocket for four of the 20 CXCL5 NMR conformers, as compared to a majority of conformers in the CXCL1, CXCL2, and CXCL8 NMR ensembles (Figure A1).

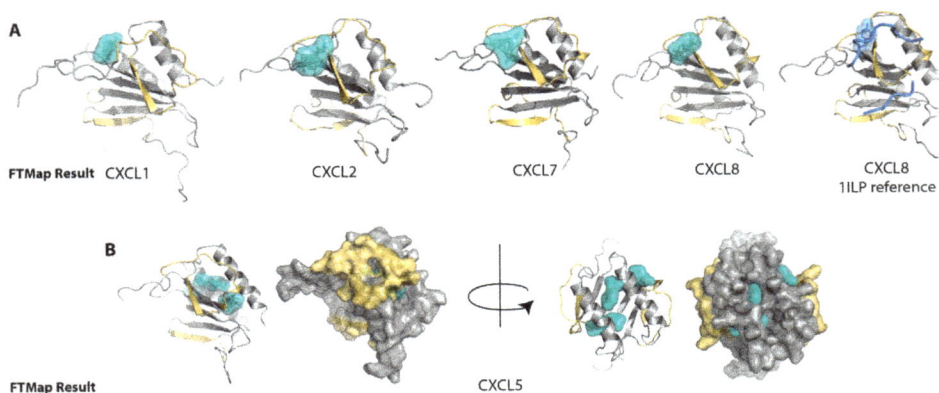

Figure 2. FTMap hot spot identification on CXCR2 chemokine ligands. The canonical sulfotyrosine-binding pocket between the N-loop and β3-strand is highlighted in yellow. The clusters that bind the pocket, each from within the top three ranking clusters, are in teal. (**A**) The clusters find the pockets for CXCL1, CXCL2, CXCL7, and CXCL8. For reference, the structure of CXCL8 bound to the CXCR1 N-terminal peptide (PDB ID: 1ILP) is shown with the peptide in blue and the tyrosine side chain revealed; (**B**) In comparison for CXCL5, the top three-ranking clusters localize to the dimer interface. The surface view is shown to underscore the lack of clusters in the binding pocket.

2.2. NMR Titration Studies with Sulfotyrosine

To further explore these results, we performed NMR titration experiments to similarly probe chemokine receptor-binding pockets with another small molecule, sulfotyrosine. We have previously shown that sulfotyrosine can be used as a surrogate for sulfated receptor peptides and is sufficient to identify the chemokine receptor sulfotyrosine-binding pocket on the chemokine ligand [16]. Using ^{1}H-^{15}N HSQC NMR spectroscopy, we monitored the spectra of CXCL5 upon titration of increasing amounts of sulfotyrosine, from 0 to 100 mM. The amino acids involved in binding were expected to show the greatest chemical shift perturbations. However, when performing these titrations with CXCL5, there were few residues that had significant chemical shift perturbations (Figure 3A, Figure A2–A). For comparison, we performed a similar titration for CXCL8 and, as predicted from our prior studies of CXCL12, there were widespread changes in the HSQC spectra throughout the course of the titration (Figure 3B, Figure A2–B). NMR HSQC experiments are superbly sensitive to changes in protein structure. For these experiments, as the only change throughout the titration was the addition of sulfotyrosine, the changes in the spectra are indicative of sulfotyrosine binding.

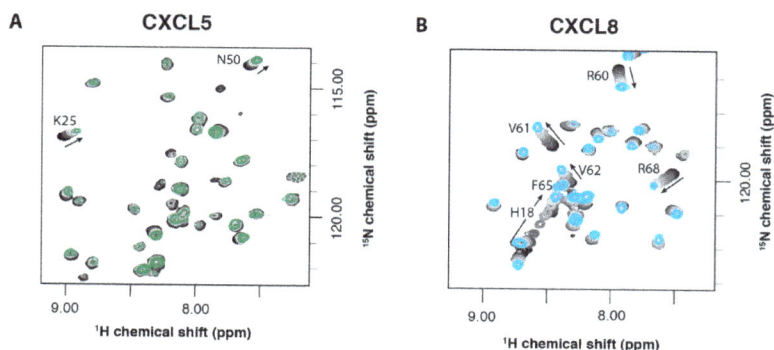

Figure 3. NMR titrations of CXCL5 and CXCL8 with sulfotyrosine (sY). Overlays of the ^{1}H-^{15}N HSQC spectra of CXCL5 (**A**) or CXCL8 (**B**) in the presence of 0 mM sY (black), 1, 5, 10, 20, 30, 40, 60, 80 and 100 mM sY (green or blue, respectively). A region of the HSQC spectra is shown to highlight that while there are some shift perturbations in (**A**); there are widespread changes in the CXCL8 (**B**) spectra.

As a measure of sulfotyrosine–chemokine interactions, total (^{1}H and ^{15}N) chemical shift perturbations can be quantified and magnitudes plotted as a function of residue number. For the CXCL5 titration, there were very minor changes in the spectra throughout the course of the titration, resulting in small chemical shift perturbations mostly within the level of noise (Figure 4A). When we mapped the amino acid residues K25 and N50 onto the structure of CXCL5 (PDB ID: 2MGS), interestingly, they do map to the edge of the sulfotyrosine-binding pocket (Figure 4C). The few, small chemical shift perturbations observed are likely due to the non-specific coordination of the negatively charged free sulfotyrosine and positively charged amino side chain of K25.

In contrast, the addition of sulfotyrosine to CXCL8 produced chemical shift perturbations indicative of specific sulfotyrosine binding [12,13]. There were regions of the N-loop and β3 strand (T12, H18, K20, and L49) encircling the canonical sulfotyrosine-binding pocket that produced significant (>0.3 ppm) chemical shift perturbations. As opposed to CXCL5, these were far above the level of noise. They closely overlap with residues that bind a CXCR1 N-terminal peptide as observed by Joseph et al., which fits a model of receptor–sulfation binding at the sulfotyrosine-binding pocket [35]. There were additional significant chemical shift perturbations in the C-terminal helix cluster (W57, V58, R60, V61, V62, F65, K67, R68, E70) adjacent to the N-loop, which may be the result of sulfotyrosine binding to the N-loop/β3 cleft or could denote a second binding site (Figure 4B,D).

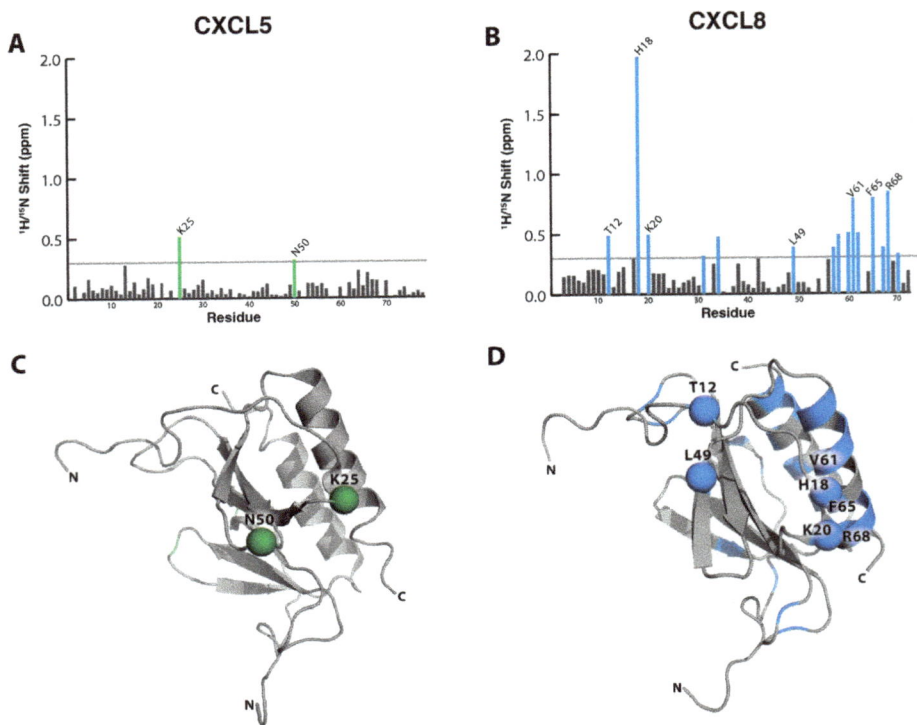

Figure 4. Total chemical shift perturbations (CSP) from 0 to 100 mM sulfotyrosine (sY) plotted for each amino acid. (**A**) CXCL5 CSP plot, residues in green reflecting CSP >0.3 ppm; (**B**) CXCL8 CSP plot, residues in blue reflecting CSP >0.3 ppm; (**C**) CXCL5 structure (PDB ID: 2MGS) with K25 and N50, residues with the largest chemical shift perturbations (>0.3 ppm) within the sY-binding pocket are highlighted with green spheres; (**D**) CXCL8 (PDB ID: 2IL8) structure highlighting residues with the highest chemical shift perturbations (>0.3 ppm) in blue. Residues of the sY-binding pockets T12, H18, K20, and L49, are shown as spheres.

2.3. Binding Affinity to Sulfotyrosine

For an NMR titration that exhibits fast exchange kinetics and reaches a point of saturation (where the addition of a ligand produces little or no spectral changes), the chemical shift perturbations at intermediate titration points reflect the fractional occupancy of a binding site, and can be used to generate a binding isotherm. Sulfotyrosine-dependent chemical shift perturbations were analyzed by nonlinear fitting to estimate the dissociation constant, K_d [30]. For CXCL5, K25 and N50 had the greatest chemical shift perturbations throughout the titration. However, using a standard ligand-depletion, saturable-binding model, the data produced a linear curve, indicating non-specific interactions between sulfotyrosine and CXCL5 (Figure 5A). While non-specific interactions may occur due to the relatively small size of sulfotyrosine and lead to observable chemical shift perturbations, even those residues that exhibited smaller perturbations did not produce a saturable binding curve (Figure A3), suggesting that CXCL5 does not bind sulfotyrosine in a specific manner. In comparison, select CXCL8 residues generated large chemical shift perturbations, resulting in saturable binding curves (Figure 5B). When calculated binding affinities were averaged, they produced a binding K_d of 35.2 ± 1.95 mM, which is comparable to other sulfotyrosine titrations [30].

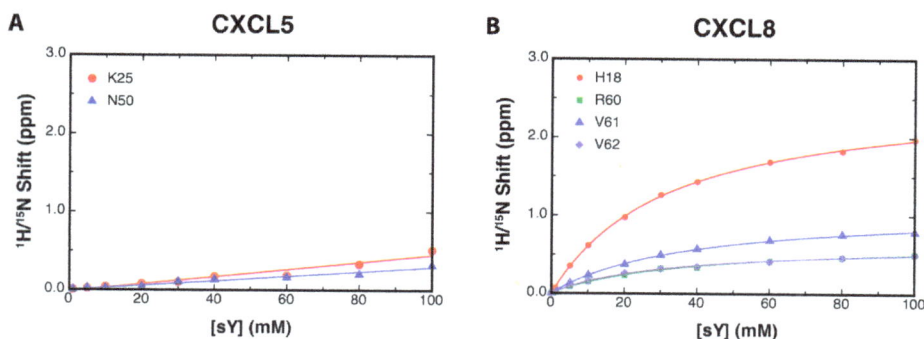

Figure 5. Sulfotyrosine–chemokine binding affinities. K_d plots of the CXCL5 (**A**) and CXCL8 (**B**) amino acids with the largest chemical shift perturbations indicating no saturable binding of sulfotyrosine (sY) to CXCL5, but did indicate saturable binding to CXCL8. The titration of sY into CXCL8 produced a K_d of 35.2 ± 1.95 mM.

3. Discussion

The mechanism by which promiscuous chemokine receptors selectively bind individual ligands remains poorly understood. A combination of factors including chemokine concentration, glycosaminoglycan (GAG) interactions, oligomerization state, and other cellular, contextual, or kinetic variables may fine-tune the propensities for chemokine–receptor interactions encoded by the amino acid sequence of each chemokine ligand. For example, CXCL5 expression was slower and more sustained compared with those of CXCL1 or CXCL8 in bacterial-infected epithelium [36,37]. This difference reveals not only the importance of chemokine expression, but also receptor selectivity, as there are often multiple ligands present simultaneously [38–40]. Post-translational modifications to the extracellular domains of the receptor are an emerging biologic paradigm that influences ligand–receptor binding kinetics, selectivity, specificity, and signaling [10,12,41,42]. The goal of the present study was to examine the potential role of N-terminal tyrosine sulfation of CXCR1 and CXCR2 in binding CXCL5 and CXCL8.

Tyrosine sulfation is an established receptor modification that we as well as others have shown to increase the affinity of a chemokine for the N-terminal domain of its cognate receptor. We used an unbiased computational solvent mapping approach to identifying hot spots on chemokine surfaces that consistently matched a known sulfotyrosine-binding site [13,16]. This same hot spot was predicted for all CXCR2 ligands, except for CXCL5. Previous studies have not only uncovered a role for chemokine receptor tyrosine sulfation, but also validated the use of sulfotyrosine as a useful molecular probe for the discovery of receptor-binding sites [16]. In striking contrast to CXCL8 and all the other chemokines tested to date [13,16,30], CXCL5 exhibited no signs of specific sulfotyrosine binding in NMR titrations. Sulfotyrosine-induced perturbations correspond closely with CXCL8 N-loop/β3 residues that shifted in a titration with a CXCR1 N-terminal peptide [35], as well as residues in the C-terminal helix that bind heparin oligosaccharides [43]. Often, there are regions of overlap between the binding of chemokine ligands with a receptor N-terminal peptide and GAGs, including for CXCL8 [35,43–46]. The pattern of shifts in both areas of CXCL8 suggests that sulfotyrosine may mimic both the modified receptor and sulfate-rich GAGs.

Sulfosite and the PSSM sulfation prediction sources predict CXCR1's tyrosine sulfation [28,29], and the PSSM predicts CXCR2's tyrosine sulfation [29]. Based on these bioinformatics analysis tools, it is likely that CXCR1 is tyrosine-sulfated, and less likely that CXCR2 is tyrosine-sulfated. However, both may be sulfated in vivo [5]. CXCL8 has a ~1–4 nM affinity at both CXCR1 and CXCR2 and is the most potent ligand at CXCR1, while CXCL5 has an affinity of ~40 and ~11 nM, respectively [22,26,47].

The data from the CXCL8 sulfotyrosine titration suggests that this may be due to the sulfation increasing its affinity, as shown previously for sulfated N-terminal receptor peptides and the following receptor/chemokine pairs: CCR2/CCL2 [10] and CCL7 [8], CCR3/CCL11 [9,11], CCL24 [11] and CCL26 [9,11], CCR5/CCL5 [14], and CXCR4/CXCL12 [12,13,15]. Thus, the binding events and affinities between the chemokines and the post-translationally modified receptors may present a nuanced form of regulation that is unique to different physiologic states and each particular chemokine.

Our FTMap analysis revealed a binding hot spot along the N-loop and β3-strand for the CXCR2-binding chemokine ligands CXCL1, CXCL2, CXCL7, and CXCL8 that corresponds to the canonical sulfotyrosine-binding pocket. This pocket identified by FTMap is compatible with a recent model of the CXCR2 N-terminal peptide bound to CXCL7, which shows the N-terminal peptide docked around the N-loop and over the β3-strand [45]. Based on this docking pose of CXCR2, its two tyrosines would face the opposite side of the chemokine around the α-helix and dimer interface. Interestingly, when the CXCR1 sequence is substituted in this model, the predicted sulfotyrosine occupies the canonical sulfotyrosine-binding site. Specifically, an alignment of CXCR1 and CXCR2 reveals that A31 of CXCR2 (A36 using the UniProtKB numbering system (entry: P25025)) corresponds to Y27 of CXCR1, which is the tyrosine predicted to be sulfated. In this model by Brown et al., A31 of CXCR2 rests in the canonical sulfotyrosine-binding pocket of CXCL7. Thus, we speculate that Y27 of CXCR1 interacts with the canonical sulfotyrosine-binding pocket of its ligands, and its sulfation increases its affinity for certain chemokines. While CXCR2 may or may not be sulfated, the N-loop/β3 cleft is predicted by FTMap as a hot spot in the site 1 interface. Taken together with the model of the CXCR2-CXCL7 complex by Brown et al., these results provide a plausible structural explanation for how tyrosine sulfation of CXCR1, but not CXCR2, might be compatible with the use of a conserved binding pocket by both receptors on promiscuous chemokine ligands.

The lack of FTMap identification of the binding pocket of CXCL5 and the differences in sulfotyrosine binding between CXCL5 and CXCL8 are due to more than differences in receptor binding as CXCL5 does bind both CXCR1 and CXCR2 (~40 vs ~11 nM, respectively) [22,26]. Sepuru et al. recognize that CXCL5 is more electrostatically neutral than any other CXCR2-activating chemokine [48]. As sulfotyrosine is a negatively charged molecule, it is likely to bind positively charged basic residues. In the region of the N-loop and β3-strand, CXCL8 has basic residues K11, K15, H18, K20, and R47, most of which are perturbed by sulfotyrosine binding or adjacent to a perturbed residue. Basic residues in this region of CXCL5 include H23, K25, and K52, which align with H18, K20, and R47 of CXCL8. Thus K11 and K15 of CXCL8 are residues that may confer sulfotyrosine specificity. Interestingly, CXCL6 is the only other ELR+ chemokine with a basic residue (R20) that corresponds to K15 of CXCL8; this position is invariably a glycine in the other CXCR2 ligands [48]. When Wolf et al. mutated R20 of CXCL6 to G, they found a loss of signaling at CXCR1, with no change in effect at CXCR2 [22], and furthermore, when Jiang et al. mutated K15 of a CXCL8 peptide to A, they found a greater than six-fold decrease in binding affinity to a CXCR1 peptide, as measured by surface plasmon resonance (SPR) [49]. These results are consistent with a specific role for R20 of CXCL6 and K15 of CXCL8 in sulfotyrosine recognition, and their higher potency as CXCR1 agonists relative to the other ELR+ ligands. The more electrostatically neutral, and less basic N-loop/β3 pocket of CXCL5 may account for the lack of sulfotyrosine binding, lack of probe binding between the N-loop and the β3-strand in FTMap, and the overall weaker potency at CXCR1 and CXCR2, more so than any other CXCR2-activating chemokine [26].

These results highlight the complexity of post-translational modifications as regulators of chemokine signaling. CXCL5 may employ a different combination of site 1 interactions with its receptors than the other chemokine ligands for CXCR1 and CXCR2. We had previously shown that there are differences in sulfated tyrosine affinities amongst multiple tyrosines on the same *receptor* N-terminus [15]. Our results suggest that, for a particular chemokine *ligand*, the sulfation of a tyrosine on its cognate receptor may not play an important role, and supports a novel paradigm in which sulfotyrosine may not universally increase the affinity of the chemokine receptor for its cognate ligand.

For promiscuous receptors, this may be a mechanism to distinguish binding between different ligands. There have long been generalizations about chemokine receptor binding and activation; however, as the intricacies of the system become more apparent, the redundancies fade in favor of subtle differences between chemokine ligands. The absence of a sulfotyrosine-binding site distinguishes CXCL5 from the other chemokines that have been examined and may confer unique functional attributes among the ELR+ subfamily.

4. Materials and Methods

4.1. FTMap

The available structures for CXCR1 and CXCR2 chemokine ligands (CXCL1-PDBID: 1MSH, CXCL2-PDB ID: 1QNK, CXCL5-PDB ID: 2MGS, CXCL7-PDB ID: 1NAP, CXCL8-PDB ID: 2IL8, 5D14) as well as CCL21 (PDB ID: 2L4N, 5EKI) and CXCL12 monomer and dimer with CXCR4 sulfopeptide (PDB IDs: 2KEC and 2K05 respectively) as a reference for chemokines that bind sulfotyrosine were downloaded from the RCSB Protein Data Bank (www.pdb.org) [50]. Using PyMOL (Schrodinger, LLC, New York, NY, Version 1.7) [51], the NMR solution structures (PDB IDs: 1MSH, 1QNK, 2MGS, 2IL8) were separated into PDB files of individual states. These and the crystal structures (PDB IDs: 1NAP, 5D14, 5EKI) were submitted to FTMap computational solvent mapping web server (ftmap.bu.edu) to identify potential binding pockets by small molecule sampling [32]. The results were downloaded and analyzed via PyMOL [51].

4.2. Protein Expression and Purification

Uniformly labeled ^{15}N-CXCL5 was expressed and purified as previously described [52]. ^{15}N-CXCL8 was supplied by Protein Foundry, LLC (Milwaukee, WI, USA).

4.3. NMR Spectroscopy

Concentrated stock solutions of ^{15}N-CXCL5 or ^{15}N-CXCL8 in H_2O were diluted to 250 μM in a solution containing 50 mM deuterated acetic acid (pH 5.0 for CXCL5, pH 5.2 for CXCL8), 10% (v/v) D_2O, 0.02% (w/v) NaN_3. All data were collected on a Bruker Avance 600 MHz spectrometer equipped with a ^{1}H/^{15}N/^{13}C cryoprobe. ^{1}H-^{15}N Heteronuclear Single Quantum Coherence experiments were used to monitor a CXCL5 or CXCL8 sample titrated with 0, 1, 5, 10, 20, 30, 40, 60, 80, and 100 mM sulfotyrosine dissolved in the same buffer as above. Spectra were processed using NMRPipe [53]. Using chemical shift assignments from the solved structures [48,54], peaks were tracked using CARA [55]. Total ^{1}H-^{5}N chemical shift perturbations were computed as $[(5\Delta\delta_{NH})^2 + (\Delta\delta_N)^2]^{1/2}$, where $\Delta\delta_{NH}$ and $\Delta\delta_N$ were the total changes in backbone amide ^{1}H and ^{15}N chemical shifts in ppm, respectively, from 0 to 100 mM sulfotyrosine. Concentration-dependent chemical shift perturbations for CXCL8 residues H18, R60, V61, and V62 upon titration with sulfotyrosine were fit to the following equation, which accounts for ligand depletion:

$$\Delta\delta = \Delta\delta_{\max} \times \frac{(K_d + [CXCL8] + x) - \sqrt{(K_d + [CXCL8] + x)^2 - 4[CXCL8]x}}{2[CXCL8]}$$

where $\Delta\delta$ is the chemical shift perturbation, $\Delta\delta_{\max}$ is the maximum chemical shift perturbation at 100% bound CXCL8, K_d is the CXCL8 sY dissociation constant, and x is the sY concentration. There were no changes in pH for the CXCL8 titration, thus, these changes in chemical shifts were due solely to the addition of sulfotyrosine. Using pro Fit 6.2 and the above equation, the K_d values and their respective errors were calculated and averaged to produce the reported affinity and error. Amino acids with the highest chemical shift perturbations were mapped onto the structure of CXCL8 using PyMOL. The same process was attempted for CXCL5; however, the chemical shift perturbation did not fit with this equation, but rather with a linear regression model.

Int. J. Mol. Sci. **2017**, *18*, 1894

Acknowledgments: This work is supported in part by grants from the National Institutes of Health including F30 CA210587 to Natasha A. Moussouras, and AI058072 and GM097381 to Brian F. Volkman. Natasha A. Moussouras is a member of the Medical Scientist Training Program at MCW, which is partially supported by a training grant from NIGMS T32-GM080202.

Author Contributions: Brian F. Volkman, Natasha A. Moussouras, and Anthony E. conceived and designed the experiments; Natasha A. Moussouras and Anthony E. Getschman performed the experiments and analyzed the data; Emily R. Lackner and Christopher T. Veldkamp contributed reagents/materials; Natasha A. Moussouras, Brian F. Volkman, and Michael B. Dwinell wrote the paper.

Conflicts of Interest: Brian F. Volkman and Michael B. Dwinell are co-founders and have ownership interests in Protein Foundry, LLC. The other authors declare no conflict of interest.

Abbreviations

CXCL	CXC ligand
CXCR	CXC receptor
CCL	CC ligand
GPCR	G-protein Coupled Receptor
sY	Sulfotyrosine
NMR	Nuclear Magnetic Resonance
HSQC	Heteronuclear Single Quantum Coherence
CSP	Chemical Shift Perturbation
ELR+	Glutamate-leucine-arginine positive
GAG	Glycosaminoglycan
SPR	Surface Plasmon Resonance

Appendix

CXCL1

Cross Cluster	Cluster Color	Number of Fragments
1*	blue	17
2#	lime green	14
3#	magenta	14
4	orange	10
5*	red	9
6#	yellow	7
7*	deep salmon	5
8	purple blue	3
9	deep purple	3
10*	deep teal	3
11*	pale cyan	3
12	white	3
13#	pale green	2
Total sY pocket (*)		37
Total dimer interface (#)		37
Total other		19

CXCL2

Cross Cluster	Cluster Color	Number of Fragments
1*	blue	18
2	lime green	16
3	magenta	12
4#	orange	12
5*	red	11
6#	yellow	5
7#	deep salmon	5
8	purple blue	5
9*	deep purple	3
10#	deep teal	3
11	pale cyan	2
12#	white	2
Total sY pocket (*)		32
Total dimer interface (#)		27
Total other		35

CXCL5

Cross Cluster	Cluster Color	Number of Fragments
1#	blue	22
2#	lime green	21
3	magenta	11
4#	orange	11
5	red	7
6#	yellow	6
7#	deep salmon	5
8#	purple blue	4
9	deep purple	3
10	deep teal	2
11#	pale cyan	1
Total sY pocket (*)		0
Total dimer interface (#)		70
Total other		23

CXCL7

Cross Cluster	Cluster Color	Number of Fragments
1	blue	15
2#	lime green	15
3*	magenta	14
4	orange	11
5*	red	10
6#	yellow	9
7#	deep salmon	6
8#	purple blue	4
9*	deep purple	4
10	deep teal	3
11#	pale cyan	2
12	white	2
Total sY pocket (*)		28
Total dimer interface (#)		36
Total other		31

CXCL8

Cross Cluster	Cluster Color	Number of Fragments
1*	blue	14
2*	lime green	13
3	magenta	13
4#	orange	12
5#	red	12
6	yellow	12
7#	deep salmon	8
8#	purple blue	7
9*	deep purple	2
Total sY pocket (*)		29
Total dimer interface (#)		39
Total other		25

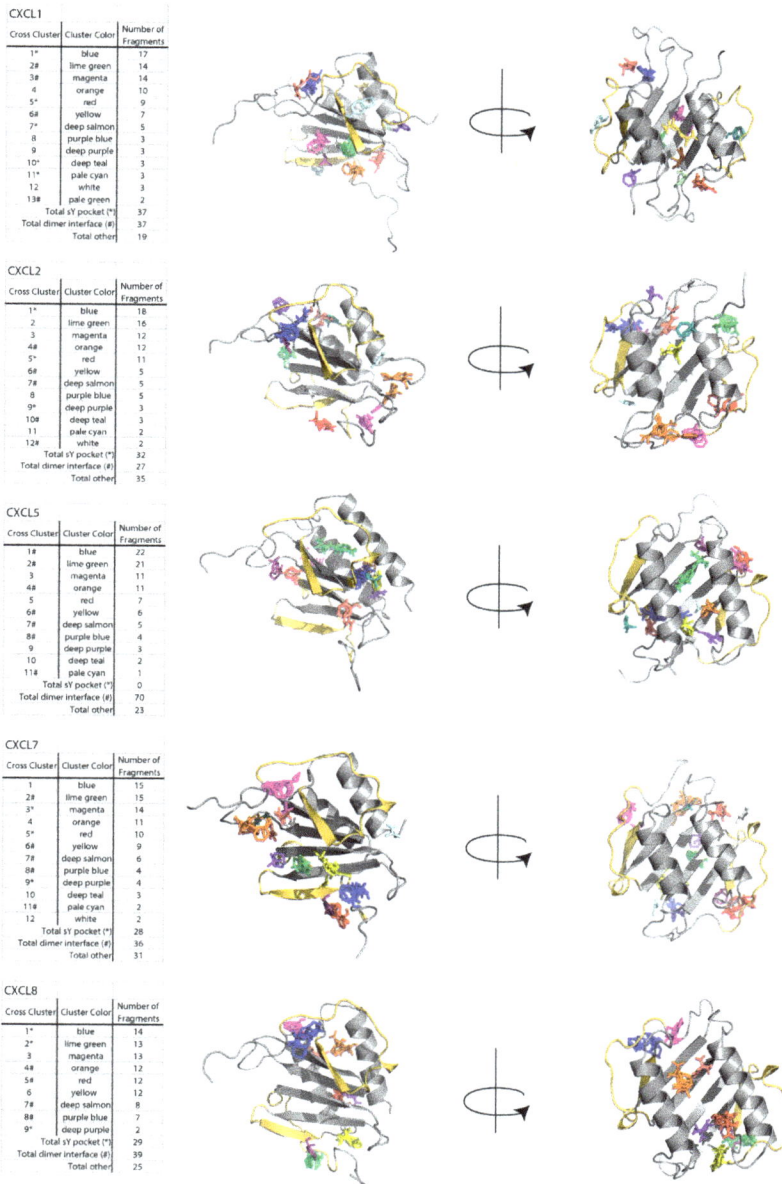

Figure A1. Complete FTMap results. All FTMap clusters are shown on the structures from Figure 2. The higher the number of probes, or fragments, in each cluster, the higher the ranking of that hot spot. Clusters that bind the sulfotyrosine binding pocket are noted with an asterisk (*), and totaled at the bottom of the table. Clusters that bind the dimer interface are noted with a number sign (#), and totaled. The remaining clusters are also totaled at the bottom of the table.

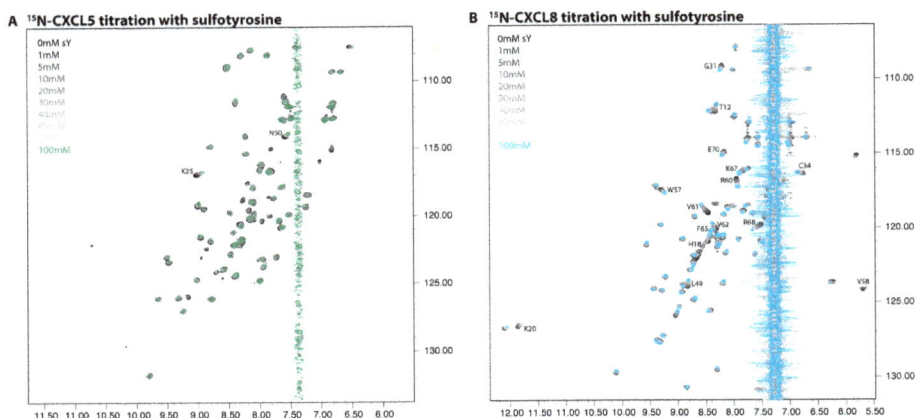

Figure A2. Complete HSQC overlays of titrations of sulfotyrosine (sY) into CXCL5 (**A**) or CXCL8 (**B**) from 0 (black) to 100 mM (green or blue, respectively). The streak around 7.4 ppm is due to increasing concentrations of sY, which are indicated in the figure. Residues with CSPs >0.3 ppm are labeled (see also Figure 4A,B).

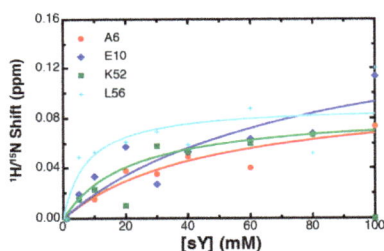

Figure A3. K_d plot showing curves with the lowest error from the titration of sY into CXCL5. These data further suggest CXCL5 had no saturable, specific binding.

References

1. Zlotnik, A.; Yoshie, O. Chemokines: A new classification system and their role in immunity. *Immunity* **2000**, *12*, 121–127. [CrossRef]
2. Zlotnik, A.; Yoshie, O.; Nomiyama, H. The chemokine and chemokine receptor superfamilies and their molecular evolution. *Genome Biol.* **2006**, *7*, 243. [CrossRef] [PubMed]
3. Griffith, J.W.; Sokol, C.L.; Luster, A.D. Chemokines and chemokine receptors: Positioning cells for host defense and immunity. *Annu. Rev. Immunol.* **2014**, *32*, 659–702. [CrossRef] [PubMed]
4. Kufareva, I.; Salanga, C.L.; Handel, T.M. Chemokine and chemokine receptor structure and interactions: Implications for therapeutic strategies. *Immunol. Cell Biol.* **2015**, *93*, 372–383. [CrossRef] [PubMed]
5. Stone, M.J.; Chuang, S.; Hou, X.; Shoham, M.; Zhu, J.Z. Tyrosine sulfation: An increasingly recognised post-translational modification of secreted proteins. *New Biotechnology* **2009**, *25*, 299–317. [CrossRef] [PubMed]
6. Ludeman, J.P.; Stone, M.J. The structural role of receptor tyrosine sulfation in chemokine recognition. *Br. J. Pharmacol.* **2014**, *171*, 1167–1179. [CrossRef] [PubMed]
7. Seibert, C.; Veldkamp, C.T.; Peterson, F.C.; Chait, B.T.; Volkman, B.F.; Sakmar, T.P. Sequential tyrosine sulfation of cxcr4 by tyrosylprotein sulfotransferases. *Biochemistry* **2008**, *47*, 11251–11262. [CrossRef] [PubMed]

3. Jen, C.H.; Leary, J.A. A competitive binding study of chemokine, sulfated receptor, and glycosaminoglycan interactions by nano-electrospray ionization mass spectrometry. *Anal. Biochem.* **2010**, *407*, 134–140. [CrossRef] [PubMed]

9. Simpson, L.S.; Zhu, J.Z.; Widlanski, T.S.; Stone, M.J. Regulation of chemokine recognition by site-specific tyrosine sulfation of receptor peptides. *Chem. Biol.* **2009**, *16*, 153–161. [CrossRef] [PubMed]

10. Tan, J.H.; Ludeman, J.P.; Wedderburn, J.; Canals, M.; Hall, P.; Butler, S.J.; Taleski, D.; Christopoulos, A.; Hickey, M.J.; Payne, R.J.; et al. Tyrosine sulfation of chemokine receptor ccr2 enhances interactions with both monomeric and dimeric forms of the chemokine monocyte chemoattractant protein-1 (mcp-1). *J. Biol. Chem.* **2013**, *288*, 10024–10034. [CrossRef] [PubMed]

11. Zhu, J.Z.; Millard, C.J.; Ludeman, J.P.; Simpson, L.S.; Clayton, D.J.; Payne, R.J.; Widlanski, T.S.; Stone, M.J. Tyrosine sulfation influences the chemokine binding selectivity of peptides derived from chemokine receptor ccr3. *Biochemistry* **2011**, *50*, 1524–1534. [CrossRef] [PubMed]

12. Veldkamp, C.T.; Seibert, C.; Peterson, F.C.; De la Cruz, N.B.; Haugner, J.C., 3rd; Basnet, H.; Sakmar, T.P.; Volkman, B.F. Structural basis of cxcr4 sulfotyrosine recognition by the chemokine sdf-1/cxcl12. *Sci. Signal.* **2008**, *1*. [CrossRef] [PubMed]

13. Veldkamp, C.T.; Seibert, C.; Peterson, F.C.; Sakmar, T.P.; Volkman, B.F. Recognition of a cxcr4 sulfotyrosine by the chemokine stromal cell-derived factor-1alpha (sdf-1alpha/cxcl12). *J. Mol. Biol.* **2006**, *359*, 1400–1409. [CrossRef] [PubMed]

14. Duma, L.; Haussinger, D.; Rogowski, M.; Lusso, P.; Grzesiek, S. Recognition of rantes by extracellular parts of the ccr5 receptor. *J. Mol. Biol.* **2007**, *365*, 1063–1075. [CrossRef] [PubMed]

15. Ziarek, J.J.; Getschman, A.E.; Butler, S.J.; Taleski, D.; Stephens, B.; Kufareva, I.; Handel, T.M.; Payne, R.J.; Volkman, B.F. Sulfopeptide probes of the cxcr4/cxcl12 interface reveal oligomer-specific contacts and chemokine allostery. *ACS Chem. Biol.* **2013**, *8*, 1955–1963. [CrossRef] [PubMed]

16. Ziarek, J.J.; Heroux, M.S.; Veldkamp, C.T.; Peterson, F.C.; Volkman, B.F. Sulfotyrosine recognition as marker for druggable sites in the extracellular space. *Int. J. Mol. Sci.* **2011**, *12*, 3740–3756. [CrossRef] [PubMed]

17. Millard, C.J.; Ludeman, J.P.; Canals, M.; Bridgford, J.L.; Hinds, M.G.; Clayton, D.J.; Christopoulos, A.; Payne, R.J.; Stone, M.J. Structural basis of receptor sulfotyrosine recognition by a CC chemokine: The N-terminal region of CCR3 bound to CCL11/Eotaxin-1. *Structure* **2014**, *22*, 1571–1581. [CrossRef] [PubMed]

18. Stillie, R.; Farooq, S.M.; Gordon, J.R.; Stadnyk, A.W. The functional significance behind expressing two IL-8 receptor types on pmn. *J. Leukoc. Biol.* **2009**, *86*, 529–543. [CrossRef] [PubMed]

19. Baggiolini, M.; Dewald, B.; Moser, B. Interleukin-8 and related chemotactic cytokines—CXC and CC chemokines. *Adv. Immunol.* **1994**, *55*, 97–179. [PubMed]

20. Dwinell, M.B.; Kagnoff, M.F. Mucosal immunity. *Curr. Opin. Gastroenterol.* **1999**, *15*, 33–38. [CrossRef] [PubMed]

21. Kagnoff, M.F.; Eckmann, L. Epithelial cells as sensors for microbial infection. *J. Clin. Invest.* **1997**, *100*, 6–10. [CrossRef] [PubMed]

22. Wolf, M.; Delgado, M.B.; Jones, S.A.; Dewald, B.; Clark-Lewis, I.; Baggiolini, M. Granulocyte chemotactic protein 2 acts via both il-8 receptors, cxcr1 and cxcr2. *Eur. J. Immunol.* **1998**, *28*, 164–170. [CrossRef]

23. Koch, A.E.; Kunkel, S.L.; Harlow, L.A.; Mazarakis, D.D.; Haines, G.K.; Burdick, M.D.; Pope, R.M.; Walz, A.; Strieter, R.M. Epithelial neutrophil activating peptide-78: A novel chemotactic cytokine for neutrophils in arthritis. *J. Clin. Invest.* **1994**, *94*, 1012–1018. [CrossRef] [PubMed]

24. Chavey, C.; Lazennec, G.; Lagarrigue, S.; Clape, C.; Iankova, I.; Teyssier, J.; Annicotte, J.S.; Schmidt, J.; Mataki, C.; Yamamoto, H.; et al. Cxc ligand 5 is an adipose-tissue derived factor that links obesity to insulin resistance. *Cell. Metab.* **2009**, *9*, 339–349. [CrossRef] [PubMed]

25. Dawes, J.M.; Calvo, M.; Perkins, J.R.; Paterson, K.J.; Kiesewetter, H.; Hobbs, C.; Kaan, T.K.; Orengo, C.; Bennett, D.L.; McMahon, S.B. Cxcl5 mediates uvb irradiation-induced pain. *Sci Transl. Med.* **2011**, *3*. [CrossRef] [PubMed]

26. Ahuja, S.K.; Murphy, P.M. The CXC chemokines growth-regulated oncogene (gro) alpha, grobeta, grogamma, neutrophil-activating peptide-2, and epithelial cell-derived neutrophil-activating peptide-78 are potent agonists for the type b, but not the type a, human interleukin-8 receptor. *J. Biol. Chem.* **1996**, *271*, 20545–20550. [CrossRef] [PubMed]

27. Monigatti, F.; Gasteiger, E.; Bairoch, A.; Jung, E. The sulfinator: Predicting tyrosine sulfation sites in protein sequences. *Bioinformatics* **2002**, *18*, 769–770. [CrossRef] [PubMed]

28. Chang, W.C.; Lee, T.Y.; Shien, D.M.; Hsu, J.B.; Horng, J.T.; Hsu, P.C.; Wang, T.Y.; Huang, H.D.; Pan, R.L. Incorporating support vector machine for identifying protein tyrosine sulfation sites. *J. Comput. Chem.* **2009**, *30*, 2526–2537. [CrossRef] [PubMed]

29. Liu, J.; Louie, S.; Hsu, W.; Yu, K.M.; Nicholas, H.B., Jr.; Rosenquist, G.L. Tyrosine sulfation is prevalent in human chemokine receptors important in lung disease. *Am. J. Respir. Cell. Mol. Biol.* **2008**, *38*, 738–743. [CrossRef] [PubMed]

30. Smith, E.W.; Lewandowski, E.M.; Moussouras, N.A.; Kroeck, K.G.; Volkman, B.F.; Veldkamp, C.T.; Chen, Y. Crystallographic structure of truncated CCL21 and the putative sulfotyrosine-binding site. *Biochemistry* **2016**, *55*, 5746–5753. [CrossRef] [PubMed]

31. Smith, E.W.; Nevins, A.M.; Qiao, Z.; Liu, Y.; Getschman, A.E.; Vankayala, S.L.; Kemp, M.T.; Peterson, F.C.; Li, R.; Volkman, B.F.; et al. Structure-based identification of novel ligands targeting multiple sites within a chemokine-g-protein-coupled-receptor interface. *J. Med. Chem.* **2016**, *59*, 4342–4351. [CrossRef] [PubMed]

32. Kozakov, D.; Grove, L.E.; Hall, D.R.; Bohnuud, T.; Mottarella, S.E.; Luo, L.; Xia, B.; Beglov, D.; Vajda, S. The ftmap family of web servers for determining and characterizing ligand-binding hot spots of proteins. *Nat. Protoc.* **2015**, *10*, 733–755. [CrossRef] [PubMed]

33. Kozakov, D.; Hall, D.R.; Chuang, G.Y.; Cencic, R.; Brenke, R.; Grove, L.E.; Beglov, D.; Pelletier, J.; Whitty, A.; Vajda, S. Structural conservation of druggable hot spots in protein-protein interfaces. *Proc. Natl. Acad. Sci. USA* **2011**, *108*, 13528–13533. [CrossRef] [PubMed]

34. Skelton, N.J.; Quan, C.; Reilly, D.; Lowman, H. Structure of a cxc chemokine-receptor fragment in complex with interleukin-8. *Structure* **1999**, *7*, 157–168. [CrossRef]

35. Joseph, P.R.; Rajarathnam, K. Solution nmr characterization of wt cxcl8 monomer and dimer binding to cxcr1 n-terminal domain. *Protein Sci.* **2015**, *24*, 81–92. [CrossRef] [PubMed]

36. Yang, S.K.; Eckmann, L.; Panja, A.; Kagnoff, M.F. Differential and regulated expression of c-x-c, c-c, and c-chemokines by human colon epithelial cells. *Gastroenterology* **1997**, *113*, 1214–1223. [CrossRef] [PubMed]

37. Johanesen, P.A.; Dwinell, M.B. Flagellin-independent regulation of chemokine host defense in campylobacter jejuni-infected intestinal epithelium. *Infect. Immun.* **2006**, *74*, 3437–3447. [CrossRef] [PubMed]

38. Murdoch, E.L.; Karavitis, J.; Deburghgraeve, C.; Ramirez, L.; Kovacs, E.J. Prolonged chemokine expression and excessive neutrophil infiltration in the lungs of burn-injured mice exposed to ethanol and pulmonary infection. *Shock* **2011**, *35*, 403–410. [CrossRef] [PubMed]

39. Proost, P.; De Wolf-Peeters, C.; Conings, R.; Opdenakker, G.; Billiau, A.; Van Damme, J. Identification of a novel granulocyte chemotactic protein (gcp-2) from human tumor cells. In vitro and in vivo comparison with natural forms of gro, IP-10, and IL-8. *J. Immunol.* **1993**, *150*, 1000–1010. [PubMed]

40. Kunkel, S.L.; Lukacs, N.; Strieter, R.M. Expression and biology of neutrophil and endothelial cell-derived chemokines. *Semin. Cell. Biol.* **1995**, *6*, 327–336. [CrossRef]

41. Kiermaier, E.; Moussion, C.; Veldkamp, C.T.; Gerardy-Schahn, R.; de Vries, I.; Williams, L.G.; Chaffee, G.R.; Phillips, A.J.; Freiberger, F.; Imre, R.; et al. Polysialylation controls dendritic cell trafficking by regulating chemokine recognition. *Science* **2016**, *351*, 186–190. [CrossRef] [PubMed]

42. Bannert, N.; Craig, S.; Farzan, M.; Sogah, D.; Santo, N.V.; Choe, H.; Sodroski, J. Sialylated o-glycans and sulfated tyrosines in the NH2-terminal domain of cc chemokine receptor 5 contribute to high affinity binding of chemokines. *J. Exp. Med.* **2001**, *194*, 1661–1673. [CrossRef] [PubMed]

43. Joseph, P.R.; Mosier, P.D.; Desai, U.R.; Rajarathnam, K. Solution nmr characterization of chemokine cxcl8/il-8 monomer and dimer binding to glycosaminoglycans: Structural plasticity mediates differential binding interactions. *Biochem. J.* **2015**, *472*, 121–133. [CrossRef] [PubMed]

44. Sepuru, K.M.; Nagarajan, B.; Desai, U.R.; Rajarathnam, K. Molecular basis of chemokine CXCL5-glycosaminoglycan interactions. *J. Biol. Chem.* **2016**, *291*, 20539–20550. [CrossRef] [PubMed]

45. Brown, A.J.; Sepuru, K.M.; Rajarathnam, K. Structural basis of native CXCL7 monomer binding to CXCR2 receptor n-domain and glycosaminoglycan heparin. *Int. J. Mol. Sci.* **2017**, *18*. [CrossRef] [PubMed]

46. Sepuru, K.M.; Rajarathnam, K. CXCL1/MGSA is a novel glycosaminoglycan (gag)-binding chemokine: Structural evidence for two distinct non-overlapping binding domains. *J. Biol. Chem.* **2016**, *291*, 4247–4255. [CrossRef] [PubMed]

47. Wuyts, A.; Proost, P.; Lenaerts, J.P.; Ben-Baruch, A.; Van Damme, J.; Wang, J.M. Differential usage of the cxc chemokine receptors 1 and 2 by interleukin-8, granulocyte chemotactic protein-2 and epithelial-cell-derived neutrophil attractant-78. *Eur. J. Biochem.* **1998**, *255*, 67–73. [CrossRef] [PubMed]

48. Sepuru, K.M.; Poluri, K.M.; Rajarathnam, K. Solution structure of cxcl5–a novel chemokine and adipokine implicated in inflammation and obesity. *PLoS ONE* **2014**, *9*. [CrossRef] [PubMed]

49. Jiang, S.J.; Liou, J.W.; Chang, C.C.; Chung, Y.; Lin, L.F.; Hsu, H.J. Peptides derived from cxcl8 based on in silico analysis inhibit cxcl8 interactions with its receptor cxcr1. *Sci. Rep.* **2015**, *5*, 18638. [CrossRef] [PubMed]

50. Berman, H.M.; Westbrook, J.; Feng, Z.; Gilliland, G.; Bhat, T.N.; Weissig, H.; Shindyalov, I.N.; Bourne, P.E. The protein data bank. *Nucleic. Acids Res.* **2000**, *28*, 235–242. [CrossRef] [PubMed]

51. Schrodinger, LLC. The pymol molecular graphics system. version 1.7.0.3. 2010.

52. Veldkamp, C.T.; Koplinski, C.A.; Jensen, D.R.; Peterson, F.C.; Smits, K.M.; Smith, B.L.; Johnson, S.K.; Lettieri, C.; Buchholz, W.G.; Solheim, J.C.; et al. Production of recombinant chemokines and validation of refolding. *Methods Enzymol.* **2016**, *570*, 539–565. [PubMed]

53. Delaglio, F.; Grzesiek, S.; Vuister, G.W.; Zhu, G.; Pfeifer, J.; Bax, A. Nmrpipe: A multidimensional spectral processing system based on unix pipes. *J. Biomol. NMR* **1995**, *6*, 277–293. [CrossRef] [PubMed]

54. Grasberger, B.L.; Gronenborn, A.M.; Clore, G.M. Analysis of the backbone dynamics of interleukin-8 by 15n relaxation measurements. *J. Mol. Biol.* **1993**, *230*, 364–372. [CrossRef] [PubMed]

55. Keller, R.L.J. (Ed.) *The Computer Aided Resonance Assignment/Tutorial*, 1st ed.; CANTINA Verlag: Goldau, Switzerland, 2004.

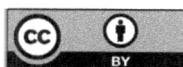

International Journal of
Molecular Sciences

MDPI

Article

CCR7 Sulfotyrosine Enhances CCL21 Binding

Andrew J. Phillips [1], Deni Taleski [2], Chad A. Koplinski [3], Anthony E. Getschman [3], Natasha A. Moussouras [4], Amanda M. Richard [1], Francis C. Peterson [3], Michael B. Dwinell [4], Brian F. Volkman [3], Richard J. Payne [2] and Christopher T. Veldkamp [1,*]

[1] Department of Chemistry, University of Wisconsin-Whitewater, Whitewater, WI 53190, USA; andrew.phillips@unmc.edu (A.J.P.); RichardAM08@uww.edu (A.M.R.)
[2] School of Chemistry, University of Sydney, Sydney 2006, Australia; deni.taleski@gmail.com (D.T.); richard.payne@sydney.edu.au (R.J.P.)
[3] Department of Biochemistry, Medical College of Wisconsin, Milwaukee, WI 53226, USA; ckoplinski@mcw.edu (C.A.K.); agetschman@mcw.edu (A.E.G.); fpeterso@mcw.edu (F.C.P.); bvolkman@mcw.edu (B.F.V.)
[4] Department of Microbiology and Immunology, Medical College of Wisconsin, Milwaukee, WI 53226, USA; nmoussouras@mcw.edu (N.A.M.); mdwinell@mcw.edu (M.B.D.)
* Correspondence: veldkamc@uww.edu; Tel.: +1-262-472-5267

Received: 27 July 2017; Accepted: 22 August 2017; Published: 25 August 2017

Abstract: Chemokines are secreted proteins that direct the migration of immune cells and are involved in numerous disease states. For example, CCL21 (CC chemokine ligand 21) and CCL19 (CC chemokine ligand 19) recruit antigen-presenting dendritic cells and naïve T-cells to the lymph nodes and are thought to play a role in lymph node metastasis of CCR7 (CC chemokine receptor 7)-expressing cancer cells. For many chemokine receptors, N-terminal posttranslational modifications, particularly the sulfation of tyrosine residues, increases the affinity for chemokine ligands and may contribute to receptor ligand bias. Chemokine sulfotyrosine (sY) binding sites are also potential targets for drug development. In light of the structural similarity between sulfotyrosine and phosphotyrosine (pY), the interactions of CCL21 with peptide fragments of CCR7 containing tyrosine, pY, or sY were compared using protein NMR (nuclear magnetic resonance) spectroscopy in this study. Various N-terminal CCR7 peptides maintain binding site specificity with Y8-, pY8-, or sY8-containing peptides binding near the α-helix, while Y17-, pY17-, and sY17-containing peptides bind near the N-loop and β3-stand of CCL21. All modified CCR7 peptides showed enhanced binding affinity to CCL21, with sY having the largest effect.

Keywords: chemokines; chemokine receptors; NMR; sulfotyrosine; CCL21; CCL19; CCR7; cancer metastasis; posttranslational modification

1. Introduction

Chemokines are small, secreted proteins that traffic immune cells in the body through functioning as chemoattractants [1]. There are approximately 50 chemokines and 20 chemokine receptors, of which many are involved in diseases, including inflammatory diseases like rheumatoid arthritis, viral diseases like human immunodeficiency virus-1 (HIV-1)/acquired immune deficiency syndrome (AIDS), and cancer metastasis [2]. The chemokine receptor CCR7 and its chemokine ligands CCL21 and, less so, CCL19, recruit circulating metastatic cancer cells to lymphatic tissue [3–6]. Chemokine receptors, like CCR7, are integral membrane proteins belonging to the rhodopsin-like or class A family of G protein-coupled receptors [1]. After synthesis, many chemokine receptors are post-translationally modified in the Golgi apparatus by tyrosylprotein sulfotransferase (TPST) enzymes, including the receptors CCR2, CCR3, CCR5, CCR8, CXC chemokine receptor 3 (CXCR3), CXCR4, and CX_3C chemokine receptor 1 (CX_3CR1) [7–13]. Tyrosine sulfation of chemokine receptor N-termini generally enhances affinity and encodes specificity between the chemokine and the receptor [10,13–19]. Chemokine receptor activation by balanced chemokine ligands generally leads to intracellular signaling through G protein- and β-arrestin-dependent pathways. Importantly, receptor activation by more than one or naturally modified ligands can lead to the reduction or absence of either pathway with a striking biological effect, which is described as "ligand" bias [20]. Lefkowitz et al. first showed CCR7 to a have biased signaling response to its two native ligands CCL21 and CCL19 [21].

Depending on the chemokine and the receptor, the receptor activation often results in intracellular signaling pathways involving the activation of intracellular kinases, of which many are serine/threonine kinases and some are tyrosine kinases [20]. Since TPST enzymes are located in the Golgi and modify tyrosine residues in certain integral membrane and secreted proteins [7], while tyrosine kinases are cytosolic enzymes, sulfotyrosine (sY) and phosphotyrosine (pY) are spatially segregated to different cellular locations. Given the single atom difference between sY and pY, it seems appropriate to ask if there are significant functional differences between the two posttranslational modifications. Others have investigated this question and have observed differing results. Hirudin, an anticoagulant, normally contains a sY at position 63 that is important for thrombin binding [22]. Replacement of sY63 in hirudin with pY showed no difference in thrombin binding and inhibition of coagulation, suggesting that sY and pY are potentially interchangeable posttranslational modifications [22]. However, sY and pY modifications are not equivalent in other systems. Sulfation of tyrosines in the N-termini of CCR5, a co-receptor for HIV-1, facilitates HIV-1 cell entry [23,24] and chemokine binding [25]. Peptides fragments of the CCR5 N-terminus containing sY residues bound envelope glycoprotein (gp)-120/CD4 complexes, while those containing tyrosine or pY residues did not [26]. Other examples have shown that sY and pY modifications are somewhat interchangeable, with SH2 domains binding much less tightly to sY versus native pY containing ligands [27,28]. Recent molecular dynamics studies investigating the structure of the chemokine CXC chemokine ligand 12 (CXCL12) bound to the sY-modified CXCR4 N-terminus predicted that substituting pY would increase the affinity of the CXCL12 and CXCR4 interaction [29]. Stone and colleagues have also demonstrated that inorganic phosphate can modulate the recognition of sulfotyrosine residues in a CCR2 receptor mimic by the CCL2 chemokine [30]. These reports suggest there are no particular trends and comparisons of the effects of sY and pY posttranslational modifications on binding that would need to be carried out on a case by case basis.

Chemokines are hypothesized to bind to and activate their receptors through a two site-two state binding and activation model [31,32]. The extracellular, sulfotyrosine-containing N-terminus of the chemokine receptor binds to the chemokine domain first, site one, which is followed by binding of the chemokine N-terminus to a second site on the receptor that results in a receptor conformational change and in activation. Due to their demonstrated role in receptor binding and specificity, we and others have focused on using the sY-chemokine interaction as a way to identify and target druggable "hotspots" on the chemokine. The CXCR4 sY21 and sY12 binding sites on CXCL12 have successfully been targeted with inhibitory small molecules [33–38]. These inhibitors are presumed to disrupt CXCL12's interaction with the CXCR4 N-terminus, and this has prompted a comparison of sulfotyrosine and phosphotyrosine modifications in the context of CCL21 binding to its receptor, CCR7. The CCR7 N-terminus contains two tyrosines at positions 8 and 17 which are predicted to be sulfated by the bioinformatics program SulfoSite [39], while only tyrosine 8 is predicted to be sulfated by Sulfinator [40]. Here we use sY-containing CCR7 N-terminal peptides to identify putative sY8 and sY17 binding regions on CCL21 and compare the impact of tyrosine sulfation versus phosphorylation or the absence of posttranslational modification on binding specificity and affinity.

2. Results

2.1. A CCR7 N-Terminal Peptide Binds CCL21

As chemokines are thought to bind and activate their receptors through a two-step, two-site binding and activation model [31,32], peptides corresponding to the receptor N-terminus have historically been used to mimic the site 1 interaction. To determine which residues in the CCR7 N-terminus may be important for binding to CCL21 as a part of site 1, a titration of a uniformly ^{15}N-labeled CCR7 1–30 C24A peptide with increasing concentrations of CCL21 was monitored using ^{15}N-^{1}H heteronuclear single quantum coherence (HSQC) spectroscopy (Figure 1A). The CCR7 peptide contained a C24A mutation to prevent oxidative dimer formation. CCL21 caused chemical shift perturbations in the CCR7 N-terminus that included residues adjacent to both Y8 and Y17 (Figure 1B). Given that sulfotyrosines in other chemokine receptors increase affinity for the chemokine ligand [10,13–19], these CCR7 chemical shift perturbations guided our design and synthesis of CCR7 N-terminal peptides to investigate tyrosine modifications at Y8 or Y17 (Figure 2). The Y8 modification was explored using CCR7 peptides containing residues 5–11 and either Y8, pY8, or sY8, while the Y17 modification was studied using CCR7 peptides containing residues 11–30 and either Y17, pY17, or sY17.

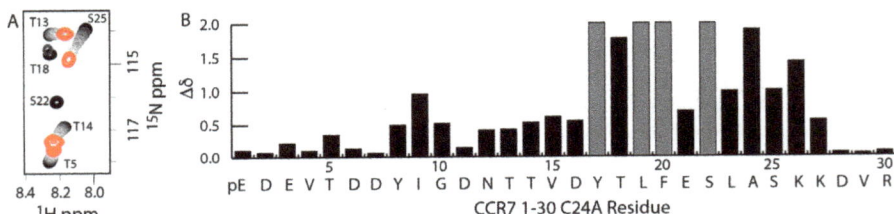

Figure 1. CCL21-induced chemical shift perturbations in the CCR7 N-terminus including tyrosine 8 and 17 and adjacent amino acids. (**A**) ^{15}N-^{1}H HSQC spectra of 200 µM U-^{15}N/^{13}C CCR7 1–30 C24A in the absence (black) and with increasing concentrations of CCL21 (grays) at 1:2.5 CCR7:CCL21 molar ratio (red); (**B**) CCL21-induced CCR7 1–30 C24A chemical shift perturbations. A portion of glutamine 1 of CCR7 1–30 C24A spontaneously reacts to form pyroglutamate; hence, the pE or pyroglutamate label at position 1. CCR7 residues that broadened beyond detection during the titration are indicated in gray with a chemical shift of 2.

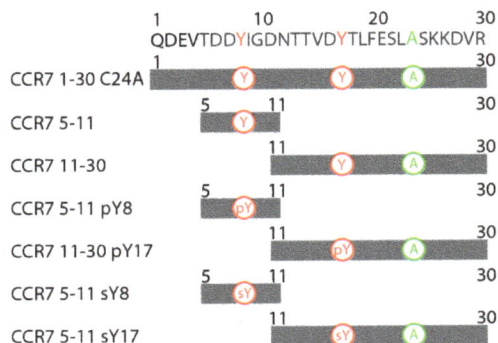

Figure 2. Schematic of the various CCR7 N-terminal peptides used in this study. CCR7 peptides correspond to the sequence of the mature CCR7 N-terminus. Those peptides including residue 24 have a C24A mutation to prevent oxidative peptide dimer formation. Tyrosine posttranslational modifications are as indicated.

2.2. CCR7 N-Terminal Peptides Maintain Binding Site Specificity upon Tyrosine Modification

Site one interactions form long, extended binding epitopes that can encompass significant amounts of the chemokine surface. To observe the important differences between modifications, U-^{15}N labeled CCL21 was titrated with the various CCR7 N-terminal peptides and NMR experiments performed. Regardless of the tyrosine modification on the CCR7(5–11) or CCR7(11–30) N-terminal peptides, binding site specificity on CCL21 was maintained, with CCR7 5–11 peptides binding alongside the alpha helix and CCR7 11–30 peptides binding to the N-loop and β3-strand of CCL21. Representative data showing overlays from a portion of the ^{15}N-^{1}H HSQC spectra of CCL21 titrated with increasing concentrations of CCR7 5–11 sY8 or CCR7 11–30 sY17 are shown in Figure 3A,B. With the exception of the CCR7 11–30 sY17 peptide, binding was in fast exchange and CCL21 assignments could be transferred by inspection. The majority of CCL21 residues bound in fast exchange upon titration with the CCR7 11–30 sY17 peptide, but a small number of residues broadened beyond detection during the titration, indicative of intermediate exchange. Residues that broadened beyond detection are indicated with a maximum chemical shift perturbation value in Figure 3D. A plot of CCL21 chemical shift perturbations at the highest CCL21: peptide molar ratio of 1:10 for peptides containing sY, or 1:30 for peptides containing Y or pY, is shown in Figure 3C for the CCR7 5–11 peptides and in Figure 3D for the CCR7 11–30 peptides. Identical residues and/or similar regions of the CCL21 structure show perturbations suggesting binding site specificity is retained regardless of the type of or the absence of tyrosine modification.

2.3. Sulfotyrosine or Phosphotyrosine Modification Increase the Affinity of CCR7 N-Terminal Peptides for CCL21

As the size of a chemical shift perturbation does not necessarily correlate with affinity, concentration-dependent CCL21 chemical shift perturbations were used to calculate the binding affinity of CCL21 for the various CCR7 peptides. Figure 4 shows representative nonlinear fitting data and dissociation constant (K_d) values for the representative residue only. Figure 4A shows the nonlinear fitting of normalized, combined amide-proton chemical shift perturbations of a representative CCL21 residue, K69, plotted versus CCR7 peptide concentrations for CCR7 5–11, CCR7 5–11 pY8, or CCR7 5–11 sY8. The nonlinear fitting of normalized, combined amide-proton chemical shift perturbations for CCL21 A53, a representative residue, plotted versus CCR7 peptide concentration for CCR7 11–30, CCR7 11–30 pY17, or CCR7 sY17 is shown in Figure 4B. Average dissociation constants obtained from the non-linear fitting of chemical shift changes for all CCL21 residues with significant peptide perturbations are reported in Table 1. Sulfated CCR7 N-terminal peptides had the highest affinity for CCL21, followed by those containing pY and, finally, the peptides with unmodified tyrosine residues. For the CCR7 5–11 peptides, a pY modification increased affinity to nearly the same extent as sY, 240 ± 60 μM versus 140 ± 40 μM K_d values, respectively. However, the pY17 modification in the CCR7 11–30 peptide ($K_d = 1700 \pm 400$ μM) did not increase affinity to CCL21 as dramatically as a sY17 modification ($K_d = 480 \pm 70$ μM). Interestingly, the CCR7 5–11 peptides exhibited higher affinities for CCL21 than their corresponding CCR7 11–30 counterparts, despite inducing smaller chemical shift perturbations.

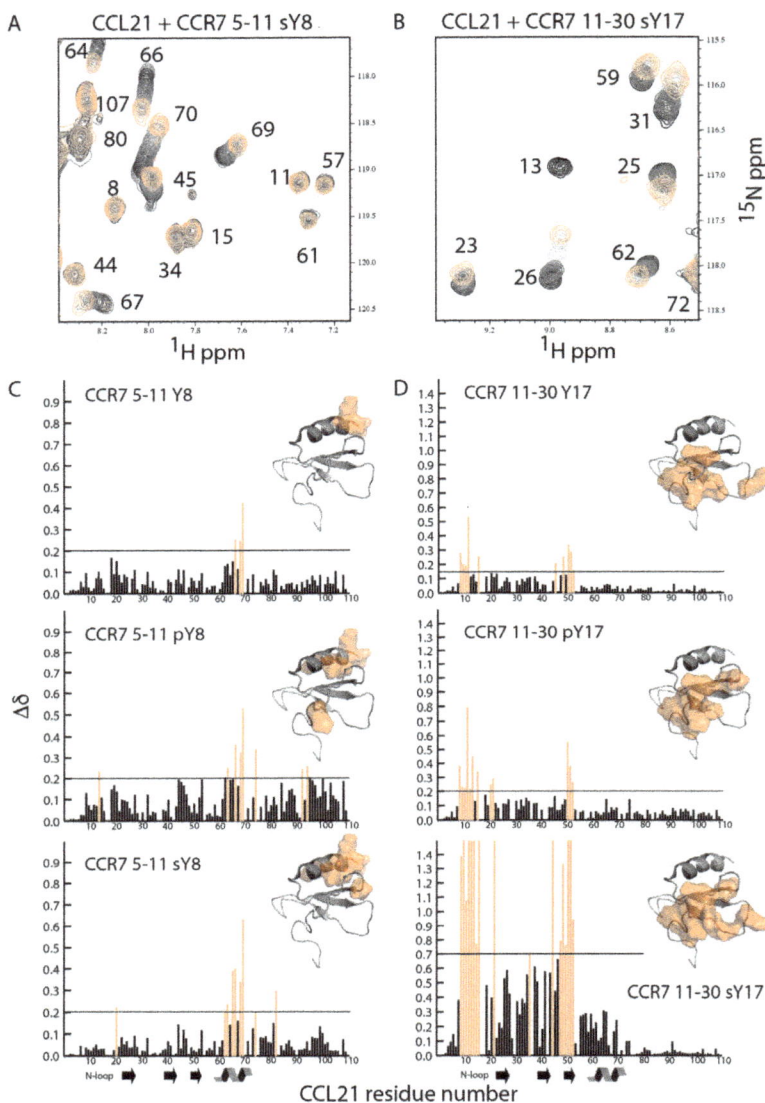

Figure 3. CCR7 N-terminal peptides maintain binding site specificity regardless of tyrosine modification. (**A**) ^{15}N-^{1}H HSQC spectra of 100 μM U-^{15}N CCL21 (black) with increasing concentrations of CCR7 5–11 sY8 in gray and orange (1:10 molar ratio); (**B**) ^{15}N-^{1}H HSQC spectra of 100 μM U-^{15}N CCL21 (black) with increasing concentrations of CCR7 11–30 sY17 in gray and orange (1:10 molar ratio); (**C**) CCL21 chemical shift perturbations and chemical shift mapping for CCR7 5–11 Y8, pY8, and sY8; (**D**) CCL21 chemical shift perturbations and chemical shift mapping for CCR7 11–30 Y17, pY17, and sY17. Residues with a chemical shift perturbation above 1.4 broadened beyond detection during the titration indicative of intermediate exchange. For clarity residues with significant chemical shift perturbations that were mapped onto the structure of CCL21-lacking residues 71–111, an extended and unstructured C-terminus, which was present [41]. CCL21 prolines and any unobservable backbone amides have chemical shift perturbations of zero.

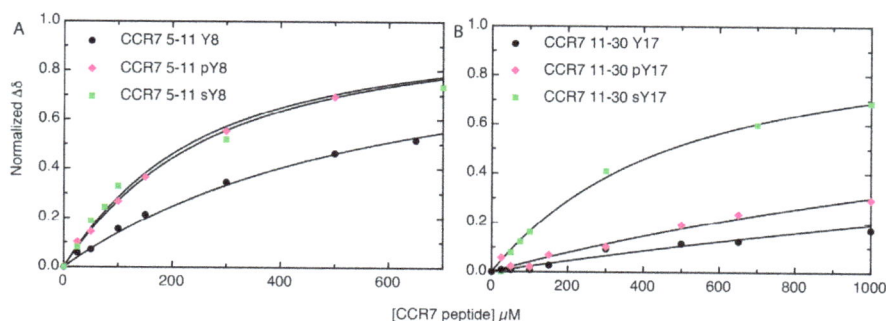

Figure 4. Tyrosine modification increases affinity of CCR7 N-terminal peptides for CCL21. Nonlinear fitting of residues with significant chemical shift perturbations was used for dissociation constant (K_d) determination. Nonlinear fitting also provided the maximum chemical shift, which was normalized to 1 in the figure for better visual comparison. (**A**) Nonlinear fitting of normalized, combined amide chemical shift perturbations for CCL21 K69, a representative residue, plotted versus CCR7 peptide concentration. For this residue only, the K_d values were as follows: CCR7 5–11 K_d = 530 ± 40 μM, CCR7 5–11 pY8 K_d = 240 ± 90 μM, CCR7 5–11 sY8 K_d = 180 ± 40 μM; (**B**) Nonlinear fitting of normalized, combined amide chemical shift perturbations for CCL21 A53, a representative residue, plotted versus CCR7 peptide concentration. For this residue only, the K_d values were as follows: CCR7 11–30 K_d = 4100 ± 900 μM, CCR7 11–30 pY17 K_d = 2200 ± 200 μM, and CCR7 11–30 sY17 K_d = 420 ± 80 μM.

Table 1. CCR7 N-terminal modifications enhance CCL21 binding affinity.

CCR7	K_d (μM) [1] ± CI [2]
5–11	700 ± 300
5–11 pY8	240 ± 60
5–11 sY8	140 ± 40
11–30	6,800 ± 500
11–30 pY17	1,700 ± 400
11–30 sY17	480 ± 70

[1] K_d values here are from the fitting of the combination of all CCL21 residues that had significant chemical shift perturbations, as indicated in Figure 3. In the case of the CCR7 11–30 sY17, the K_d value is derived from only residues with a significant chemical shift that did not broaden beyond detection. [2] CI is the confidence interval at a 95% confidence level.

3. Discussion

Our previous NMR studies defined the 3D structure of full-length CCL21 and mapped the interaction surface of a peptide corresponding to the N-terminal 30 residues of CCR7 [41]. The unsulfated CCR7 1–30 peptide induced significant chemical shift perturbations in the N-loop and β3 strand of CCL21. We separated the CCR7 N-terminal domain into two fragments corresponding to residues 5–11 and 11–30, each of which contained a tyrosine that may be a substrate for sulfation by TPST enzymes. While each peptide interacted with CCL21, the shifts induced by CCR7 11–30 binding were very similar to the pattern observed in the previous titration with CCR7 1–30. The CCR7 5–11 peptides induced smaller chemical shifts in the α-helix of CCL21. Small chemical shifts in the α-helix of CCL21 were also observed with unsulfated CCR7 1–30, but these shifts were dwarfed by those in the N-loop and the β3 strand of CCL21. A comparison of CCL21 chemical shift perturbations for CCR7 5–11 sY8, CCR7 11–30 sY17, and CCR7 1–30 in Figure 5 indicates that CCR7 5–11 and CCR7 11–30 perturbations could potentially be found in those observed for the longer CCR7 1–30 peptide. This suggests that the CCR7 site 1 interaction with CCL21 may be somewhat modular as it can be dissected into two parts, potentially suggesting that small molecule ligands could be developed to target each part and later linked. Also, as the CCR7 5–11 peptides all have higher affinity for CCL21 than the correspondingly modified CCR7 11–30 peptides (Table 1), CCR7 residues 5–11 may contribute significantly to CCL21 recognition. Phosphorylation or sulfation of either tyrosine 8 or 17 enhanced the binding of CCR7 N-terminal receptor peptides to CCL21, but sulfation of tyrosine 17 had the largest effect, increasing the affinity of CCR7 11–30 by more than 10-fold (Table 1). While there is no consensus sequence for tyrosine sulfation, proximity to one or more acidic amino acids increases the likelihood of sulfation [39,40]. Tyrosine 17 is next to aspartate 16 suggesting it may be a poorer TPST substrate than tyrosine 8, which follows aspartate 6 and 7. This is interesting as sulfotyrosine 17 has the greater impact in this analysis.

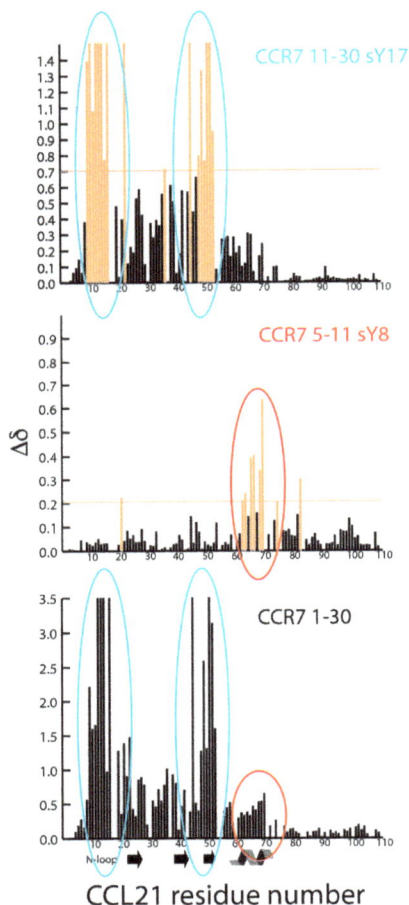

Figure 5. CCR7 site 1 is potentially modular with respect to CCL21 binding. CCL21 chemical shift perturbations are shown for CCR7 11–30 sY17 (top), CCR7 5–11 sY8 (middle), and CCR7 1–30 (bottom), adapted from Love et al. [41]. For CCR7 11–30 sY17 and CCR7 1–30, residues whose signal broadens beyond detection during titration are indicated with the highest chemical shift perturbation value. CCR7 11–30 sY17 and other CCR7 11–30 peptides induce chemical shift perturbations in the N-loop and β3 strand (circled in blue) with similar perturbations observed for CCR7 1–30, as indicated by blue ovals. CCR7 5–11 sY8 and other CCR7 5–11 peptides induce chemical shift perturbations in CCL21's α-helix with potentially similar perturbations observed for CCR7 1–30, as indicated with the red ovals.

Binding of CCL19 or CCL21 to CCR7 leads to differential activation of GRKs and recruitment of β-arrestin, resulting in different cellular responses for the two chemokine ligands [21,42]. For example, only CCL19 activation of CCR7 results in receptor internalization and desensitization [21,42]. A truncated version of CCL21, in which CCL21's unique, glycosaminoglycan-binding C-terminal tail has been proteolytically removed by plasmin, also results in signaling that is unique compared to CCL19 and full length CCL21 [43–46]. This ligand bias likely results from different CCR7 conformations in the presence of CCL19 and either full length or truncated CCL21 [43], but tyrosine sulfation in CCR7 could also be a contributing factor. While we have only investigated the interaction of CCL21 with CCR7 sulfopeptides here, Stone and colleagues have shown for CCR3 N-terminal peptides that different receptor tyrosine sulfation patterns impact which of the three chemokine ligands, CCL11, CCL24, or CCL26, the receptor prefers to bind [13,19]. It is plausible that that the degree of tyrosine sulfation or the ratio of sY8 to sY17 may impact affinity of CCR7 for its various ligands and thereby contribute to ligand bias. It should be noted that we attempted to use sodium chlorate, which has been reported to inhibit TPSTs and thus tyrosine sulfation [7], to determine if reducing CCR7 tyrosine sulfation impacted CCR7 signaling. However, treatment with sodium chlorate altered CCR7 surface expression levels, making results uninterpretable.

In addition to potential tyrosine sulfation, CCR7 is also posttranslationally modified through glycosylation. Sixt and colleagues report that polysialic acid is essential for the activation of CCR7 in dendritic cells by full length CCL21, while CCL19 and C-terminally truncated CCL21 can activate CCR7 independent of the polysialylation status of the receptor [47]. Legler and colleagues have reported distinct *N*-glycosylation patterns capped with sialic acid for specific cell types, for example B-cells and expanded T-cells, and that glycosylation inhibits chemokine activation of CCR7 unless removed by glycosidases [46]. One of the *N*-glycosylation and polysialylation sites is N12 of the mature CCR7 N-terminus (N36 if the signal sequence is included in the residue numbering) [46,47]. Interestingly, the CCR7 5–11 sY8 peptide induced chemical shifts located in the α-helix of CCL21 that are similar to those induced by polysialic acid as seen by Sixt and colleagues [47]. This further suggests a possible role for receptor sulfotyrosine in CCR7 ligand bias.

Here we show that that sulfotyrosine or phosphotyrosine increase the affinity of N-terminal CCR7 peptides for CCL21 with the sulfotyrosine modification having the largest effect. We also observe that CCR7 peptide binding specificity remains the same regardless of whether tyrosine residues are modified or not. Given that ligand bias is observed in CCR7 signaling and given the impact of posttranslational modifications like glycosylation or polysialylation [46,47], we hypothesize that the sulfotyrosine modification will also have an impact on biased signaling. A better understanding of biased signaling in CCR7 could allow for the selective targeting of only CCL19 or CCL21 signaling, which may be therapeutically beneficial for various disease states. Future studies will continue to focus on the impact of CCR7 N-terminal posttranslational modifications on binding to CCL21 and will also incorporate C-terminally truncated CCL21. These future studies will also seek to assess whether TPSTs can sulfate CCR7 Y8 and Y17 and move toward the inclusion of the full length CCR7 receptor through incorporating cell-based assays.

4. Materials and Methods

4.1. Recombinant Protein Purification and Peptide Synthesis

CCL21 was expressed and purified as previously described [48]. CCR7 1–30 C24A (QDEVTDDYIGDNTTVDYTLFESLASKKDVR), a peptide corresponding to the sequence of the N-terminus of mature CCR7 [49] (with the exception of a C24A mutation to prevent oxidative dimer formation), was expressed recombinantly and purified as follows. DNA coding for a SMT3-CCR7 1–30 C24A fusion was cloned into the BamHI and HindIII sites of pQE30. This pQE30-SMT3-CCR7 1–30 C24A was transformed into SG13009 [pREP4] *E. coli*. Cells were grown at 37 °C in 1L of U-^{15}N/^{13}C M9 minimal media to an optical density at 600 nm (OD$_{600}$) of 0.6, at which time expression was induced with 1 mM isopropyl β-D-1-thiogalactopyranoside. After 5 h, cell pellets were collected by centrifugation (3000× g for 30 min) and stored at −80 °C until processing. Cells were resuspended and lysed by sonication in buffer A (50 mM sodium phosphate, 300 mM sodium chloride, 10 mM imidazole, pH 8.0) containing 0.1% (*v/v*) β-mercaptoethanol and 1 mM phenylmethanylsulfonyl fluoride. The lysate was clarified by centrifugation (15,000× g for 15 min) and the supernatant containing the His$_6$-SMT3-CCR7 1–30 C24A fusion was applied to 2 mL of His60 nickel resin. The column was washed with 40 mL of buffer A and eluted with buffer B (50 mM sodium phosphate, 300 mM sodium chloride, 500 mM imidazole, pH 8.0). The eluent containing the His$_6$-SMT3-CCR7 1–30 C24A fusion was dialyzed (MWCO 3,000) twice against 4 L of 20 mM TRIS, pH 8.0, at 4 °C with stirring. The dialysate was transferred to a 50 mL conical vial and digested with 400 μg of His$_6$-Ubiquitin like protease 1 (His$_6$-ULP1) with stirring at 4 °C until complete cleavage of the His$_6$-SMT3-CCR7 1–30 C24A fusion was achieved based on SDS-PAGE. To separate the His$_6$-ULP1 and His$_6$-SMT3 from CCR7 1–30 C24A, the digestion was applied to 2 mL of His60 nickel resin. The column flow through and one 10 mL buffer A contained the CCR7 1–30 C24A was filtered (0.2 μm), and CCR7 1–30 C24A was further purified by reverse-phase HPLC using a 30 min 0–70% (*v/v*) acetonitrile gradient in aqueous 0.1% (*v/v*) triflouroacetic acid.

CCR7 sulfotyrosine-containing peptides (CCR7 5–11 sY8, NH$_2$-TDDsYIGD-CONH$_2$ and CCR7 11–30 sY17, NH$_2$-DNTTVDsYTLFESLASKKDVR-CONH$_2$) were synthesized and purified as previously described [12]. CCR7 phosphotyrosine-containing peptides (CCR7 5–11 pY8, NH$_2$-TDDpYIGD-CONH$_2$ and CCR7 11–30 pY17, NH$_2$-DNTTVDpYTLFESLASKKDVR-CONH$_2$) and CCR7 peptides lacking a posttranslational modification (CCR7 5–11 Y8, NH$_2$-TDDYIGD-CONH$_2$ and CCR7 11–30 Y17, NH$_2$-DNTTVDYTLFESLASKKDVR-CONH$_2$) were purchased from a commercial vendor.

4.2. Protein NMR

NMR spectroscopic data were collected at the NMR facility at the Medical College of Wisconsin on a Bruker Avance 600 MHz spectrometer equipped with ^{1}H/^{13}C/^{15}N Cryoprobe® at 25 °C. Chemical shift assignments for CCR7 1–30 C24A (H, N, C, C$^\alpha$, and most side chain carbons) were determined by standard techniques [50] using 1.05 mM U-^{15}N/^{13}C labeled CCR7 1–30 C24A in NMR buffer (25 mM deuterated MES, 10% D$_2$O, 0.2% NaN$_3$, pH 6.0). To determine CCR7 N-terminal residues likely involved in CCL21 binding, 200 μM U-^{15}N/^{13}C CCR7 1–30 C24A in NMR buffer was monitored using ^{15}N-^{1}H HSQC spectra while titrating with increasing CCL21 concentrations (molar ratios of 1:0, 1:0.25, 1:0.5, 1:0.75, 1:1, 1:1.5, 1:2 and 1:2.5 of CCR7:CCL21). Under these conditions the majority of CCR7 residues bind CCL21 in fast exchange, allowing for chemical shift assignments to be transferred by inspection, while some residues broadened beyond detection during the titration.

To identify the impact of CCR7 tyrosine modification on CCL21 binding, 100 μM of U-^{15}N CCL21 in NMR buffer was titrated with increasing concentrations of the indicated CCR7 peptides and monitored using ^{15}N-^{1}H HSQC spectra, as previously described [51,52]. Molar ratio for CCL21 to CCR7 5–11, CCR7 5–11 pY8, CCR7 11–30, or CCR7 11–30 pY17 were as follows: 1:0, 1:0.25, 1:0.5, 1:1, 1:1.5, 1:3, 1:6.5, 1:10, 1:15, 1:25, and 1:30. Molar ratios for CCL21 to CCR7 5–11 sY8 or CCR7 11–30 sY17 were as follows: 1:0, 1:0.25, 1:0.5, 1:0.75, 1:1, 1:3, 1:7, and 1:10. Under these conditions most CCL21 residues bind the various CCR7 peptides in fast exchange, allowing chemical shift assignments [41] to be transferred by inspection. Combined amide chemical shift perturbations (Δδ) were computed as $[(5\Delta\delta_H)^2+(\Delta\delta_N)^2]^{1/2}$, where $\Delta\delta_H$ and $\Delta\delta_N$ are the changes in backbone amide ^{1}H and ^{15}N chemical shifts in ppm, respectively. Dose-dependent changes in chemical shift perturbations upon titration with the various CCR7 peptides were used to determine dissociation constant (K$_d$) values through nonlinear fitting to an equation that takes into account ligand depletion, as previously described [41,52].

Acknowledgments: This work was supported by the National Institutes of Health through grant 1R15CA159202-01 to Christopher T. Veldkamp and grant F30CA210587 to Natasha A. Moussouras.

Author Contributions: Christopher T. Veldkamp and Andrew J. Phillips conceived and designed the experiments; Christopher T. Veldkamp and Andrew J. Phillips performed the experiments; Christopher T. Veldkamp and

Andrew J. Phillips analyzed the data; Andrew J. Phillips, Chad A. Koplinski, Anthony E. Getschman, Deni Taleski, Natasha A. Moussouras, Amanda M. Richard, Francis C. Peterson, Michael B. Dwinell, Richard J. Payne, and Brian F. Volkman contributed reagents/materials/analysis.

Conflicts of Interest: The authors declare no conflict of interest. The funding sponsors had no role in the design of the study; in the collection, analyses, or interpretation of data; in the writing of the manuscript, and in the decision to publish the results.

Abbreviations

CCL21	CC chemokine ligand 21
CCL19	CC chemokine ligand 19
CCR7	CC chemokine receptor 7
NMR	Nuclear magnetic resonance
sY	Sulfotyrosine
pY	Phosphotyrosine

References

1. Baggiolini, M. Chemokines in pathology and medicine. *J. Intern. Med.* **2001**, *250*, 91–104. [CrossRef] [PubMed]
2. Proudfoot, A.E. Chemokine receptors: Multifaceted therapeutic targets. *Nat. Rev. Immunol.* **2002**, *2*, 106–115. [CrossRef] [PubMed]
3. Ben-Baruch, A. Organ selectivity in metastasis: Regulation by chemokines and their receptors. *Clin. Exp. Metastasis* **2008**, *25*, 345–356. [CrossRef] [PubMed]
4. Wiley, H.E.; Gonzalez, E.B.; Maki, W.; Wu, M.T.; Hwang, S.T. Expression of CC chemokine receptor-7 and regional lymph node metastasis of B16 murine melanoma. *J. Natl. Cancer Inst.* **2001**, *93*, 1638–1643. [CrossRef] [PubMed]
5. Oliveira-Neto, H.H.; de Souza, P.P.; da Silva, M.R.; Mendonca, E.F.; Silva, T.A.; Batista, A.C. The expression of chemokines CCL19, CCL21 and their receptor CCR7 in oral squamous cell carcinoma and its relevance to cervical lymph node metastasis. *Tumour Biol.* **2013**, *34*, 65–70. [CrossRef] [PubMed]
6. Legler, D.F.; Uetz-von Allmen, E.; Hauser, M.A. CCR7: Roles in cancer cell dissemination, migration and metastasis formation. *Int. J. Biochem. Cell Biol.* **2014**, *54*, 78–82. [CrossRef] [PubMed]
7. Moore, K.L. The biology and enzymology of protein tyrosine O-sulfation. *J. Biol. Chem.* **2003**, *278*, 24243–24246. [CrossRef] [PubMed]
8. Moore, K.L. Protein tyrosine sulfation: A critical posttranslation modification in plants and animals. *Proc. Natl. Acad. Sci. USA* **2009**, *106*, 14741–14742. [CrossRef] [PubMed]
9. Seibert, C.; Sanfiz, A.; Sakmar, T.P.; Veldkamp, C.T. Preparation and analysis of N-terminal chemokine receptor sulfopeptides using tyrosylprotein sulfotransferase enzymes. *Methods Enzymol.* **2016**, *570*, 357–388. [PubMed]
10. Seibert, C.; Sakmar, T.P. Toward a framework for sulfoproteomics: Synthesis and characterization of sulfotyrosine-containing peptides. *Biopolymers* **2008**, *90*, 459–477. [CrossRef] [PubMed]
11. Stone, M.J.; Chuang, S.; Hou, X.; Shoham, M.; Zhu, J.Z. Tyrosine sulfation: An increasingly recognised post-translational modification of secreted proteins. *New Biotechnol.* **2009**, *25*, 299–317. [CrossRef]
12. Stone, M.J.; Payne, R.J. Homogeneous sulfopeptides and sulfoproteins: Synthetic approaches and applications to characterize the effects of tyrosine sulfation on biochemical function. *Acc. Chem. Res.* **2015**, *48*, 2251–2261. [CrossRef] [PubMed]
13. Ludeman, J.P.; Stone, M.J. The structural role of receptor tyrosine sulfation in chemokine recognition. *Br. J. Pharmacol.* **2014**, *171*, 1167–1179. [CrossRef] [PubMed]
14. Farzan, M.; Babcock, G.J.; Vasilieva, N.; Wright, P.L.; Kiprilov, E.; Mirzabekov, T.; Choe, H. The role of post-translational modifications of the cxcr4 amino terminus in stromal-derived factor 1 α association and HIV-1 entry. *J. Biol. Chem.* **2002**, *277*, 29484–29489. [CrossRef] [PubMed]
15. Veldkamp, C.T.; Seibert, C.; Peterson, F.C.; Sakmar, T.P.; Volkman, B.F. Recognition of a CXCR4 sulfotyrosine by the chemokine stromal cell-derived factor-1α (SDF-1α/CXCL12). *J. Mol. Biol.* **2006**, *359*, 1400–1409. [CrossRef] [PubMed]

16. Seibert, C.; Veldkamp, C.T.; Peterson, F.C.; Chait, B.T.; Volkman, B.F.; Sakmar, T.P. Sequential tyrosine sulfation of CXCR4 by tyrosylprotein sulfotransferases. *Biochemistry* **2008**, *47*, 11251–11262. [CrossRef] [PubMed]

17. Millard, C.J.; Ludeman, J.P.; Canals, M.; Bridgford, J.L.; Hinds, M.G.; Clayton, D.J.; Christopoulos, A.; Payne, R.J.; Stone, M.J. Structural basis of receptor sulfotyrosine recognition by a CC chemokine: The N-terminal region of CCR3 bound to CCL11/eotaxin-1. *Structure* **2014**, *22*, 1571–1581. [CrossRef] [PubMed]

18. Tan, J.H.; Ludeman, J.P.; Wedderburn, J.; Canals, M.; Hall, P.; Butler, S.J.; Taleski, D.; Christopoulos, A.; Hickey, M.J.; Payne, R.J.; et al. Tyrosine sulfation of chemokine receptor CCR2 enhances interactions with both monomeric and dimeric forms of the chemokine monocyte chemoattractant protein-1 (MCP-1). *J. Biol. Chem.* **2013**, *288*, 10024–10034. [CrossRef] [PubMed]

19. Zhu, J.Z.; Millard, C.J.; Ludeman, J.P.; Simpson, L.S.; Clayton, D.J.; Payne, R.J.; Widlanski, T.S.; Stone, M.J. Tyrosine sulfation influences the chemokine binding selectivity of peptides derived from chemokine receptor CCR3. *Biochemistry* **2011**, *50*, 1524–1534. [CrossRef] [PubMed]

20. Amarandi, R.M.; Hjorto, G.M.; Rosenkilde, M.M.; Karlshoj, S. Probing biased signaling in chemokine receptors. *Methods Enzymol.* **2016**, *570*, 155–186. [PubMed]

21. Zidar, D.A.; Violin, J.D.; Whalen, E.J.; Lefkowitz, R.J. Selective engagement of G protein coupled receptor kinases (GRKs) encodes distinct functions of biased ligands. *Proc. Natl. Acad. Sci. USA* **2009**, *106*, 9649–9654. [CrossRef] [PubMed]

22. Hofsteenge, J.; Stone, S.R.; Donella-Deana, A.; Pinna, L.A. The effect of substituting phosphotyrosine for sulphotyrosine on the activity of hirudin. *Eur. J. Biochem.* **1990**, *188*, 55–59. [CrossRef] [PubMed]

23. Farzan, M.; Mirzabekov, T.; Kolchinsky, P.; Wyatt, R.; Cayabyab, M.; Gerard, N.P.; Gerard, C.; Sodroski, J.; Choe, H. Tyrosine sulfation of the amino terminus of CCR5 facilitates HIV-1 entry. *Cell* **1999**, *96*, 667–676. [CrossRef]

24. Liu, X.; Malins, L.R.; Roche, M.; Sterjovski, J.; Duncan, R.; Garcia, M.L.; Barnes, N.C.; Anderson, D.A.; Stone, M.J.; Gorry, P.R.; et al. Site-selective solid-phase synthesis of a CCR5 sulfopeptide library to interrogate HIV binding and entry. *ACS Chem. Biol.* **2014**, *9*, 2074–2081. [CrossRef] [PubMed]

25. Farzan, M.; Chung, S.; Li, W.; Vasilieva, N.; Wright, P.L.; Schnitzler, C.E.; Marchione, R.J.; Gerard, C.; Gerard, N.P.; Sodroski, J.; et al. Tyrosine-sulfated peptides functionally reconstitute a CCR5 variant lacking a critical amino-terminal region. *J. Biol. Chem.* **2002**, *277*, 40397–40402. [CrossRef] [PubMed]

26. Cormier, E.G.; Persuh, M.; Thompson, D.A.; Lin, S.W.; Sakmar, T.P.; Olson, W.C.; Dragic, T. Specific interaction of CCR5 amino-terminal domain peptides containing sulfotyrosines with HIV-1 envelope glycoprotein GP120. *Proc. Natl. Acad. Sci. USA* **2000**, *97*, 5762–5767. [CrossRef] [PubMed]

27. Ju, T.; Niu, W.; Cerny, R.; Bollman, J.; Roy, A.; Guo, J. Molecular recognition of sulfotyrosine and phosphotyrosine by the SRC homology 2 domain. *Mol. Biosyst.* **2013**, *9*, 1829–1832. [CrossRef] [PubMed]

28. Ju, T.; Niu, W.; Guo, J. Evolution of SRC homology 2 (SH2) domain to recognize sulfotyrosine. *ACS Chem. Biol.* **2016**, *11*, 2551–2557. [CrossRef] [PubMed]

29. Rapp, C.; Klerman, H.; Levine, E.; McClendon, C.L. Hydrogen bond strengths in phosphorylated and sulfated amino acid residues. *PLoS ONE* **2013**, *8*. [CrossRef] [PubMed]

30. Ludeman, J.P.; Nazari-Robati, M.; Wilkinson, B.L.; Huang, C.; Payne, R.J.; Stone, M.J. Phosphate modulates receptor sulfotyrosine recognition by the chemokine monocyte chemoattractant protein-1 (MCP-1/CCL2) *Org. Biomol. Chem.* **2015**, *13*, 2162–2169. [CrossRef] [PubMed]

31. Crump, M.P.; Gong, J.H.; Loetscher, P.; Rajarathnam, K.; Amara, A.; Arenzana-Seisdedos, F.; Virelizier, J.L.; Baggiolini, M.; Sykes, B.D.; Clark-Lewis, I. Solution structure and basis for functional activity of stromal cell-derived factor-1; dissociation of CXCR4 activation from binding and inhibition of HIV-1. *EMBO J.* **1997**, *16*, 6996–7007. [CrossRef] [PubMed]

32. Kleist, A.B.; Getschman, A.E.; Ziarek, J.J.; Nevins, A.M.; Gauthier, P.A.; Chevigne, A.; Szpakowska, M.; Volkman, B.F. New paradigms in chemokine receptor signal transduction: Moving beyond the two-site model. *Biochem. Pharmacol.* **2016**, *114*, 53–68. [CrossRef] [PubMed]

33. Veldkamp, C.T.; Ziarek, J.J.; Peterson, F.C.; Chen, Y.; Volkman, B.F. Targeting SDF-1/CXCL12 with a ligand that prevents activation of CXCR4 through structure-based drug design. *J. Am. Chem. Soc.* **2010**, *132*, 7242–7243. [CrossRef] [PubMed]

34. Smith, E.W.; Liu, Y.; Getschman, A.E.; Peterson, F.C.; Ziarek, J.J.; Li, R.; Volkman, B.F.; Chen, Y. Structural analysis of a novel small molecule ligand bound to the CXCL12 chemokine. *J. Med. Chem.* **2014**, *57*, 9693–9699. [CrossRef] [PubMed]

35. Smith, E.W.; Nevins, A.M.; Qiao, Z.; Liu, Y.; Getschman, A.E.; Vankayala, S.L.; Kemp, M.T.; Peterson, F.C.; Li, R.; Volkman, B.F.; et al. Structure-based identification of novel ligands targeting multiple sites within a chemokine-G-protein-coupled-receptor interface. *J. Med. Chem.* **2016**, *59*, 4342–4351. [CrossRef] [PubMed]

36. Smith, E.W.; Lewandowski, E.M.; Moussouras, N.A.; Kroeck, K.G.; Volkman, B.F.; Veldkamp, C.T.; Chen, Y. Crystallographic structure of truncated CCL21 and the putative sulfotyrosine-binding site. *Biochemistry* **2016**, *55*, 5746–5753. [CrossRef] [PubMed]

37. Ziarek, J.J.; Kleist, A.B.; London, N.; Raveh, B.; Montpas, N.; Bonneterre, J.; St-Onge, G.; DiCosmo-Ponticello, C.J.; Koplinski, C.A.; Roy, I.; et al. Structural basis for chemokine recognition by a G protein-coupled receptor and implications for receptor activation. *Sci. Signal.* **2017**, *10*. [CrossRef] [PubMed]

38. Ziarek, J.J.; Liu, Y.; Smith, E.; Zhang, G.; Peterson, F.C.; Chen, J.; Yu, Y.; Chen, Y.; Volkman, B.F.; Li, R. Fragment-based optimization of small molecule CXCL12 inhibitors for antagonizing the CXCL12/CXCR4 interaction. *Curr. Top. Med. Chem.* **2012**, *12*, 2727–2740. [CrossRef] [PubMed]

39. Chang, W.C.; Lee, T.Y.; Shien, D.M.; Hsu, J.B.; Horng, J.T.; Hsu, P.C.; Wang, T.Y.; Huang, H.D.; Pan, R.L. Incorporating support vector machine for identifying protein tyrosine sulfation sites. *J. Comput. Chem.* **2009**, *30*, 2526–2537. [CrossRef] [PubMed]

40. Monigatti, F.; Gasteiger, E.; Bairoch, A.; Jung, E. The sulfinator: Predicting tyrosine sulfation sites in protein sequences. *Bioinformatics* **2002**, *18*, 769–770. [CrossRef] [PubMed]

41. Love, M.; Sandberg, J.L.; Ziarek, J.J.; Gerarden, K.P.; Rode, R.R.; Jensen, D.R.; McCaslin, D.R.; Peterson, F.C.; Veldkamp, C.T. Solution structure of CCL21 and identification of a putative CCR7 binding site. *Biochemistry* **2012**, *51*, 733–735. [CrossRef] [PubMed]

42. Hauser, M.A.; Legler, D.F. Common and biased signaling pathways of the chemokine receptor CCR7 elicited by its ligands CCL19 and CCL21 in leukocytes. *J. Leukoc. Biol.* **2016**, *99*. [CrossRef] [PubMed]

43. Hjorto, G.M.; Larsen, O.; Steen, A.; Daugvilaite, V.; Berg, C.; Fares, S.; Hansen, M.; Ali, S.; Rosenkilde, M.M. Differential CCR7 targeting in dendritic cells by three naturally occurring CC-chemokines. *Front. Immunol.* **2016**, *7*, 568. [CrossRef] [PubMed]

44. Lorenz, N.; Loef, E.J.; Kelch, I.D.; Verdon, D.J.; Black, M.M.; Middleditch, M.J.; Greenwood, D.R.; Graham, E.S.; Brooks, A.E.; Dunbar, P.R.; et al. Plasmin and regulators of plasmin activity control the migratory capacity and adhesion of human T cells and dendritic cells by regulating cleavage of the chemokine CCL21. *Immunol. Cell Biol.* **2016**, *94*, 955–963. [CrossRef] [PubMed]

45. Barmore, A.J.; Castex, S.M.; Gouletas, B.A.; Griffith, A.J.; Metz, S.W.; Muelder, N.G.; Populin, M.J.; Sackett, D.M.; Schuster, A.M.; Veldkamp, C.T. Transferring the C-terminus of the chemokine CCL21 to CCL19 confers enhanced heparin binding. *Biochem. Biophys. Res. Commun.* **2016**, *477*, 602–606. [CrossRef] [PubMed]

46. Hauser, M.A.; Kindinger, I.; Laufer, J.M.; Spate, A.K.; Bucher, D.; Vanes, S.L.; Krueger, W.A.; Wittmann, V.; Legler, D.F. Distinct CCR7 glycosylation pattern shapes receptor signaling and endocytosis to modulate chemotactic responses. *J. Leukoc. Biol.* **2016**, *99*, 993–1007. [CrossRef] [PubMed]

47. Kiermaier, E.; Moussion, C.; Veldkamp, C.T.; Gerardy-Schahn, R.; de Vries, I.; Williams, L.G.; Chaffee, G.R.; Phillips, A.J.; Freiberger, F.; Imre, R.; et al. Polysialylation controls dendritic cell trafficking by regulating chemokine recognition. *Science* **2016**, *351*, 186–190. [CrossRef] [PubMed]

48. Veldkamp, C.T.; Koplinski, C.A.; Jensen, D.R.; Peterson, F.C.; Smits, K.M.; Smith, B.L.; Johnson, S.K.; Lettieri, C.; Buchholz, W.G.; Solheim, J.C.; et al. Production of recombinant chemokines and validation of refolding. *Methods Enzymol.* **2016**, *570*, 539–565. [PubMed]

49. Birkenbach, M.; Josefsen, K.; Yalamanchili, R.; Lenoir, G.; Kieff, E. Epstein-barr virus-induced genes: First lymphocyte-specific G protein-coupled peptide receptors. *J. Virol.* **1993**, *67*, 2209–2220. [PubMed]

50. Markley, J.L.; Ulrich, E.L.; Westler, W.M.; Volkman, B.F. Macromolecular structure determination by NMR spectroscopy. *Methods Biochem. Anal.* **2003**, *44*, 89–113. [PubMed]

51. Veldkamp, C.T.; Peterson, F.C.; Pelzek, A.J.; Volkman, B.F. The monomer-dimer equilibrium of stromal cell-derived factor-1 (CXCL12) is altered by PH, phosphate, sulfate, and heparin. *Protein Sci.* **2005**, *14*, 1071–1081. [CrossRef] [PubMed]

52. Veldkamp, C.T.; Kiermaier, E.; Gabel-Eissens, S.J.; Gillitzer, M.L.; Lippner, D.R.; DiSilvio, F.A.; Mueller, C.J.; Wantuch, P.L.; Chaffee, G.R.; Famiglietti, M.W.; et al. Solution structure of CCL19 and identification of overlapping CCR7 and PSGL-1 binding sites. *Biochemistry* **2015**, *54*, 4163–4166. [CrossRef] [PubMed]

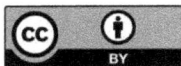

International Journal of
Molecular Sciences

MDPI

Article

The Chemokine Receptor CXCR6 Evokes Reverse Signaling via the Transmembrane Chemokine CXCL16

Vivian Adamski [1], Rolf Mentlein [2], Ralph Lucius [2], Michael Synowitz [1], Janka Held-Feindt [1,†] and Kirsten Hattermann [2,*,†]

[1] Department of Neurosurgery, University Medical Center Schleswig-Holstein UKSH, Campus Kiel, D-24105 Kiel, Germany; Vivian.adamski@uksh.de (V.A.); Michael.synowitz@uksh.de (M.S.); Janka.held-feindt@uksh.de (J.H.-F.)

[2] Department of Anatomy, University of Kiel, D-24118 Kiel, Germany; rment@anat.uni-kiel.de (R.M.); rlucius@anat.uni-kiel.de (R.L.)

* Correspondence: k.hattermann@anat.uni-kiel.de; Tel.: +49(0)431-880-2460
† These authors contributed equally to this work.

Received: 31 May 2017; Accepted: 6 July 2017; Published: 8 July 2017

Abstract: Reverse signaling is a signaling mechanism where transmembrane or membrane-bound ligands transduce signals and exert biological effects upon binding of their specific receptors, enabling a bidirectional signaling between ligand and receptor-expressing cells. In this study, we address the question of whether the transmembrane chemokine (C-X-C motif) ligand 16, CXCL16 is able to transduce reverse signaling and investigate the biological consequences. For this, we used human glioblastoma cell lines and a melanoma cell line as as in vitro models to show that stimulation with recombinant C-X-C chemokine receptor 6 (CXCR6) or CXCR6-containing membrane preparations induces intracellular (reverse) signaling. Specificity was verified by RNAi experiments and by transfection with expression vectors for the intact CXCL16 and an intracellularly-truncated form of CXCL16. We showed that reverse signaling via CXCL16 promotes migration in CXCL16-expressing melanoma and glioblastoma cells, but does not affect proliferation or protection from chemically-induced apoptosis. Additionally, fast migrating cells isolated from freshly surgically-resected gliomas show a differential expression pattern for CXCL16 in comparison to slowly-migrating cells, enabling a possible functional role of the reverse signaling of the CXCL16/CXCR6 pair in human brain tumor progression in vivo.

Keywords: chemokine; chemokine receptor; reverse signaling; cellular communication; brain tumor; glioma; tumor cell migration

1. Introduction

Cellular communication is frequently mediated by more or less specific binding of a ligand to its corresponding receptor, exerting intracellular signaling cascades and downstream effects in the receptor-expressing cell. However, transmembrane or membrane-bound ligands can also serve as signaling "receptors" and thus enable a bidirectional cellular communication. This signaling mode is termed "reverse signaling" and has so far been described for members of some (super)families of transmembrane ligands including the tumor necrosis factor-α (TNFα) superfamily, the ephrin ligand family and the semaphorins; for a review, see [1–3]. Reverse signaling depends on the intracellular domains of the ligands and/or associated molecules. This intracellular communication is involved in immune regulation and modulation [1,4,5], development and maintenance of the nervous system including axon guidance and synaptic plasticity [2,3,6,7], bone remodeling [8] and vascular morphogenesis and angiogenesis [9].

Recently, we were able to report another alternative signaling mode that is mediated via the transmembrane chemokines CXCL16 and CX3CL1 (chemokine (C-X3-C motif) ligand 1). In this process, upon shedding by matrix metalloproteinases (a disintegrin and metalloproteinase (ADAM) 10 and ADAM17), the chemokine domain can be released from the transmembrane stack [10–12], binds to the transmembrane form and elicits intracellular extracellular signal-regulated kinase $\frac{1}{2}$ (ERK1/2, p42/p44) and Akt signaling followed by downstream proliferative and anti-apoptotic effects in glioma cell lines and primary human meningioma cells [13,14]. Apart from this novel signaling mode, the soluble forms of CXCL16 and CX3CL1, of course, evoke effects via their known receptors. CXCL16 is a ligand for the chemokine receptor and HIV (human immunodeficiency virus) co-receptor CXCR6/Bonzo [15] and recruits immune cells, e.g., in rheumatoid arthritis [16]. However, CXCL16 and/or CXCR6 are also overexpressed in several types of tumors, including breast, prostate and gastrointestinal cancers, and benign and malignant tumors of the nervous system [17–22]. Within these tumors, the CXCL16/CXCR6 axis plays a multifaceted role by promoting proliferation and migration of tumor cells [17–19,21] and attraction and modulation of immune cells supporting immune-mediated tumor control [23–25].

Thus, regarding the facts that (1) reverse signaling via transmembrane ligands has been reported for a considerable number of ligand-receptor pairs and (2) we recently could show that transmembrane CXCL16 can transduce signals via its intracellular domain upon binding of its soluble form ("inverse signaling"), we wondered if reverse signaling may also take place in the interaction between transmembrane CXCL16 and its known receptor CXCR6.

To investigate intracellular signaling of CXCL16 upon stimulation with CXCR6, initially, we used human glioblastoma cell lines (known to express transmembrane CXCL16, but not CXCR6) and applied CXCR6 in different forms. The specificity of reverse signaling was proven by silencing experiments, as well as by transfection experiments using a CXCL16-negative, CXCR6-negative melanoma cell line to investigate intracellular signaling and biological effects upon stimulation with CXCR6.

2. Results

2.1. Expression of CXCL16 and CXCR6 in Native and Stably-Transfected Human Tumor Cell Lines

From our recent investigations, we know that CXCL16 is highly expressed in different human gliomas, while the corresponding receptor CXCR6 is restricted to a small subset of glioma cells with stem cell characteristics [20]. To investigate a putative reverse signaling mediated by transmembrane CXCL16, we used CXCL16-positive and CXCR6-negative glioblastoma cell lines. We verified the expression of CXCL16 and the lack of CXCR6 in human glioblastoma cell lines A172, LN229, T98G and U251MG on mRNA level by quantitative reverse transcription polymerase chain reaction (qRT-PCR) and on protein level by immunocytochemistry (ICC) for cell lines used in the following sections (Figure 1A; compare also [13] for independent results on T98G and A172).

To prove specificity, we used stable transfected LOX melanoma cell clones. LOX melanoma cells do not endogenously express CXCL16, nor CXCR6, and so, we generated LOX clones expressing transmembrane CXCL16 (LOX-CXCL16) or a C–terminally truncated version of transmembrane CXCL16 (LOX-ΔCXCL16) and a clone from the empty expression vector (LOX-pcDNA) [13]. To verify the expression of CXCL16 (and CXCR6) of the LOX cell clones used for the following assays, we performed qRT-PCR and immunocytochemistry (Figure 1B). Additionally, we used LOX melanoma cells to generate stable clones expressing CXCR6 (LOX-CXCR6). For controls, the empty control vector was inserted (LOX-pCMV), and we confirmed CXCR6 expression by immunocytochemistry and Western blot (Figure 1C).

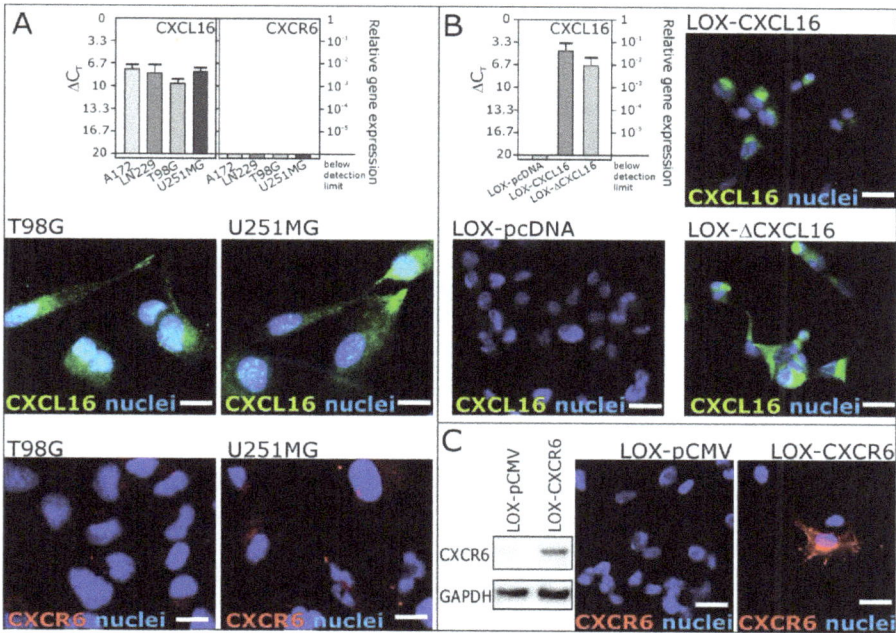

Figure 1. Expression of CXCL16 and CXCR6 mRNA and protein in glioblastoma cells and stably transfected LOX melanoma cell clones by quantitative reverse transcription polymerase chain reaction (qRT-PCR) and immunocytochemistry (ICC). (**A**) Expression of CXCL16 and CXCR6 was investigated in glioblastoma cell lines A172, LN229, T98G and U251MG (for biological independent results of A172 and T98G, compare also [13]). CXCL16 was detected at moderate to high extends, whereas CXCR6 was undetectable or yielded just background staining; (**B**) expression of CXCL16 was investigated in clones from natively CXCL16-negative, CXCR6-negative LOX melanoma cells. While the LOX-pcDNA clone was CXCL16 negative, the LOX-CXCL16 clone showed CXCL16 at the mRNA and protein level. A C-terminally truncated version of CXCL16 (in LOX-ΔCXCL16 cells) was also detectable at the mRNA and protein level (for verification of truncation, see [13]); (**C**) Expression of CXCR6 was investigated in LOX melanoma cell clones. While the LOX-pCMV clone was CXCR6 negative, a LOX-CXCR6 transfected clone yielded positive staining for CXCR6 and a specific signal at about 43 kDa in Western blot experiments. Values of qRT-PCR are shown as ΔC_T, meaning that a 3.33 higher ΔC_T indicates a 10-fold lower mRNA expression. $n = 3$ independent experiments; examples shown for immunocytochemistry. Scale bars indicate 20 μm, respectively.

2.2. Recombinant CXCR6 Induces ERK1/2 Phosphorylation via CXCL16 in Glioblastoma Cells

To investigate a putative reverse signaling of transmembrane CXCL16 upon binding of its known receptor CXCR6, for the first approach, we used different CXCL16-positive, CXCR6-negative glioblastoma cell lines and stimulated them with 25 ng/mL recombinant CXCR6 for 10 or 15 min. As shown in Figure 2A, this stimulation yields a phosphorylation of ERK1/2 in glioblastoma cells (T98G, U251MG). This effect drastically decreased when glioblastoma cells were transfected with siRNAs specifically targeting CXCL16 prior to stimulation with recombinant CXCR6 (Figure 2B, in comparison to control siRNA transfections), indicating a specific signaling mechanism via CXCL16. The efficiency of siRNA-mediated reduction of CXCL16 was proven by qRT-PCR and immunoblotting for each independent experiment (Figure 2B, lower part).

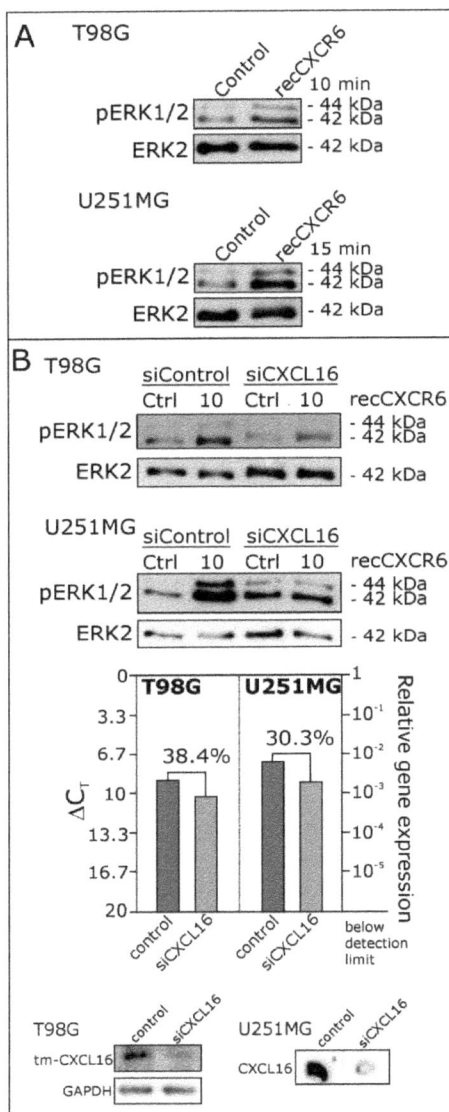

Figure 2. Phosphorylation of the extra cellular-regulated kinases ERK1/2 upon stimulation with recombinant CXCR6 in glioblastoma cells. (**A**) T98G and U251MG glioblastoma cells were stimulated with 25 ng/mL recombinant (rec) CXCR6 for 10 or 15 min, respectively, and phosphorylation of ERK1/2 was investigated by Western blot; equal loading was ensured by reprobing of the membranes with antibodies for the non-phosphorylated kinase ERK2. Stimulation with recombinant CXCR6 yielded a clear phosphorylation signal for both cell lines; (**B**) when CXCL16 expression was reduced in T98G and U251MG cells to 30–40% by CXCL16-specific siRNA (siCXCL16) as proven by qRT-PCR and Western or dot blotting, ERK1/2 phosphorylation after 10 minutes of stimulation with recombinant CXCR6 was clearly diminished in comparison to control siRNA transfections. Examples of *n* = 3 independent experiments.

2.3. Signaling of Recombinant and Membrane-Expressed CXCR6 Depends on the Expression of Intact Transmembrane CXCL16

In the next step, we stimulated stably CXCL16 expressing LOX melanoma cells (LOX-CXCL16) with recombinant CXCR6 and observed again an activation of ERK1/2 (Figure 3A, upper part). Additionally, we extracted membranes from stably CXCR6 expressing LOX cells (LOX-CXCR6) and used these for stimulations yielding also the activation of ERK1/2 signaling, while stimulation with control membranes from LOX-pCMV failed to induce phosphorylation. As a control, we repeated stimulation experiments with LOX-pcDNA control cells that are negative for CXCL16 (and also CXCR6), and neither recombinant, nor membrane expressed CXCR6 could activate ERK1/2 signaling (Figure 3B). Furthermore, we stimulated LOX melanoma cells stably expressing a CXCL16 variant that lacks the cytoplasmic tail due to truncation (LOX-ΔCXCL16) with recombinant and membrane expressed CXCR6, as well as control membrane fractions and did not observe any ERK1/2 phosphorylation either (Figure 3C). As a further control, to exclude unspecific reaction of a recombinant receptor preparation, we stimulated LOX-CXCL16 and LOX-pcDNA cells also with recombinant CX3CR1. CX3CR1 is the receptor for the transmembrane chemokine CX3CL1, which is not expressed by LOX clones. CX3CR1 does not bind to CXCL16, so that recCX3CR1 may serve as an unrelated recombinant receptor control. Accordingly, stimulation with recCX3CR1 did not yield any activation of the ERK1/2 pathway (compare Figure S1).

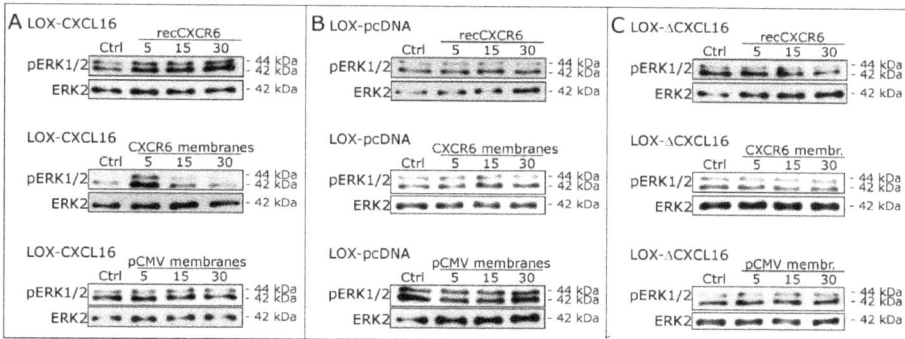

Figure 3. Phosphorylation of ERK1/2 upon stimulation with recombinant CXCR6 or membrane preparations of CXCR6-expressing and control LOX clones. (**A**) In LOX-CXCL16 clones, stimulation with 25 ng/mL recombinant (rec) CXCR6 (upper panel), as well as with membranes from CXCR6-expressing LOX cells (CXCR6 membranes, 5 μg/mL membrane preparation, middle panel) induced a robust phosphorylation of ERK1/2, while stimulation with control membranes lacking CXCR6 (pCMV membranes, lower panel) failed to activate ERK1/2; (**B**) in LOX-pcDNA cells that are CXCL16-negative and CXCR6-negative, stimulation with neither recombinant CXCR6, nor CXCR6 membranes, nor pCMV membranes yielded ERK1/2 phosphorylation; (**C**) LOX-ΔCXCL16 cells lacking the intracellular domain of the transmembrane CXCL16 also did not show any activation of the ERK1/2 signaling pathway upon stimulation with recombinant or membrane expressed CXCR6. Examples of *n* = 3 independent experiments.

These results indicate that signaling upon CXCR6 stimulation specifically depends on the expression of CXCL16 including its intracellular domain and may physiologically occur upon exposition of transmembrane CXCL16 to CXCR6-expressing membranes.

2.4. Biological Effects of Reverse Signaling via CXCL16

To investigate which biological consequences might result from the reverse signaling of the CXCL16-CXCR6 axis, we first referred to the effects observed with inverse signaling in glioma cells [13] and tested the proliferative and anti-apoptotic effects in LOX-CXCL16 and corresponding control clones. However, in these CXCL16-transfected melanoma cells, we did not observe any regulation of proliferation upon stimulation with recombinant CXCR6 (Figure 4A), nor could we detect less cleavage of poly(ADP ribose) polymerase (PARP, Figure 4B) after induction of apoptosis with 0.1 µg/mL camptothecin. Additionally, we did not observe any proliferative or anti-apoptotic effects in endogenously CXCL16-expressing glioblastoma cells (Figure 4A,B).

Next, we investigated the migratory potential of LOX-CXCL16 cells in comparison to LOX-pcDNA (control) and LOX-ΔCXCL16 (C-terminally truncated) and of T98G glioblastoma cells in a scratch assay with or without stimulation with recombinant CXCR6 (Figure 4C). Here, we could show that CXCR6 stimulation enhanced the migration into the cell free area in a time span of 8 h for LOX-CXCL16 and T98G glioblastoma cells, while there was no significant difference in migration between unstimulated and CXCR6-stimulated cultures in LOX-pcDNA and LOX-ΔCXCL16 cells.

Interestingly, when we investigated the expression of CXCL16 in fast migrating in comparison to slowly-migrating cells isolated from freshly-dissected glioblastomas, as described previously [26], we could show that in most investigated glioblastomas, CXCL16 expression was elevated in fast migrating cells in comparison to slowly-migrating ones (Figure 4D), which may indicate that high CXCL16 levels might favor migratory potential in glioblastomas.

Summarizing, our data show that transmembrane CXCL16 transduces signals upon stimulation with its known receptor CXCR6, activating intracellular ERK1/2 signaling. This reverse signaling depends on the intracellular domain of CXCL16 and promotes migration in CXCL16-expressing melanoma and glioblastoma cells in vitro. Additionally, we could show that fast migrating glioblastoma cells isolated from freshly-dissected glioblastomas express CXCL16 at higher levels in comparison to slowly-migrating cells, giving a first hint that reverse signaling might also contribute to glioblastoma migration processes in vivo.

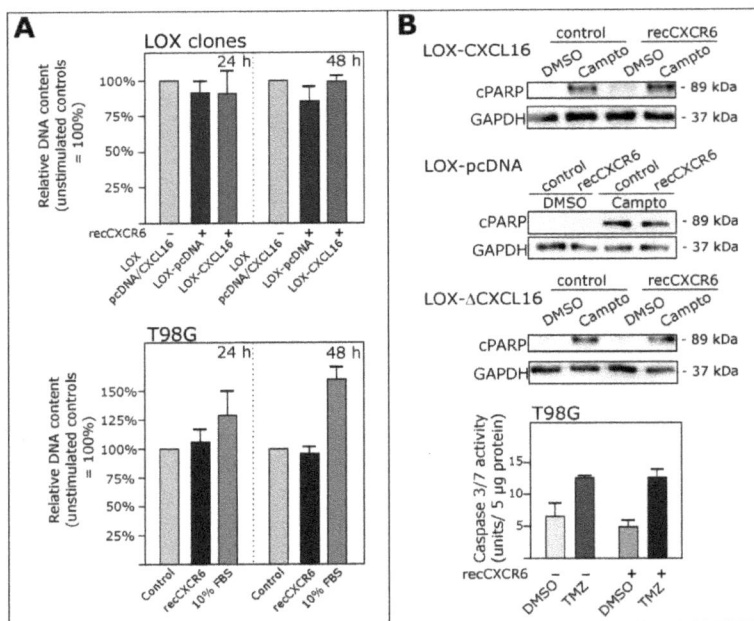

Figure 4. *Cont.*

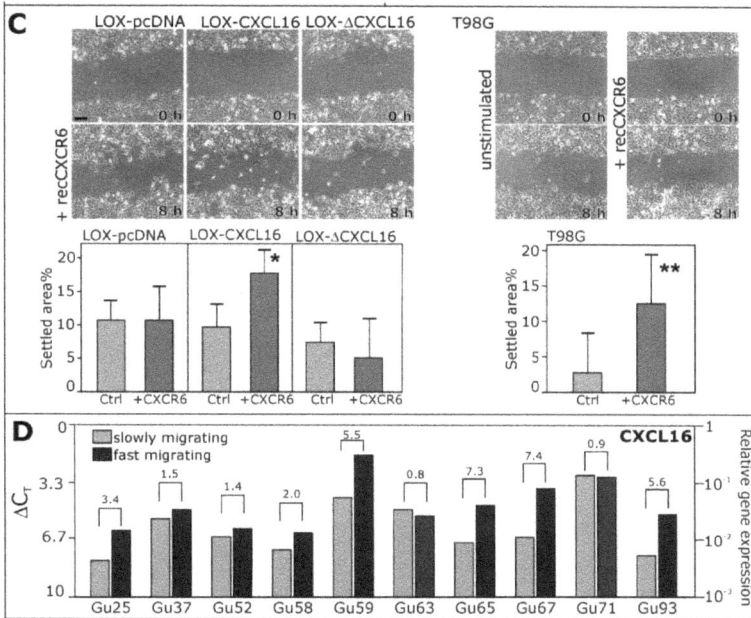

Figure 4. Biological effects of reverse signaling via the CXCR6-CXCL16-axis. (**A**) To investigate effects on proliferation, DNA contents were measured in LOX-CXCL16 and as a control in LOX-pcDNA cells stimulated (or not) with 50 ng/mL recombinant (rec) CXCR6 for 24 or 48 h (upper part). Corresponding experiments were also performed with T98G glioblastoma cells (lower part); 10% fetal bovine serum (FBS) served as the positive control for proliferation. Unstimulated controls were set to 100%, respectively, and stimulation with CXCR6 did not yield any significant induction or reduction of DNA content. Mean ± SD from $n = 3$ independent experiments; (**B**) apoptosis was induced with 0.1 µg/mL camptothecin (Campto), in comparison to equal volumes of solvent control dimethylsulfoxide (DMSO) for 18 h in LOX-CXCL16, LOX-pcDNA and LOX-ΔCXCL16 cells or for 48 h in T98G glioblastoma cells, and simultaneous stimulation with 50 ng/mL recCXCR6 did not reduce cleavage of PARP (cPARP) as detected by Western blot or caspase 3/7 activity as determined by fluorimetric measurement of substrate cleavage, both indicating apoptosis. For Western blotting, equal loading was ensured by reprobing of the membrane with a glyceraldehyde 3-phosphate dehydrogenase (GAPDH)-specific antibody. Examples (Western blot) or mean values (caspase activity) of $n = 3$ independent experiments; (**C**) to investigate migration, scratch assays were performed with LOX clones LOX-CXCL16, LOX-pcDNA and LOX-ΔCXCL16 or T98G glioblastoma cells stimulated with 50 ng/mL recCXCR6 or left unstimulated for controls. Scratch areas were measured at the beginning and after 8 h, and settled areas were determined as the percentage of the initial scratch area. Stimulation with 50 ng/mL CXCR6 promotes migration of LOX-CXCL16 and T98G cells, but not LOX-pcDNA or LOX-ΔCXCL16 cells. Mean ± SD from $n = 4$ independent experiments; exemplary images are shown with equal magnifications, respectively; scale bar indicates 50 µm; * $p < 0.05$, ** $p < 0.01$; (**D**) fast migrating glioblastoma cells from freshly-dissected glioblastomas mostly show higher CXCL16 mRNA expression levels than the slowly migrating cells of the same tumor preparation. ΔC_T levels are shown in a logarithmic scale (a 3.33 higher ΔC_T value indicates a 10-fold lower mRNA expression), and numbers above the brackets indicate the (linearized) x-fold expression difference between fast and slowly-migrating cells of ten different primary and secondary glioblastoma samples.

3. Discussion

Physiologically, transmembrane CXCL16 is among others expressed by immune and endothelial cells and can be induced in inflammatory conditions [11,15,16,27]. The chemokine domain is shed from the transmembrane protein by the matrix metalloproteinases ADAM 10 and 17 [10–12] and promotes trafficking of immune cells [15]. Additionally, CXCL16 has been shown to increase proliferation, e.g., of glial precursor cells [28] and endothelial cells [29]. Interestingly, the transmembrane form of CXCL16 mediates firm adhesion contacts between ligand and CXCR6 receptor-expressing cells indicating that also transmembrane CXCL16 may bind to CXCR6 and does not afford an activation of CXCR6 [27].

However, recently, we showed that CXCL16 can also induce signals independently from CXCR6 by a mechanism we termed inverse signaling. In this signaling mode, the chemokine domain of CXCL16 binds to the transmembrane form of CXCL16, induces intracellular ERK1/2 and Akt signaling and promotes proliferation and rescue from chemically-induced apoptosis [13,14]. In the present study, we demonstrated that the transmembrane form of CXCL16 may also transduce signals upon stimulation with CXCR6 resulting in the activation of ERK1/2 followed by increased migration in the ligand-bearing cell. Additionally, as previously shown for inverse signaling, reverse signaling and downstream effects depend on the intact intracellular domain of CXCL16. In glioblastomas, CXCR6 is expressed by a small subset of tumor cells with stem cell properties [20], so that direct cell contacts might enable reverse signaling via CXCL16.

Regarding effects via transmembrane ligands in a more general view, the reverse signaling is often involved in modulating the balance in dynamic changing systems and plasticity, like for example the Eph (erythropoietin-producing human hepatocellular receptors)/ephrin interactions in the formation and maintenance of synapses [2], in angiogenesis [9] and in bone remodelling [8], TNF family members as co-stimulators and direct effectors in the adaptive and innate immune system [1,30] and the semaphorins in a variety of processes including axonal guidance, angiogenesis and immune response [31]. These interactions often evoke cell cytoskeleton rearrangement and migratory processes and involve a multitude of signaling pathways including, e.g., the ERK1/2, Akt and STAT3 (Signal transducer and activator of transcription 3) pathways [6,9,32,33]. Apart from its role in physiological development and homeostasis, reverse signaling has also been described in tumor progression showing diverse effects, for example breast cancer-associated angiogenesis [34] and increased glioma cell motility via ephrin-B2 [35]. Interestingly, the semaphorin Sema5A has been shown to inhibit glioma cell motility [36], while this and other semaphorins seem to promote cancer growth and metastasis [31].

Thus, reverse signaling contributes to tumor biology in a multifaceted way. We were able to show now that the transmembrane chemokine CXCL16 can also mediate reverse signaling and promotes migration in the tumor context. In this line, we observed that fast migrating glioblastoma cells show higher CXCL16 expression levels in comparison to slowly-migrating cells of the same tumors.

4. Materials and Methods

4.1. Cell Cultures and Freshly-Isolated Glioma Cells

The human glioblastoma multiforme (GBM) cell lines A172 (ECACC 880624218), U251MG (ECACC 89081403; formerly known as U373MG), T98G (ECACC 92090213) and LN229 (ATCC-CRL-2611) were obtained from the European Collection of Cell Cultures (ECACC, Salisbury, UK) or the American Type Culture Collection (ATCC, Manassas, VA, USA) and cultured as described before [26]. Fast and slowly-migrating native human GBM cells were isolated as mentioned previously [26] and in accordance with the Helsinki Declaration of 1975 with approval of the ethics committee of the University of Kiel, Germany, after written informed consent of donors (file reference: D 408/14). For an overview of clinical data available for these samples, please refer to [26]. Different GBM cells were checked for purity by immunostaining with markers specific for GBM cultures (glial fibrillary acidic protein (GFAP) and fibronectin [37,38]; compare Figure S2) and for the absence of *Mycoplasma* contamination. LOX melanoma cells were a gift from Udo Schumacher, Department of

Anatomy, University of Hamburg, Germany [39]. Cell lines' identity was proven routinely by short tandem repeat profiling at the Department of Forensic Medicine (Kiel, Germany) using the Powerplex HS Genotyping Kit (Promega, Madison, WC, USA) and the 3500 Genetic Analyser (Thermo Fisher Scientific, Waltham, MA, USA).

4.2. Stable Transfected Cell Lines

Stable transfected LOX-pcDNA, LOX-CXCL16 and intracellularly truncated LOX-ΔCXCL16 clones were generated as described previously [13].

Expression vectors for CXCR6 (CXCR6 ORF with C-terminal GFP-tag in a pCMV backbone, pCMV6-CXCR6-GFP, RG206517) and pCMV (pCMV-AC-GFP, PS100010) were obtained from OriGene (Herford, Germany), and transfection of LOX melanoma cells (250,000 cells) was performed with TurboFect (Fermentas, Sankt Leon-Rot, Germany) in serum-free Dulbecco's Modified Eagle's Medium (dulbecco's modified eagle's medium (DMEM); Invitrogen, Carlsbad, CA, USA) without antibiotics using 3 μg of the respective expression vectors and 3 μL TurboFect in a total volume of 1 mL. After 6 h, cells were rinsed, and normal growth medium (RPMI + 10% fetal bovine serum (FBS)) was added. Successful transfection was controlled by immunocytochemistry and quantitative real-time PCR (qRT-PCR). Stable clones were generated by selection with 0.8 mg/mL G418 (Calbiochem, Merck Company, Darmstadt, Germany), and colonies were picked after 10–20 days, amplified and checked for expression by qRT-PCR and immunocytochemistry.

4.3. Immunocytochemistry

Glioblastoma cell lines and different stably-transfected LOX melanoma cells grown on glass cover slips were prepared as described before [40]. Cells were incubated with primary and secondary antibodies; nuclei were stained; and slides were analyzed using a Zeiss fluorescence microscope and a Zeiss camera (Zeiss, Oberkochen, Germany). Primary antibodies were anti-CXCL16 (1:200, 500-P200, rabbit; Peprotech, Hamburg, Germany) and anti-CXCR6 (1:100, MAB699, mouse; R&D Systems, Systems, Minneapolis, MN, USA). Primary antibodies were omitted for negative controls. As secondary antibodies, donkey anti-mouse or anti-rabbit IgGs labeled with Alexa Fluor 488 or Alexa Fluor 555 (1:1000; Invitrogen, Carlsbad, CA, USA) were used.

4.4. Reverse Transcription and Quantitative Real-Time PCR

RNA of the different cell types was isolated with the TRIzol® Reagent (Invitrogen, Carlsbad, CA, USA) or with the ARCTURUS® PicoPure® RNA Isolation Kit (Applied Biosystems, Waltham, MA, USA) according to the manufacturer's instructions. DNase digestion, cDNA synthesis and qRT-PCR were performed as described before [38] using TaqMan primer probes (Applied Biosystems): CXCL16 (Hs00222859_m1), CXCR6 (Hs00174843_m1), glyceraldehyde 3-phosphate dehydrogenase (GAPDH) (Hs99999905_m1). Cycles of threshold (C_T) were determined, and ΔC_T values of each sample were calculated as $C_{T\,gene\,of\,interest} - C_{T\,GAPDH}$. A ΔC_T of 3.33 corresponds to a 10-fold lower expression compared to GAPDH. For statistical analysis, the relative gene expression compared to GAPDH ($2^{-\Delta C_T}$) was employed. The induction of gene expression upon stimulation is displayed as relative gene expression; n-fold expression changes were calculated as $\Delta\Delta C_T$ values = $2^{\Delta C_T\,control - \Delta C_T\,stimulus}$.

4.5. RNAi Silencing

After cultivation of human glioblastoma cell lines in DMEM plus 10% FBS in 6-well dishes (180,000 cells/well) for 24 h, cells were transfected with siCXCL16 RNA (CXCL16 siRNA ID: s33808; 20 nM/well; Life Technologies, Darmstadt, Germany) dissolved in a mixture of Opti-MEM medium and lipofectamine (Life Technologies) for 5 h as described before [13]. In parallel, a transfection with silencer select negative control siRNA (Life technologies) was performed under the same conditions. After transfection, cell culture medium was changed, and glioblastoma cells were cultured for another 24 h in DMEM plus 10% FBS. Then, cells were applied for Western blot experiments as described below. For controlling the knockdown efficiency, the RNA of transfected cells were purified in parallel with the PicoPure RNA Isolation Kit (Applied Biosystems, Waltham, MA, USA), and qRT-PCR using CXCL16 TaqMan primer probes (Applied Biosystems) was performed as described above. Additionally, cell lysates were also analyzed for CXCL16 protein expression by Western or dot blotting as described below.

4.6. Membrane Isolation

For isolation of cell membranes, stable transfected LOX-CXCR6 and LOX-pCMV clone cells were lysed in 5 mM HEPES buffer, then 200 mM HEPES buffer containing 1.4 mM sodium chloride was added, and the mixture was centrifuged at 800 rpm for 8 min at 4 °C. Supernatants were transferred into a new tube and centrifuged once again at 14,000 rpm for 60 min at 4 °C. The remaining pellets were resuspended with 50 μL of 20 mM HEPES buffer including 0.14 mM sodium chloride, and membranes were kept at 4 °C until usage.

4.7. Western Blot

Western blotting was performed as described [38]. Briefly, native, sicontrol and siCXCL16 transfected glioblastoma cells, as well as LOX-CXCL16, LOX-pcDNA and truncated LOX-ΔCXCL16 clones were stimulated either with 25 ng/mL recombinant CXCR6 protein (BIOZOL, Eching, Germany), 25 ng/mL recombinant CX3CR1 protein (BIOZOL, as a control) or with 5 μg/mL of LOX-CXCR6 and LOX-pCMV (control) cell membranes for 5–30 min, respectively, and cell lysates were separated by electrophoresis using 10% acrylamide gels. Then, lysates were transferred to polyvinylidene fluoride (PVDF) membranes by blotting, blocked with 5% bovine serum albumin and incubated with a rabbit anti-phospho-ERK1/2 primary antibody (1:1000, Cell Signaling Technology, Danvers, MA, USA, #9101), a rabbit anti-CXCR6 antibody (1:250, Acris, Herford, Germany, SP1286P) or a rabbit anti-CXCL16 antibody (1:250, PeproTech, Hamburg, Germany, #500-P200), and afterwards, the addition of a horseradish-peroxidase labeled secondary antibody (donkey anti-rabbit, Santa Cruz Biotechnology, Santa Cruz, CA, USA) followed by chemo-luminescence detection (GE Healthcare, Munich, Germany or Millipore, Darmstadt, Germany) was performed. To ensure equal loading amounts, membranes were reactivated with methanol, stripped with ReBlot Plus Strong Antibody Strip Solution (Millipore) and re-probed with an antibody against the non-phosphorylated protein (mouse anti-ERK2, 1:200, Santa Cruz Biotechnology, sc1647) or GAPDH (mouse anti-GAPDH, 1:250, Santa Cruz Biotechnology, sc47724). For CXCL16 dot blotting, cell lysates were directly applied to PVDF membranes, blocked, incubated with anti-CXCL16, and signals were detected as described above.

4.8. Proliferation Assay

Proliferation assays were performed as described [21]. Briefly, LOX-CXCL16, LOX-pcDNA (1×10^5) and T98G glioblastoma cells (5×10^4) were grown for one day in 10% FBS-supplemented DMEM and stimulated in DMEM plus 0.5% FBS (LOX clones) or 2% FBS (T98G cells) with 50 ng/mL recombinant CXCR6 protein (BIOZOL) for 24 h up to 48 h. In parallel, control groups without stimulation were used. Then, 250 μL of CyQUANT GR dye/cell-lysis buffer and 2.5 μL RNase (CyQUANT® Cell Proliferation Assay Kit (C-7026); Thermo Fisher Scientific, Waltham, MA, USA) were added to the cells, and lysates were scraped off, briefly centrifuged and added 250 μL 2× CyQUANT GR. Sample fluorescence was measured using a fluorescence microplate reader (CM Genios, Tecan, Männedorf, Switzerland) with filters appropriate for 480-nm excitation and 520-nm emission maxima. Results were calculated in ng DNA as the percentage of unstimulated controls.

4.9. Anti-Apoptosis Assay

Apoptosis was induced in LOX-CXCL16, LOX-pcDNA and truncated LOX-ΔCXCL16 clones by the addition of 0.1 μg/mL camptothecin (Sigma-Aldrich, St. Louis, MO, USA) applied in a stock solution in DMSO, in the presence or absence of 50 ng/mL recombinant CXCR6 (BIOZOL, Eching,

Germany). The final solvent concentration of 0.1% DMSO in camptothecin-treated cultures was also used in controls. After stimulation, cleavage of poly(ADP Ribose) polymerase (PARP) was measured by Western blot (150,000 cells/25 mm^2 flask, grown for 30 h and stimulated for 18 h) as described above using an antibody specifically detecting cleaved PARP (Asp124, 1:500, Cell Signaling Technology, Danvers, MA, USA). An antibody against GAPDH (1: 500; Santa Cruz Biotechnology, Santa Cruz, CA, USA) served as the loading control.

In T98G glioblastoma cells (250,000 cells/25 mm^2 flask, grown for 24 h), apoptosis was induced with 400 μg/mL TMZ (solved in DMSO) for 48 h in the presence or absence of 50 ng/mL recombinant CXCR6 (BIOZOL, Eching, Germany). Cells were lysed, and caspase 3/7 activity was measured as previously described [13] and normalized using a caspase 7 standard (Enzo Life Science, Lörrach, Germany).

4.10. Migration Assay

Migration was analyzed in wound healing assays (scratch assay; compare [13]). Briefly, 1.5×10^5–1.8×10^5 LOX-CXCL16, LOX-pcDNA, truncated LOX-ΔCXCL16 clones or T98G glioblastoma cells/well were seeded on 6-well dishes, grown to confluence, scratched with a pipet tip, washed and supplemented (or not for controls) with 50 ng/mL recombinant CXCR6 protein (BIOZOL). In each experiment, three scratch regions were photographed at 0 and 8 h. Scratch areas were measured, and differences between 8 and 0 h were determined (yielding the settled area). Stimuli were normalized to non-stimulated controls.

4.11. Statistical Analysis

For statistical analysis, a two-tailed Student's *t*-test was used. Significance levels were $p < 0.05$ (indicated by *), $p < 0.01$ (indicated by **) and $p < 0.001$ (indicated by ***).

5. Conclusions

In this study, we could show that the transmembrane chemokine CXCL16 can mediate intracellular signaling upon stimulation with its receptor CXCR6 in the ligand expressing cell. This signaling mechanism has previously been reported for other transmembrane ligands like ephrins, semaphorins and TNF family members and was termed reverse signaling. We now observed that reverse signaling via the transmembrane chemokine CXCL16 promotes migration in the tumor context, but does not affect proliferation or rescue from apoptosis in melanoma or glioblastoma cells. In this line, we could detect that fast migrating glioblastoma cells show higher CXCL16 expression levels in comparison to slowly-migrating cell fractions of the same tumor.

Taken together, being produced as a transmembrane ligand, CXCL16 harbors a broad range of para- and autocrine communication options that may be regulated via expression levels of ligand and receptor (e.g., in inflammation) and via cleavage and release of the chemokine domain by ADAMs. Apart from the classical forward signaling via CXCR6, the transmembrane CXCL16 form may also mediate signaling on its own, either upon binding its soluble CXCL16 (inverse signaling) or upon binding of its receptor CXCR6 (reverse signaling), inducing proliferation and survival, as well as migration in tumor cells.

Supplementary Materials: Supplementary materials can be found at www.mdpi.com/1422-0067/18/7/1468/s1.

Acknowledgments: We thank Judith Becker, Martina Burmester, Fereshteh Ebrahim and Brigitte Rehmke for expert technical assistance and Udo Schumacher (Anatomy, University of Hamburg, Germany) for kindly providing the LOX melanoma cells. This work was supported by the "Deutsche Forschungsgemeinschaft (ME 758/10-1, HE3400/5-1)", by the popgen 2.0 network (P2N; supported by a grant from the German Ministry for Education and Research (01EY1103)) and an intramural grant of the Medical Faculty of the University of Kiel ("Forschungsförderung 2016").

Author Contributions: Rolf Mentlein, Janka Held-Feindt and Kirsten Hattermann conceived of and designed the study; Vivian Adamski, Janka Held-Feindt and Kirsten Hattermann performed the experiments and analyzed the data; Ralph Lucius and Michael Synowitz contributed materials and data and assisted in data analysis; Janka Held-Feindt and Kirsten Hattermann wrote the paper. All authors revised the manuscript.

Conflicts of Interest: The authors declare no conflict of interest.

Abbreviations

ADAM	A disintegrin and metalloproteinase
DMEM	Dulbecco's Modified Eagle's Medium
DMSO	Dimethylsulfoxide
ERK	Extracellular signal-regulated kinase (p42/p44)
FBS	Fetal bovine serum
GAPDH	Glyceraldehyde 3-phosphate dehydrogenase
GBM	Glioblastoma multiforme
ICC	Immunocytochemistry
qRT-PCR	Quantitative reverse transcription polymerase chain reaction

References

1. Eissner, G.; Kolch, W.; Scheurich, P. Ligands working as receptors: Reverse signaling by members of the TNF superfamily enhance the plasticity of the immune system. *Cytokine Growth Factor Rev.* **2004**, *1*, 353–366 [CrossRef] [PubMed]
2. Klein, R. Bidirectional modulation of synaptic functions by Eph/ephrin signaling. *Nat. Neurosci.* **2009**, *12*, 15–20. [CrossRef] [PubMed]
3. Zhou, Y.; Gunput, R.A.; Pasterkamp, R.J. Semaphorin signaling: Progress made and promises ahead. *Trends Biochem. Sci.* **2008**, *33*, 161–170. [CrossRef] [PubMed]
4. Juhasz, K.; Buzas, K.; Duda, E. Importance of reverse signaling of the TNF superfamily in immune regulation. *Expert Rev. Clin. Immunol.* **2013**, *9*, 335–348. [CrossRef] [PubMed]
5. Shao, Z.; Schwarz, H. CD137 ligand, a member of the tumor necrosis factor family, regulates immune responses via reverse signal transduction. *J. Leukoc. Biol.* **2011**, *89*, 21–29. [CrossRef] [PubMed]
6. Xu, N.J.; Henkemeyer, M. Ephrin reverse signaling in axon guidance and synaptogenesis. *Semin. Cell Dev. Biol.* **2012**, *23*, 58–64. [CrossRef] [PubMed]
7. Yu, L.; Zhou, Y.; Cheng, S.; Rao, Y. Plexin A-Semaphorin-1a reverse signaling regulates photoreceptor axon guidance in Drosophila. *J. Neurosci.* **2011**, *30*, 12151–12156. [CrossRef] [PubMed]
8. Matsuo, K.; Otaki, N. Bone cell interactions through Eph/ephrin: Bone modeling, remodeling and associated diseases. *Cell Adh. Migr.* **2012**, *6*, 148–156. [CrossRef] [PubMed]
9. Sawamiphak, S.; Seidel, S.; Essmann, C.L.; Wilkinson, G.A.; Pitulescu, M.E.; Acker, T.; Acker-Palmer, A. Ephrin-B2 regulates VEGFR2 function in developmental and tumour angiogenesis. *Nature* **2010**, *465*, 487–491. [CrossRef] [PubMed]
10. Garton, K.J.; Gough, P.J.; Blobel, C.P.; Murphy, G.; Greaves, D.R.; Dempsey, P.J.; Raines, E.W. Tumor necrosis factor-α-converting enzyme (ADAM17) mediates the cleavage and shedding of fractalkine (CX3CL1). *J. Biol. Chem.* **2001**, *276*, 37993–38001. [PubMed]
11. Abel, S.; Hundhausen, C.; Mentlein, R.; Schulte, A.; Berkhout, T.A.; Broadway, N.; Hartmann, D.; Sedlacek, R.; Dietrich, S.; Muetze, B.; et al. The transmembrane CXC-chemokine ligand 16 is induced by IFN-γ and TNF-α and shed by the activity of the disintegrin-like metalloproteinase ADAM10. *J. Immunol.* **2004**, *172*, 6362–6372. [CrossRef] [PubMed]
12. Ludwig, A.; Schulte, A.; Schnack, C.; Hundhausen, C.; Reiss, K.; Brodway, N.; Held-Feindt, J.; Mentlein, R. Enhanced expression and shedding of the transmembrane chemokine CXCL16 by reactive astrocytes and glioma cells. *J. Neurochem.* **2005**, *93*, 1293–1303. [CrossRef] [PubMed]
13. Hattermann, K.; Gebhardt, H.; Krossa, S.; Ludwig, A.; Lucius, R.; Held-Feindt, J.; Mentlein, R. Transmembrane chemokines act as receptors in a novel mechanism termed inverse signaling. *Elife* **2016**, *5*, e10820. [CrossRef] [PubMed]

14. Hattermann, K.; Bartsch, K.; Gebhardt, H.; Mehdorn, H.M.; Synowitz, M.; Schmitt, A.D.; Mentlein, R.; Held-Feindt, J. "Inverse signaling" of the transmembrane chemokine CXCL16 contributes to proliferative and anti-apoptotic effects in cultured human meningioma cells. *Cell Commun. Signal.* **2016**, *14*, 26. [CrossRef] [PubMed]

15. Matloubian, M.; David, A.; Engel, S.; Ryan, J.E.; Cyster, J.G. A transmembrane CXC chemokine is a ligand for HIV-coreceptor Bonzo. *Nat. Immunol.* **2000**, *1*, 298–304. [CrossRef] [PubMed]

16. Van der Voort, R.; van Lieshout, A.W.; Toonen, L.W.; Slöetjes, A.W.; van den Berg, W.B.; Figdor, C.G.; Radstake, T.R.; Adema, G.J. Elevated CXCL16 expression by synovial macrophages recruits memory T cells into rheumatoid joints. *Arthritis Rheum.* **2005**, *52*, 1381–1391. [CrossRef] [PubMed]

17. Xiao, G.; Wang, X.; Wang, J.; Zu, L.; Cheng, G.; Hao, M.; Sun, X.; Xue, Y.; Lu, J.; Wang, J. CXCL16/CXCR6 chemokine signaling mediates breast cancer progression by pERK1/2-dependent mechanisms. *Oncotarget* **2015**, *6*, 14165–14178. [CrossRef] [PubMed]

18. Singh, R.; Kapur, N.; Mir, H.; Singh, N.; Lillard, J.W., Jr.; Singh, S. CXCR6-CXCL16 axis promotes prostate cancer by mediating cytoskeleton rearrangement via Ezrin activation and $\alpha_v \beta_3$ integrin clustering. *Oncotarget* **2016**, *7*, 7343–7353. [PubMed]

19. Takiguchi, G.; Nishita, M.; Kurita, K.; Kakeji, Y.; Minami, Y. Wnt5a-Ror2 signaling in mesenchymal stem cells promotes proliferation of gastric cancer cells by activating CXCL16-CXCR6 axis. *Cancer Sci.* **2016**, *107*, 290–297. [CrossRef] [PubMed]

20. Hattermann, K.; Held-Feindt, J.; Ludwig, A.; Mentlein, R. The CXCL16-CXCR6 chemokine axis in glial tumors. *J. Neuroimmunol.* **2013**, *260*, 47–54. [CrossRef] [PubMed]

21. Held-Feindt, J.; Rehmke, B.; Mentlein, R.; Hattermann, K.; Knerlich, F.; Hugo, H.-H.; Ludwig, A.; Mehdorn, H.M. Overexpression of CXCL16 and its receptor CXCR6/Bonzo promotes growth of human schwannomas. *Glia* **2008**, *56*, 764–774. [CrossRef] [PubMed]

22. Li, G.; Hattermann, K.; Mentlein, R.; Mehdorn, H.M.; Held-Feindt, J. The transmembrane chemokines CXCL16 and CX3CL1 and their receptors are expressed in human meningiomas. *Oncol. Rep.* **2013**, *29*, 563–570. [PubMed]

23. Veinotte, L.; Gebremeskel, S.; Johnston, B. CXCL16-positive dendritic cells enhance invariant natural killer T cell-dependent IFNγ production and tumor control. *Oncoimmunology* **2016**, *5*, e1160979. [CrossRef] [PubMed]

24. Yoon, M.S.; Pham, C.T.; Phan, M.T.; Shin, D.J.; Jang, Y.Y.; Park, M.H.; Kim, S.K.; Kim, S.; Cho, D. Irradiation of breast cancer cells enhances CXCL16 ligand expression and induces the migration of natural killer cells expressing the CXCR6 receptor. *Cytotherapy* **2016**, *18*, 1532–1542. [CrossRef] [PubMed]

25. Kee, J.Y.; Ito, A.; Hojo, S.; Hashimoto, I.; Igarashi, Y.; Tsuneyama, K.; Tsukada, K.; Irimura, T.; Shibahara, N.; Takasaki, I.; Inujima, A.; et al. CXCL16 suppresses liver metastasis of colorectal cancer by promoting TNF-α-induced apoptosis by tumor-associated macrophages. *BMC Cancer* **2014**, *14*, 949. [CrossRef] [PubMed]

26. Adamski, V.; Schmitt, A.D.; Flüh, C.; Synowitz, M.; Hattermann, K.; Held-Feindt, J. Isolation and characterization of fast-migrating human glioma cells in the progression of malignant gliomas. *Oncol. Res.* **2016**, *25*, 341–353. [CrossRef] [PubMed]

27. Shimaoka, T.; Nakayama, T.; Fukumoto, N.; Kume, N.; Takahashi, S.; Yamaguchi, J.; Minami, M.; Hayashida, K.; Kita, T.; Ohsumi, J.; et al. Cell surface-anchored SR-PSOX/CXC chemokine ligand 16 mediates firm adhesion of CXC chemokine receptor 6-expressing cells. *J. Leukoc. Biol.* **2004**, *75*, 267–274. [CrossRef] [PubMed]

28. Hattermann, K.; Ludwig, A.; Gieselmann, V.; Held-Feindt, J.; Mentlein, R. The chemokine CXCL16 induces migration and invasion of glial precursor cells via its receptor CXCR6. *Mol. Cell. Neurosci.* **2008**, *39*, 133–141. [CrossRef] [PubMed]

29. Zhuge, X.; Murayama, T.; Arai, H.; Yamauchi, R.; Tanaka, M.; Shimaoka, T.; Yonehara, S.; Kume, N.; Yokode, M.; Kita, T. CXCL16 is a novel angiogenic factor for human umbilical vein endothelial cells. *Biochem. Biophys. Res. Commun.* **2005**, *331*, 1295–1300. [CrossRef] [PubMed]

30. Sun, M.; Fink, P.J. A new class of reverse signaling costimulators belongs to the TNF family. *J. Immunol.* **2007**, *179*, 4307–4312. [CrossRef] [PubMed]

31. Battistini, C.; Tamagnone, L. Transmembrane semaphorins, forward and reverse signaling: Have a look both ways. *Cell. Mol. Life Sci.* **2016**, *73*, 1609–1622. [CrossRef] [PubMed]

32. Daar, I.O. Non-SH2/PDZ reverse signaling by ephrins. *Semin. Cell. Dev. Biol.* **2012**, *23*, 65–74. [CrossRef] [PubMed]

33. Kisiswa, L.; Osorio, C.; Erice, C.; Vizard, T.; Wyatt, S.; Davies, A.M. TNFα reverse signaling promotes sympathetic axon growth and target innervation. *Nat. Neurosci.* **2012**, *16*, 865–875. [CrossRef] [PubMed]
34. Noren, N.K.; Lu, M.; Freeman, A.L.; Koolpe, M.; Pasquale, E.B. Interplay between EphB4 on tumor cells and vascular ephrin-B2 regulates tumor growth. *Proc. Natl. Acad. Sci. USA* **2004**, *101*, 5583–5588. [CrossRef] [PubMed]
35. Nakada, M.; Anderson, E.M.; Demuth, T.; Nakada, S.; Reavie, L.B.; Drake, K.L.; Hoelzinger, D.B.; Berens, M.E. The phosphorylation of ephrin-B2 ligand promotes glioma cell migration and invasion. *Int. J. Cancer* **2010**, *126*, 1155–1165. [CrossRef] [PubMed]
36. Li, X.; Law, J.W.; Lee, A.Y. Semaphorin 5A and plexin-B3 regulate human glioma cell motility and morphology through Rac1 and the actin cytoskeleton. *Oncogene* **2012**, *31*, 595–610. [CrossRef] [PubMed]
37. Jones, T.R.; Rouslathi, E.; Schold, S.C.; Bigner, D.D. Fibronectin and glial fibrillary acidic protein expression in normal brain and anaplastic human gliomas. *Cancer Res.* **1982**, *42*, 168–177. [PubMed]
38. Nishiguchi, D.J.; Stephens, R.E.; Yates, A.J. Application of flow cytometry to analyses of cultured human glioma and fetal brain cells. *J. Neuropathol. Exp. Neurol.* **1985**, *44*, 254–267. [CrossRef] [PubMed]
39. Thies, A.; Mauer, S.; Fodstad, O.; Schumacher, U. Clinically proven markers of metastasis predict metastatic spread of human melanoma cells engrafted in scid mice. *Br. J. Cancer* **2007**, *96*, 609–616. [CrossRef] [PubMed]
40. Hattermann, K.; Held-Feindt, J.; Lucius, R.; Sebens Müerköster, S.; Penfold, M.E.; Schall, T.J.; Mentlein, R. The chemokine receptor CXCR7 is highly expressed in human glioma cells and mediates anti-apoptotic effects. *Cancer Res.* **2010**, *70*, 3299–3308. [CrossRef] [PubMed]

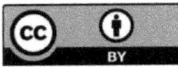

International Journal of
Molecular Sciences

MDPI

Article

Biophysical and Computational Studies of the vCCI:vMIP-II Complex

Anna F. Nguyen [1], Nai-Wei Kuo [1], Laura J. Showalter [1], Ricardo Ramos [1], Cynthia M. Dupureur [2], Michael E. Colvin [1] and Patricia J. LiWang [1,*]

[1] Departments of Molecular Cell Biology and Chemistry and Chemical Biology, and the Health Sciences Research Institute, University of California Merced 5200 North Lake Rd, Merced, CA 953402, USA; aankirskaia@ucmerced.edu (A.F.N.); nicolekuo2010@gmail.com (N.-W.K.); lshowalter@ucmerced.edu (L.J.S.); rramos4@ucmerced.edu (R.R.); mcolvin@ucmerced.edu (M.E.C.)

[2] Department of Chemistry & Biochemistry, University of Missouri-St. Louis, St. Louis, MO 63121, USA; dupureurc@umsl.edu

* Correspondence: pliwang@ucmerced.edu; Tel.: +1-209-228-4568

Received: 20 July 2017; Accepted: 9 August 2017; Published: 16 August 2017

Abstract: Certain viruses have the ability to subvert the mammalian immune response, including interference in the chemokine system. Poxviruses produce the chemokine binding protein vCCI (viral CC chemokine inhibitor; also called 35K), which tightly binds to CC chemokines. To facilitate the study of vCCI, we first provide a protocol to produce folded vCCI from *Escherichia coli* (*E. coli*.) It is shown here that vCCI binds with unusually high affinity to viral Macrophage Inflammatory Protein-II (vMIP-II), a chemokine analog produced by the virus, human herpesvirus 8 (HHV-8). Fluorescence anisotropy was used to investigate the vCCI:vMIP-II complex and shows that vCCI binds to vMIP-II with a higher affinity than most other chemokines, having a K_d of 0.06 ± 0.006 nM. Nuclear magnetic resonance (NMR) chemical shift perturbation experiments indicate that key amino acids used for binding in the complex are similar to those found in previous work. Molecular dynamics were then used to compare the vCCI:vMIP-II complex with the known vCCI:Macrophage Inflammatory Protein-1β/CC-Chemokine Ligand 4 (MIP-1β/CCL4) complex. The simulations show key interactions, such as those between E143 and D75 in vCCI/35K and R18 in vMIP-II. Further, in a comparison of 1 μs molecular dynamics (MD) trajectories, vMIP-II shows more overall surface binding to vCCI than does the chemokine MIP-1β. vMIP-II maintains unique contacts at its N-terminus to vCCI that are not made by MIP-1β, and vMIP-II also makes more contacts with the vCCI flexible acidic loop (located between the second and third beta strands) than does MIP-1β. These studies provide evidence for the basis of the tight vCCI:vMIP-II interaction while elucidating the vCCI:MIP-1β interaction, and allow insight into the structure of proteins that are capable of broadly subverting the mammalian immune system.

Keywords: chemokine binding protein; chemokine analog; anti-inflammation; 35K; vCCI; vMIP-II; MIP-1β/CCL4; molecular dynamics

---

1. Introduction

Protein–protein interactions are critical for many aspects of biological and immunological function. Of particular interest are virally-encoded proteins that undermine the immune system, often by having the ability to promiscuously bind many targets, and therefore, help the virus evade immune surveillance. One such system targeted by viruses is the chemokine system, in which virally encoded proteins disrupt the chemokine receptor/ligand interaction [1]. Chemokines (chemotactic cytokines) are a class of small secreted proteins that mediate immune cell chemotaxis as part of the inflammatory response. There are about 18 human chemokine receptors that are activated upon binding to their cognate chemokine ligand [2]. About 50 chemokine ligands are known, spanning 4 sub-families. The two major subfamilies are CC chemokines (named for the adjacent Cys near the N-terminus of the protein) and CXC chemokines (named for having an intervening amino acid between the conserved N-terminal Cys). In general, CC chemokines (named numerically as CCL1; chemokine ligand 1, etc.) bind to and activate cognate receptors on the surfaces of monocytes, macrophages and T-cells, and these receptors are numerically named as CC receptors (e.g., CCR1, CCR2). CXC chemokines tend to have cognate receptors on the surface of neutrophils [2], with receptors such as CXCR1. Chemokines can sometimes bind multiple receptors, and receptors often have more than one cognate ligand, although CC chemokines are restricted to CC chemokine receptors, and CXC chemokines have their own CXC receptors.

Because of the central nature of the chemokine system in activating and localizing immune cells, subversion of the process may be useful to a virus. Several types of chemokine-binding proteins (CKBPs) have been identified (reviewed in [3]), including those that bind chemokines from multiple subfamilies, such as Myxoma-T7 (M-T7) from myxoma [4], M3 from γ-herpesvirus-68 [5–8], and the poxvirus-encoded smallpox virus-encoded chemokine receptor (SECRET) domain [9]. These proteins have gained interest as inflammation inhibitors, due to their ability to bind to pro-inflammatory proteins.

One of the most potent inhibitors of chemokine action is the poxvirus-encoded protein vCCI (viral CC chemokine inhibitor; also called 35K). This approximately 240 amino acid protein binds 80 CC-chemokines across several species, about 20 of which have nanomolar affinity to this inhibitor [10,11]. The protein sequence across several poxviruses shows high identity, and the structures from cowpox [12], rabbitpox [13], and mousepox [14] reveal a beta sandwich with a binding face containing several key negatively charged amino acids, as well as a long acidic loop between beta strands 2 and 3. We have carried out structural studies of vCCI in complex with MIP-1β (also called CCL4 [13]), which revealed details of the interaction between vCCI and the chemokine, including several close contacts that are critical for binding. Mutagenesis of vCCI/35K by others, in vitro and in vivo, has confirmed the importance of several of the residues suggested by the structure, including E143 and the acidic loop [14,15]. Mutagenesis studies on the chemokines themselves have also been carried out by us and others and indicate that several evolutionarily conserved, positively charged residues are important for binding to vCCI/35K [11,16,17]. In our work, with a variety of eotaxin mutants (CCL11 [11]), we showed that eotaxin's binding to vCCI was dependent on the presence of several basic residues in the chemokine.

Viruses have also evolved the ability to interfere with the chemokine system by producing chemokine homologs, small proteins that mimic the chemokine's ability to bind a chemokine receptor, thus blocking the native chemokine. Herpesvirus HHV-8 encodes several such chemokine analogs; of particular interest is the protein vMIP-II (virally encoded macrophage inflammatory protein-II), which has about 40% identity with the human CC chemokine MIP-1β, and has been shown to bind and antagonize several CC chemokine receptors (CCR1, CCR2, CCR5, though it can agonize CCR3 and CCR8), as well as at least one CXC receptor (CXCR4) [18–20]. This range of receptor binding is much greater than a typical chemokine. We have previously studied vMIP-II to elucidate its ability to bind glycosaminoglycans, and have shown that, in solution, it is a soluble monomer with a fold similar to that of MIP-1β [21,22]. Due to its nanomolar affinity to, and broad ability to bind to chemokine receptors [18,22], vMIP-II has engendered interest as an anti-inflammatory agent, with some success in rat studies involving ischemic stroke [23], spinal cord injury [24], and kidney transplant rejection [25].

vCCI and vMIP-II are therefore complementary proteins, the former having evolved to bind a large variety of CC chemokines, and the latter having evolved to be a prototypical chemokine ligand with the ability to bind many receptors. While we have studied these proteins in complex with their natural ligands [11,13,22,26], we developed the hypothesis that a significant amount of insight could be obtained by determining whether a tight complex could be formed by these proteins. In other words, we set out to study the complex between an "ideal" chemokine binding protein (vCCI) and an "ideal" chemokine homolog (vMIP-II). Due to the broad action of these proteins, an understanding of these powerful viral tools may be helpful in designing strategies to manipulate or control immune responses, and could be applicable to fields ranging from autoimmunity to traumatic brain injury.

We present a technique for producing rabbitpox vCCI from *Escherichia coli* (*E. coli*.), as well as experimental and molecular dynamics analysis of the vCCI:vMIP-II complex and the vCCI:MIP-1β complex, comparing these two complexes to explore the differences in binding between the virus-encoded chemokine analog and a natural human chemokine [13]. Our results show that the affinity of vCCI to vMIP-II is higher than that between vCCI and natural chemokines [11,18] and suggest explanations for this high affinity, as well as for previously-reported functional results.

2. Results

2.1. Folded Viral CC Chemokine Inhibitor(vCCI)/35K Can Be Produced from E. coli

Despite interest in the mechanism of affinity of vCCI, and for its possible use as a therapeutic, it has been relatively time consuming to produce in vitro, since bacterial expression results in unfolded protein. High expression of proteins from this family have been described from yeast [11–13], baculovirus [14,17], and an antibody fragment crystallizable region(Fc)-linked vCCI was produced from 293T mammalian cells [15]. Each technique is useful, but the lack of an *E. coli* expression protocol has limited study of the protein, and in particular, limited the ability of investigators to easily make a wide range of mutants. We have expressed vCCI from *E. coli*, and show that the protein can successfully be refolded. Briefly, the cells are disrupted in 6 M guanidine hydrochloride at pH 8.0 under reducing conditions, and purified with a nickel chelating column. After further reducing agent is added, the solution is slowly added to 20× volume of a cold refold buffer containing L-arginine, sucrose, and glutathione, and incubated for 1 day. The solution is then dialyzed at pH 7.4, followed by addition of a protease to allow cleavage of the fusion tag. Final purification is carried out on an anion-exchange column (see Materials and Methods for details).

The final product of refolding and purification results in a ^{15}N heteronuclear single quantum coherence (HSQC) spectrum of vCCI/35K that is essentially identical to that produced from *Pichia pastoris* yeast expression (Figure 1A and Figure S1). Further, this protein forms a complex upon addition of chemokine analog vMIP-II (Figure 1B), showing its functionality.

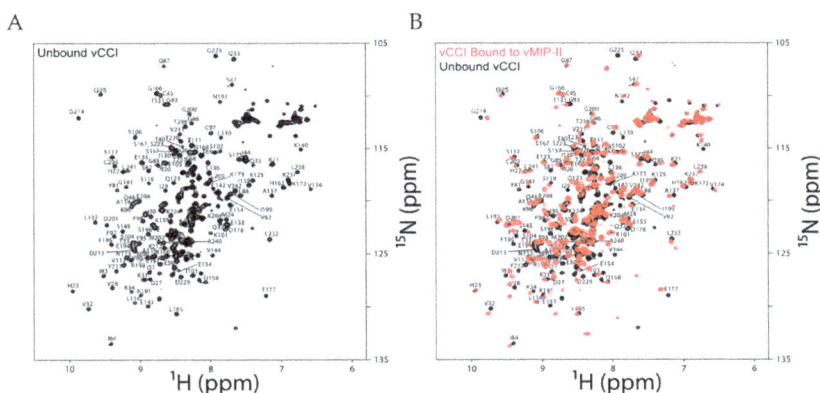

Figure 1. (**A**) ^{1}H-^{15}N heteronuclear single quantum coherence (HSQC) spectrum of unbound ^{15}N-labeled vCCI in 100 mM NaCl, 20 mM NaOP (sodium phosphate) pH 7.0, measured at 37 °C; (**B**) Overlay of the ^{1}H-^{15}N HSQC spectra of free ^{15}N-labeled viral CC chemokine inhibitor (vCCI) (black) and ^{15}N vCCI:^{14}N vMIP-II (red) with a ratio of 1:3, measured under the same conditions as in (**A**). The concentration of vCCI was 50–60 μM.

2.2. vCCI:vMIP-II Produce a High Affinity Complex

vCCI has a remarkable ability to bind almost all chemokines from the CC subfamily, and a qualitative measure of its binding with herpesvirus encoded vMIP-II has been reported [10]. To more quantitatively investigate the affinity between vCCI and vMIP-II, we used isothermal titration calorimetry, in which vMIP-II was titrated into a solution of vCCI. This technique can provide several thermodynamic parameters, and often a dissociation constant. Analysis of the titration data indicated that the K_d of the complex was below 1×10^{-10} M (Table S1). This is the lowest detectable limit of the instrument, and so an alternate method was used to obtain a more accurate binding constant.

An alternative method of obtaining affinity involves a competition technique in which vCCI is bound to a fluorescently labeled chemokine (eotaxin-1/CCL11), and the competitor (vMIP-II in this case) is titrated into the solution, with the resulting change in fluorescence anisotropy providing the dissociation constant for the interaction [11]. This showed a K_d of 0.06 ± 0.006 nM for the vCCI:vMIP-II interaction (Figure 2). This is among the tightest measured vCCI:chemokine interactions.

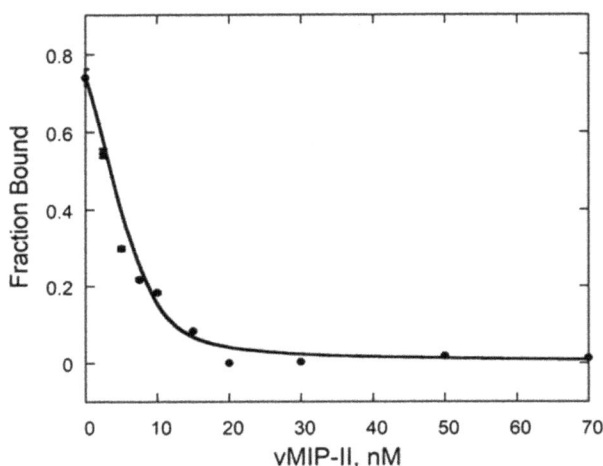

Figure 2. Competition fluorescence anisotropy of the vCCI:vMIP-II interaction. vMIP-II was added to a complex of vCCI with fluorescently labeled eotaxin-1 (CCL11) as in [11]. Error bars are shown, but are sometimes within the size of the data point.

2.3. Changes in Chemical Shift Suggest vCCI:vMIP-II Interaction Is Similar to Other vCCI:Chemokine Complexes

To determine the amino acids that are likely involved in the vCCI:vMIP-II complex, a comparison of chemical shift changes between the free and bound forms of both vCCI/35K and vMIP-II was carried out. In the case of vCCI, ^{15}N HSQC spectra in the free and bound form using ^{15}N labeled vCCI (with non-isotopically labeled vMIP-II) were measured and compared, to determine the level of peak movement upon complex formation. (Assignments of the unbound vCCI were obtained from [27] and Biological Magnetic Resonance Bank (BMRB) databank 6809.) Chemical shift changes in the ^{15}N vMIP-II HSQC spectrum upon binding non-isotopically labeled vCCI/35K were also determined. In cases where unambiguous assignment of the peak in the bound spectrum was not possible, conservative assessments of peak movements were made, indicating that actual peak movement could be greater than shown. Figure 3 shows residue-by-residue chemical shift change. See Table 1 for definitions of chemical shift perturbation categories.

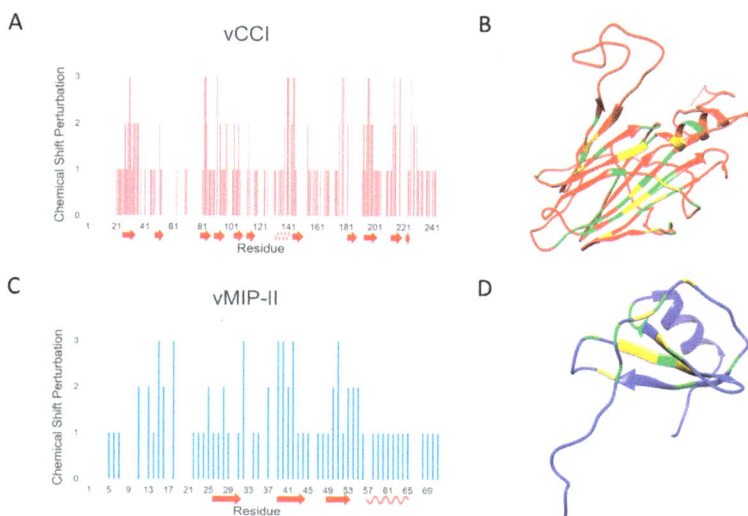

Figure 3. Changes in chemical shift upon complex formation. (**A**) Changes in chemical shift in vCCI upon binding to vMIP-II. Arrows represent beta strands while spiral lines represent alpha helices. See Table 1 for definitions of "0", "1", "2", "3"; (**B**) Structure showing changes in vCCI (Protein Data Bank code 2FFK upon binding vMIP-II. Green indicates greater than average, up to 1 standard deviation away from the average; yellow indicates over 1 standard deviation away from the average; red indicates below one standard deviation or the peak had not been discernable; (**C**) Changes in chemical shift in vMIP-II upon binding to vCCI. Secondary structure is shown by arrows and spiral lines, as in (A). See Table 1 for definitions of "0", "1", "2", "3"; (**D**) Structure showing those changes in vMIP-II upon binding vCCI (Protein Data Bank code 1VMP). Green indicates greater than average, up to 1 standard deviation away from the average; yellow indicates over 1 standard deviation away from the average; blue indicates below one standard deviation or the peak had not been discernable. All structure figures were prepared by using UCSF Chimera (UCSF Resource for Biocomputing, Visualization, and Informatics, San Francisco, CA, USA) [28].

Table 1. Definitions of the chemical shift perturbation categories in Figure 3.

Chemical Shift Perturbation	Definition	vCCI Chemical Shift	vMIP-II Chemical Shift
0	No confirmable change	No peaks visible	No peaks visible
1	Less than or equal to average	$\Delta\delta_{obs} \leq 0.045$	$\Delta\delta_{obs} \leq 0.100$
2	Greater than average, up to one standard deviation above average	$0.045 < \Delta\delta_{obs} \leq 0.086$	$0.100 < \Delta\delta_{obs} \leq 0.178$
3	Greater than one standard deviation above average	$\Delta\delta_{obs} \geq 0.086$	$\Delta\delta_{obs} \geq 0.178$

$\Delta\delta$obs: the difference in chemical shift between bound and free form of ^{15}N-labeled complexes, as defined in Methods.

As shown in Figure 3A, the areas of greatest chemical shift change for vCCI/35K upon binding to vMIP-II are located in the region of amino acids in the 80's, 140's, and 190's, with changes also observed in the 30's, 170's–180's and 220's. These areas are shown on the structure of vCCI/35K (shown without vMIP-II) in Figure 3B, and indicate a binding surface similar to those shown previously [11,13,14,27], comprised of negative charges (D141, E143, as well as likely the negatively charged loop in the 52–77 region that is not clearly assignable, likely due to flexibility) as well as interaction in the early 80's region. Figure 3C indicates that vMIP-II interacts with vCCI/35K using residues from its N-loop region (residues 12–19), and with the second beta strand in the 30's region, as well as with residues in the early 50's. Figure 3D shows vMIP-II with presumed interacting regions highlighted.

2.4. Molecular Dynamics Simulations on vCCI:vMIP-II

To further clarify the structural components and the likely interacting surfaces of the complex, and to gain insight into the extraordinarily tight binding between vCCI/35K and vMIP-II, we carried out molecular dynamics (MD) simulations to create 1 microsecond (µs) trajectories of both the vCCI:MIP-1β complex and the vCCI:vMIP-II complex. Both trajectories are based on the reported vCCI:MIP-1β structure (Protein Data Bank (PDB) ID: 2FFK), but for MIP-1β, the residues were changed to reflect the wild type chemokine, as opposed to the triple mutant used in that structure determination [13]. The vCCI:vMIP-II trajectory was created from the same complex structure, but by computationally superimposing the vMIP-II structure onto the MIP-1β chain to minimize the average difference between the corresponding Cα backbone atoms ([13]; Figure 4A,B and Figure S2). (A third simulation was also included that used the 2FFK structure directly, keeping MIP-1β as a triple mutant (K45A/R46A/K48A) instead of changing it to wild type. However, this third simulation is not emphasized in this work; see the Materials and Methods section for more details on the simulations.)

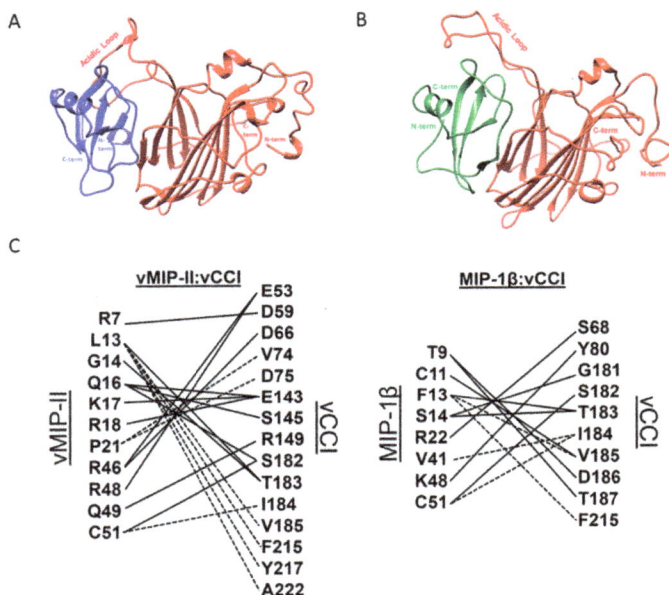

Figure 4. Complexes after 1 µs molecular dynamics simulation of vCCI:chemokine. For all figures, vCCI is in red ribbon, and the bound chemokine is either blue ribbon (vMIP-II) or green ribbon (MIP-1β). (**A**) Structure of vCCI:vMIP-II after 1 µs trajectory; (**B**) Structure of vCCI:MIP-1β in complex after 1 µs trajectory; (**C**) Interactions between residues of vCCI and vMIP-II, as well as vCCI and MIP-1β. Hydrogen bonds (solid lines) are shown if they appear in at least 50% of the last 300 ns of the molecular dynamics simulation. Dashed lines indicate non-hydrogen-bond interactions between residues. These are defined as residues whose access to solvent is occluded upon complex formation at least 50% of the time, and that are within 2.8 Å of the partner residue on the other protein in at least 50% of the structures sampled every 20 ns for the final 500 ns of the trajectory.

Analysis of the secondary structure of the complexes during the trajectory shows that all of the α-helices and β-sheets are preserved though out the 1 microsecond runs for all three complexes (see Figure S3). The root-mean-square deviation (RMSD) in the position of the backbone Cα atoms for the entire complex is less than 1 nm over the entire runs and the RMSD for the individual vCCI and MIP-1β chains is less than 0.8 nm, indicating no gross protein disordering over the simulation, although there are highly flexible regions in both the vCCI and the chemokines. The residue-level fluctuations (RMSF) are the root-mean square fluctuations of each residue around the average protein structure for a trajectory. The RMSF values plotted vs sequence location and calculated for the final 750 ns of the trajectories are shown in Figure S4. These show significant fluctuations of the vCCI N-terminal residues in all three complexes, as well as in the vCCI loop at residues 52–77. As described below, the loop acts as an "arm" that folds down on the bound chemokine. The MIP-1β structures show significant fluctuations at both the N- and C-termini, while vMIP-II shows fewer fluctuations at its termini.

Figure 5 plots the total number of interstrand (vCCI:chemokine) hydrogen bonds over the 1 microsecond simulation for each of the three complexes. The vCCI:vMIP-II complex has significantly more interstrand hydrogen bonds than either of the MIP-1β complexes while the wild type MIP-1β has more than the mutant. Figure 4C shows the hydrogen bonds formed in the vCCI complex with both vMIP-II and MIP-1β.

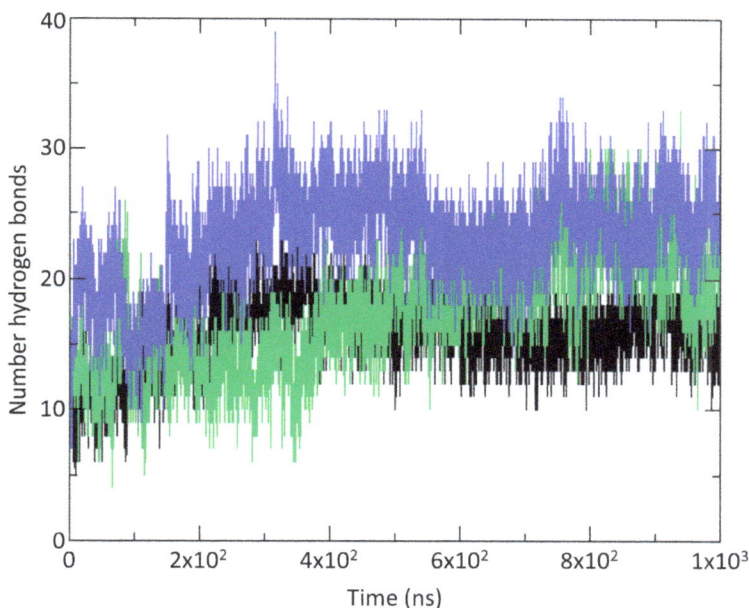

Figure 5. Number of interstrand (vCCI:chemokine) hydrogen bonds observed throughout the molecular dynamics (MD) trajectory for vCCI:vMIP-II (blue); vCCI:MIP-1β (green) and vCCI:MIP-1β-K45A/R46A/L48A (black).

We analyzed the effect of individual residues in vCCI and the chemokine ligand on solvent exposure, using the server-based program PDBePISA [29–31]. The program computes the solvent accessible surface area for both the complex and the computationally separated fragments, and reports the solvent-exposed surface area of each residue in the separated proteins, and the amount of area that is buried when the complex is formed. This analysis was performed every 10 nanoseconds for the final 500 nanoseconds of the simulation, for a total of 51 structures analyzed per complex. The three complexes show different total amounts of buried surface area, as shown in Table 2. Additionally, specific residue–residue contacts vary between the three different complexes. Figure S5 shows interactions of residues that are occluded during the simulation upon complex formation at least 50% of the time, and that are within 2.8 Å of the partner residue in at least 50% of the structures sampled every 20 ns for the final 500 ns of the trajectory.

Table 2. Buried surface area between vCCI and chemokine variants averaged over 51 structures analyzed during the final 500 ns of simulation.

Complex	vCCI Buried Surface Area (Å^2)	Chemokine Buried Surface Area (Å^2)
vCCI:vMIP-II	1473	1528
vCCI:MIP-1β wild type	1355	1392
vCCI:MIP-1β K45A/R46A/K48A (variant used in 2FFK structure determination)	1020	1060

A comparison of the dynamics trajectories of vCCI/35K binding to vMIP-II and to MIP-1β shows some striking differences, in particular, revealing several possible interactions that may account for the approximately 10-fold tighter binding for vMIP-II to vCCI/35K. First, at the end of the simulation, the total buried surface area for vMIP-II in complex is 1528 Å^2, while the buried surface area for MIP-1β in complex is 1392 Å^2. Second, as shown in Figures 5 and 4C, during the time course of the trajectory, vCCI/35K shows an overall larger number of hydrogen bonds with vMIP-II than with MIP-1β. Third, the flexible, negatively charged loop in the 52–77 region of vCCI (between beta strands 2 and 3) makes more contact, including a larger number of hydrogen bonds over the course of the trajectory, with vMIP-II than with MIP-1β. And finally, during the 1 μs trajectory, vMIP-II shows overall more interactions with vCCI than does MIP-1β, in particular, at the N-terminus of the chemokine where a large portion of that region of vMIP-II lays across the vCCI binding face, while the MIP-1β N-terminus does not.

The vCCI:vMIP-II trajectory shows several individual interactions that illuminate aspects of their binding and complementary interactions, including significant contact throughout the trajectory between residues E143 on vCCI/35K and residue R18 in vMIP-II (Figure 6A); and interaction between the negatively charged loop between strands β2 and β3 in vCCI/35K with K45/R46 in vMIP-II (Figure 6C). A similar trajectory is seen for vCCI:MIP-1β, with MIP-1β residue R18 showing interactions with E143, as well as D141 of vCCI (Figure 6B). However, vMIP-II's R18 residue also shows interaction with vCCI residue D75 for almost half the time steps in the trajectory, while no such interaction is observed with MIP-1β. The trajectories also show both vMIP-II and MIP-1β have their 24/45/46 position residues clustered together, and interacting with the vCCI loop between β2 and β3, but the interaction is much more extensive in the vCCI:vMIP-II complex (Figure 6C,D and Figure 4C). The N-terminus of each of the chemokines also behaves very differently in the trajectory. vMIP-II shows considerably more interaction with vCCI throughout its N-terminus for much of the trajectory while the MIP-1β trajectory shows an N-terminus that does not appear to interact consistently with vCCI, with main contacts to the binding partner not starting until residue 8. In total, the simulation results point to possible reasons why vCCI shows different binding constants to various partners.

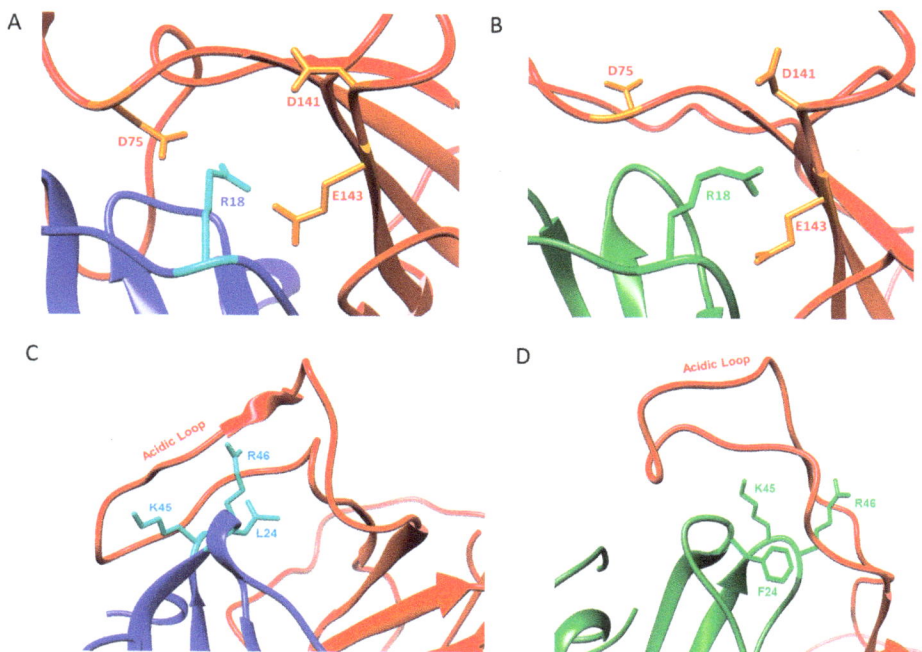

Figure 6. Interactions between vCCI and vMIP-II or MIP-1β. vCCI is in red ribbon and the bound chemokine is either blue ribbon (vMIP-II) or green ribbon (MIP-1β). (**A**) A close-up of the interaction between R18 of vMIP-II (cyan) and D75, D141, E143 of vCCI (orange); (**B**) A close-up of the interaction between R18 of MIP-1β (bright green) and D75, D141, E143 of vCCI (orange); (**C**) A close-up of the interaction between the β2 and β3 loop of vCCI (red) and K45 and R46 of vMIP-II (cyan). L24 of vMIP-II is also indicated in cyan; (**D**) A close-up of the interaction between the β2 and β3 loop of vCCI (red) and K45 and R46 of MIP-1β (bright green). F24 of MIP-1β is also indicated in bright green.

3. Discussion

The ability to modulate the immune system, and in particular, to reduce the inflammatory response, has great potential in health and medicine. Protein therapeutics have been approved for this purpose [32,33], and investigation has continued into other potential sources of anti-inflammatory proteins. Both herpesviruses and poxviruses have evolved to produce proteins that subvert the mammalian chemokine system, and these include both chemokine binding proteins as well as chemokine homologs [3,34,35]. The current work investigates the unusually high affinity interaction between the vCCI/35K chemokine binding protein from rabbitpox, and vMIP-II, a chemokine analog from herpesvirus HHV-8, with a combination of biophysical and molecular dynamics techniques.

vCCI was successfully produced and purified from *E. coli*. This fairly efficient procedure will greatly expand the range of experiments that can be carried out with vCCI, from quickly making large quantities of the protein (and any desired variants) for X-ray crystallography, to inexpensive isotopic labeling that can lead to a variety of NMR experiments, including a full structure determination. Isothermal titration calorimetry indicated a high affinity for the vCCI:vMIP-II complex, and this was confirmed by fluorescence anisotropy, which revealed a K_d of 0.06 nM ± 0.006 nM that is significantly lower than the K_d observed for vCCI with other chemokines using the same method [11]. Other groups have investigated the binding constant of vCCI with various chemokines using other methods, including early qualitative work that suggested that vCCI/35K bound vMIP-II more tightly than most other chemokines [10]. Others have used a scintillation proximity assay [35] and surface plasmon resonance [14,16,17] to show that vCCI/35K binds a variety of chemokines at levels ranging from sub-nanomolar to 20 nM.

Analysis of chemical shift perturbation by NMR indicates that vCCI/35K interacts with vMIP-II using residues similar to those that have been shown to be important in binding by vCCI to other chemokines, MIP-1β/CCL4, and eotaxin-1/CCL11 [11,13], such as acidic residues in the 141/143 area. Similarly, chemical shift perturbation of vMIP-II upon binding vCCI/35K shows chemical shift changes in generally known areas, including the region near R18, as well as the area near the so-called N-loop of the chemokine, where hydrophobic L13 is located (Figure 3). While NMR chemical shift perturbation is a powerful tool, there are two main drawbacks. First, while a perturbation suggests a locus for protein–protein interaction, and one can infer regions of interaction between proteins, it does not confirm a pairwise interaction with the binding partner. Second, 2D ^{15}N HSQC spectra can be ambiguous in terms of assigning peaks upon movement. To resolve ambiguity would require ^{13}C-labeling of the protein(s) and a series of 3D NMR experiments [11]. Therefore, we chose to pursue molecular dynamics simulations, which provide a high resolution "movie" (within certain approximations) of the structure and motions of all atoms in the protein and surrounding solvent, and can delineate specific interactions and provide insight into differences in affinity.

Atomistic classical molecular dynamics (MD) is a well-established tool for studying protein structure and dynamics [36]. In typical protein MD, the motions of all atoms are simulated using empirical force fields that approximate the forces due to bonded and non-bonded interactions. The resulting output is a high-resolution series of atomic motions that can be analyzed to characterize the structure and dynamics of the protein, and infer the energy causes of the observed behavior. With modern computers and MD software, it is feasible to routinely run simulations of moderately large proteins (including a solvation shell of water and ions) for microsecond timescales, with the largest published MD simulations reaching millisecond times [37]. The accuracy is limited by the approximate nature of the force field and the limitation that bonds are not broken or formed during the simulations (including protonation and deprotonation of acid and base sites), but MD has been shown able to accurately predict protein properties, such as the folded conformation of small proteins [38].

In the investigation of the vCCI:vMIP-II complex, a 1 μs MD trajectory was run, providing great insight into likely interactions that were not observable and/or confirmable by our NMR experiments to this point. In general, the hypothesis that these two viral proteins may be a near-ideal binding pair is supported by the MD trajectories, which show that that vCCI:vMIP-II complex has a larger buried surface area (including the vMIP-II's N-terminus) and a greater number of hydrogen bonds throughout the trajectory, including more interactions between the chemokine and the negatively charged flexible loop of vCCI than the vCCI:MIP-1β complex. The MD simulations also provide context for specific regions of interaction that may be useful in general for a vCCI:chemokine complex. For example, D141 and E143 in vCCI were observed to contact R18 in the vCCI:MIP-1β structure [13], and this R18 was found to be critical for vCCI/35K binding in other chemokines [11,13,16,17]. However, mutational studies on vCCI/35K showed E143 to be more important than D141 [15]. The MD trajectory provides an explanation, showing significant, continuous interaction between E143 (vCCI/35K) and R18 (vMIP-II), while almost no close interaction across the trajectory is observed with D141. In the vCCI:MIP-1β trajectory, significant hydrogen bonding interaction (although below the 50% threshold for Figure 4C) is observed between R18 of the chemokine and both E143 and D141 of vCCI, although the interaction with E143 predominates.

The MD trajectory also provides a possible explanation for other unexplained mutational results. In the original structure of the complex between vCCI/35K and MIP-1β/CCL4, it was observed that both Y80 and R89 in vCCI/35K appeared close in space to the 48th position of MIP-1β [13]. In many chemokines, this position contains a large, basic residue that could be expected to both sterically and electrostatically clash with those groups. It had been noted that mutation of this residue to the smaller Ala48 increased affinity for a similar chemokine MCP-1/CCL2 [16,17]. Indeed, MIP-1β was mutated from a Lys to an Ala at that position in the structure, and that mutation was attributed to tighter binding to vCCI. In an attempt to design a vCCI/35K that was better able to bind chemokines, White et al. mutated each Y80 and R89 to Ala in vaccinia vCCI/35K, hypothesizing that a smaller, uncharged residue in these positions would better interact with the large basic residue of a chemokine [15]. Interestingly, while the vCCI/35K R89A mutation did lead to a better chemokine binding ability, Y80A completely abolished the activity of the protein. The MD trajectory of Y80 in the vCCI:MIP-1β complex shows the tyrosine side chain of vCCI consistently forming a hydrogen bond with the backbone nitrogen of Lys48 of MIP-1β (Figures 4C and 7B). This Y80 hydrogen bond was not consistently observed in the vCCI:vMIP-II trajectory, although the trajectory shows consistent contact between these residues (Figure S5). In either case, the Y80 in this crowded area of the protein shows little motion and appears to be holding open the negatively charged loop in vCCI. The Y80 residue in vCCI has also been mutated by Arnold et al., who replaced tyrosine with arginine. This mutation did also lead to loss of chemokine binding ability, although in this case, the cause is likely placing a basic Arg on vCCI near the Arg48 of a chemokine [14].

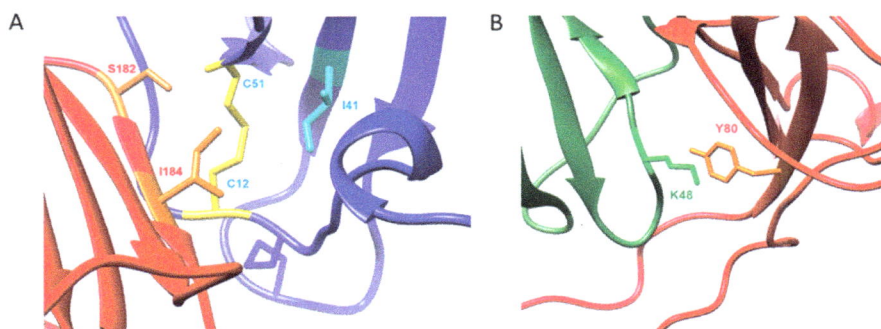

Figure 7. Interactions illuminated by molecular dynamics simulation of the vCCI:MIP-1β and vCCI:vMIP-II complex. vCCI is in red ribbon in both instances, bound vMIP-II is in blue ribbon, and bound MIP-1β is in green ribbon. (A) Interaction between I184 of vCCI (orange) and I41 of vMIP-II (cyan), as well as S182 of vCCI (orange) with the backbone of C51 of vMIP-II (yellow). C12 of vMIP-II is also indicated in yellow; (B) Interaction between Y80 of vCCI (orange) and the backbone of K48 of MIP-1β (green).

The MD trajectory has helped reveal several interesting interactions that NMR alone had difficulty explaining. Arnold et al. observed that the mutation of residues S182 and I184 (using the present vCCI numbering) resulted in substantial loss of binding activity, especially for I184 [14]. However, previous chemical shift assignments for vCCI with other chemokines [11,13] as well as the current work with vMIP-II, are unable to quantify the shifts to these residues in vCCI. The MD trajectory, however, reveals an interaction between VCCI I184 and vMIP-II Ile41 and Cys51, seemingly to help anchor vCCI to the chemokine throughout the trajectory (Figure 7A); this interaction is also seen in the vCCI:MIP-1β trajectory, explaining large chemical shift changes in chemokines in the region 39–42. vCCI Ser182, meanwhile, appears to have formed a hydrogen bond to the backbone N-H of C51 in both vMIP-II and MIP-1β. This may explain the large chemical shift changes to that region of the spectra. This was also observed in the chemical shift changes of eotaxin in the vCCI:eotaxin complex [11].

Overall, a combination of biochemical, biophysical, and computational experiments have been used to provide a comprehensive explanation of the basis for the high affinity interaction between vCCI/35K and vMIP-II. These proteins each exemplify a highly evolved mechanism to mimic and/or subvert the mammalian immune system, and an understanding of their interaction will be useful in both their development as possible therapeutics and in general protein design for immunomodulation.

4. Materials and Methods

4.1. Protein Purification

4.1.1. Purifying vCCI from *E. coli*

The gene sequence encoding the rabbit pox vCCI was slightly modified by PCR to allow for proper cleavage by enterokinase, which does not cut efficiently near proline. DNA coding for Met-Pro in the first two amino acids was replaced with DNA coding for Ala-Met-Ala. The resulting gene was cloned into the pET32a vector utilizing the restriction sites *NcoI* and *HindIII*. The plasmid was transformed into *E. coli* BL21 (DE3) (Novagen, Madison, WI, USA) competent cells and expressed in Luria broth or minimal media with $^{15}NH_4Cl$ as the sole nitrogen source. Protein production was induced when the absorbance at 600 nm reached 0.70–0.75 with the addition of isopropyl β-D-1-thiogalactopyranoside (IPTG) to 1mM and incubated with shaking at 22 °C for 20 h. The cells were then harvested by centrifugation at $4200 \times g$, 4 °C for 12 min and supernatant was discarded.

The cell pellet was resuspended in 6 M guanidine hydrochloride, 200 mM NaCl, and 50 mM Tris (pH 8.0) and was lysed by three passages through a French press and then centrifuged at $27,000 \times g$ for 1 h. The supernatant was decanted and 15 mM β-mercaptoethanol (β-ME) was added and allowed to stir at room temperature for 2 hours to reduce. The solution was then loaded onto a nickel chelating column (Qiagen, Hilden, Germany) equilibrated with the resuspension buffer containing 15 mM βME after a thorough 0.3 M imidazole wash to remove unbound nickel. The column containing the bound vCCI was washed with 10 column volumes of resuspension buffer containing 15 mM βME, and then with 10 column volumes of wash buffer (6 M Guanidinium chloride, 200 mM NaCl, 15 mM βME, 80 mM NaOP, pH 7.2). Proteins were eluted from the column using 6 M guanidine hydrochloride, 200 mM NaCl, and 60 mM NaOAc, pH 4. Fractions containing the eluted protein were identified by absorbance at 280 nm and then pooled together. βME was then added to a concentration of 25 mM. The fractions were allowed to stir for one hour at room temperature, followed by stirring for 12 hours at 4 °C overnight.

The protein was then refolded by dropwise addition to 20x volume of ice-cold refolding buffer (9.6 mM NaCl, 0.4 mM KCl, 2 mM $CaCl_2$, 2 mM $MgCl_2$, 550 mM L-arginine hydrochloride, 400 mM sucrose, 3 mM reduced glutathione (GSH), 0.3 mM oxidized glutathione (GSSG), 50 mM Tris, pH 8) and then allowed to stir 24 h at 4 °C. The solution was dialyzed 4 times into 4 liters 200 mM NaCl, 2 mM $CaCl_2$, 20 mM Tris, pH 7.4 buffer at 4 °C.

To cleave the thioredoxin fusion tag from the purified protein, the samples were incubated for 12 hours at 4 °C with 650 nM of the protease enterokinase. The samples were then dialyzed 4 times into 4 L of 20 mM Bis-Tris, 50 mM NaCl pH 7.1 and then passed through a 0.2 μm nylon filter to then be purified on a HiTrap™ Q HP Column (GE Healthcare Life Sciences, Chicago, IL, USA) using a gradient from 50 mM NaCl, 20 mM Bis-Tris pH 7.1 to 1 M NaCl, 20 mM Bis-Tris pH 7.1, to separate the cleaved tag from vCCI. The fractions were analyzed on an SDS-PAGE gel to confirm purity and then fractions containing vCCI were concentrated using the Amicon concentrators (Millipore, Billerica, MA, USA), and buffer was changed to 100 mM NaCl, 20 mM NaOP pH 7.0 with 0.02% NaN_3 for NMR studies.

4.1.2. Expression and Purification of vMIP-II

The gene for vMIP-II was placed into a pET28 vector and transformed into *Escherichia coli* BL21 (DE3) (Novagen, Madison, WI, USA) competent cells and expressed in either minimal media with $^{15}NH_4Cl$ as the sole nitrogen source for ^{15}N-labeled samples or Luria Broth for ^{14}N-labeled samples. Protein production was induced by adding IPTG to 1 mM and incubated with shaking at 37 °C for 5 h.

The cell pellet was resuspended in 6 M guanidine hydrochloride, 200 mM NaCl, 10 mM benzamidine, 50 mM Tris (pH 8.0) and were lysed by French press and then centrifuged at 27,000× *g* for 1 h. The soluble portion was then loaded onto a nickel chelating column (Qiagen, Hilden, Germany) equilibrated with the resuspension buffer. Proteins were eluted from the column using a pH gradient with 6 M guanidine hydrochloride, 200 mM NaCl, 60 mM NaOAc (pH 4) followed by addition of 10 mM βME while stirring for 2 hours at room temperature. The proteins were then refolded by dropwise addition into 10× volume of refolding buffer (550 mM L-arginine hydrochloride, 200 mM NaCl, 1 mM EDTA (Ethylenediaminetetraacetic acid), 1 mM reduced glutathione (GSH), 0.1 mM oxidized glutathione (GSSG), 50 mM Tris, pH 8), and then allowed to stir overnight at 4 °C. The solution was dialyzed three times into 4 L of 200 mM NaCl, 20 mM Tris pH 8 buffer at 4 °C.

To cleave the Small Ubiquitin-like Modifier (SUMO) fusion tag from the purified protein, the samples were incubated for 12 hours with 100 nM of the Ubl-specific protease 1 (ULP-1). The protein solution was then centrifuged to remove precipitated material and added onto a second nickel chelating column (Qiagen, Hilden, Germany), with flow-through containing the cleaved vMIP-II being collected. The samples were then dialyzed and purified on a C_4 reversed-phase chromatography column (Vydac, Hesperia, CA, USA), using an acetonitrile gradient. The fractions were analyzed on an sodium dodecyl sulfate polyacrylamide gel electrophoresis (SDS-PAGE) gel to confirm purity and lyophilized in a Labconco freeze-dry system.

The proteases used in these purifications were produced and purified in our laboratory as briefly described: ULP1 or enterokinase protease were proteins were expressed in LB medium using a pET-28b vector and the cells were collected and French pressed. The ULP1 protease from the supernatant was purified using a nickel chelating column [39]. The enterokinase was found in the inclusion body and resuspended in 6M guanidinium buffer before being purified using a nickel chelating column. Enterokinase was then dialyzed in buffer to allow for refolding and tested for activity through self-cleavage of the fusion tag (manuscript in preparation).

Proteins used in fluorescence anisotropy studies were purified as specified in [11]. vCCI for these experiments were made using a gene encoding rabbitpox virus vCCI cloned into pPIC9K plasmid and then transformed into *Pichia pastoris* strain SMD1168 (Invitrogen, Carlsbad, CA, USA) and purified as previously described [13].

4.2. Nuclear Magnetic Resonance (NMR) Spectroscopy

All NMR samples were made in 20 mM sodium phosphate buffer, 100 mM NaCl with 10% D_2O, 5 μM 2,2-dimethyl-2-silapentane-5-sulfonic acid (DSS), and 0.02% NaN_3, with a final pH of 7.0. [15]N labeled lyophilized vMIP-II was resuspended into 5 mM NaOP buffer, pH 2.8 in order to dissolve the protein, and then 10 μL was added to 340 μL NMR buffer (either alone or with 150 uM ^{14}N-vCCI) for final vMIP-II concentration of 50-60 μM. ^{14}N-vMIP-II was also resuspended into 5 mM NaOP, pH 2.8, and 10 μL was added to 340 μL NMR buffer containing ^{15}N-labeled vCCI, for a final concentration of 150 μM VMIP-II in the sample. vCCI was exchanged into NMR buffer as explained in the above sections, with final concentrations for ^{15}N samples being 50–60 μM.

All HSQC NMR data were acquired on a four-channel 600 MHz Bruker Avance III spectrometer (Bruker Corp, Billerica, MA) equipped with a (GRASP II) gradient accessory and a (TCI) cryoprobe with an actively shielded Z-gradient coil. Spectra with ^{15}N-labeled vMIP-II were measured at 25 °C; spectra with ^{15}N-labeled vCCI were measured at 37 °C. The chemical shift was referenced relative to internal DSS [40]. The data were processed using NMRPipe [41] and analyzed using PIPP [42] (Available online: https://spin.niddk.nih.gov/bax/software/NMRPipe/). For HSQC spectra, sweep width = 8474.576(^{1}H) and 1766.784 Hz (^{15}N), with 1280 points in ^{1}H and 128* (256 total) points in [15]N.

The weighted average chemical shift change of the ^{1}H and ^{15}N resonances for each residue upon binding was calculated using the equation [43]:

$$\Delta\delta_{obs} = \sqrt{\frac{\Delta\delta_H{}^2 + \left(\frac{\Delta\delta_N}{5}\right)^2}{2}} \tag{1}$$

where $\Delta\delta_H$ and $\Delta\delta_N$ are the chemical shift changes of the ^{1}H and ^{15}N dimensions, respectively. Here, the $\Delta\delta_{obs}$ is the difference between bound and free form of ^{15}N-labeled complexes. Due to lack of ^{13}C labeling, some bound peak identifications were estimates; to be conservative, the nearest residue without a clear origin were assumed to belong to the residues in question.

4.3. Isothermal Titration Calorimetry (ITC)

A Nano ITC Low Volume isothermal titration calorimeter (TA Instruments, New Castle, DE, USA) was loaded with degassed 10 uM vCCI in 20 mM NaOP, 100 mM NaCl, pH 7.0 and water in the reference cell. Twenty 2.5 µL injections of 100 µM vMIP-II also in 20 mM NaOP, 100 mM NaCl, pH 7.0 were then injected at 300 second intervals, with a 350 rpm stirring speed. Baseline selection, buffer-into-buffer blank was subtracted from the data, and peak-by-peak manual integration was performed using NanoAnalyze software (TA Instruments, New Castle, DE, USA). The data for an independent binding site model was provided by the software. The K_d was below detectable limits (10^{-10} nM).

4.4. Fluorescence Anisotropy

Fluorescence anisotropy experiments were carried out in three independent experiments as described in [11], at 25 °C and pH of 7.0 utilizing a Photon Counting (PC1) spectrofluorimeter and VINCI software (ISS, Champaign, IL, USA), with an excitation wavelength of 497 nm and emission wavelength of 524 nm. The obtained data were then fit to a system of mass conservation equations as well as the following equation:

$$\theta = \frac{[L]_{free} \times K_a}{1 + [L]_{free} \times K_a} \tag{2}$$

where θ is the fraction of bound eotaxin-K63C, $[L]_{free}$ is the concentration of unbound vCCI, and K_a is the association constant for the complex.

For the competitive binding experiment, a 1:1 ratio of the vCCI:eotaxin-K63C (both proteins were prepared and purified as described in [11], with eotaxin-K63C labeled with fluorescein-5-maleimide) complex was prepared at a concentration of 8 nM. 500 µL of this complex was then mixed with varying amounts of unlabeled vMIP-II and incubated 30 minutes at 25 °C. Anisotropy measurements were taken and the values were normalized so that 1 represents the 100% bound state. The resulting data were fit using Scientist software (Micromath, Salt Lake City, UT, USA) to a system of equations described previously [44,45].

4.5. Molecular Dynamics

All-atom molecular dynamics was performed on three vCCI:MIP complexes. All three complex structures were based on the NMR structure of the VCCI:MIP-1β complex (PDB: 2FFK), which has three mutations from the wild type MIP-1β sequence. We recreated the original wild type structure by in silico editing of the 2FFK experimental structure. The vCCI:vMIP-II starting structure was created from the vCCI:MIP-1β structure by computationally superimposing the experimental vMIP structure (PDB code 1VMP) on the MIP-1β chain, to minimize the average difference between the corresponding Cα backbone atoms (see Figure S2). The net charge (−11 vCCI:vMIP-II, −26 vCCI:MIP-1β mutant, −23 vCCI:MIP-1β wild type) on the complexes was neutralized by adding Na+ ions and additional Na$^+$/Cl$^-$ pairs (~60) were added to yield an ion concentration of approximately 70 millimolar. After short equilibration runs, a full 1 microsecond of MD simulation was run using Gromacs 5.0.7 [46–48] using the NPT ensemble, the Verlet cutoff scheme and a 2 fs timestep. All bonds to hydrogen were constrained to their equilibrium length using the LINCS algorithm [49]. Temperature was maintained at 300K using the Bussi et al. thermostat [50] and pressure at 1 bar using the Parrinello-Rahman barostat [51]. The simulations were performed using the AMBER99SB-ILDN force field for the protein [52] and the TIP3P water model [53].

4.6. Figure Preparation

All structure figures were prepared by using UCSF Chimera (UCSF Resource for Biocomputing, Visualization, and Informatics, San Francisco, CA, USA) [28].

Supplementary Materials: Supplementary materials can be found at www.mdpi.com/1422-0067/18/8/1778/s1.

Acknowledgments: Funding was provided by NIH R01AI112011 and by Army W911NF-11-1-0139. This work was partially supported by the National Science Foundation through the NSF-CREST: Center for Cellular and Bio-molecular Machines at University of California, Merced (NSF-HRD-1547848). MEC is partially supported by the Art and Fafa Kamangar Chair in Biological Science at University of California, Merced.

Author Contributions: Anna F. Nguyen, Nai-Wei Kuo, Patricia J. LiWang and Cynthia M. Dupureur designed the biophysical experiments, and Anna F. Nguyen and Nai-Wei Kuo carried them out; Laura J. Showalter and Ricardo Ramos helped produce proteins; Michael E. Colvin designed and carried out molecular dynamics simulations; Anna F. Nguyen, Patricia J. LiWang, Laura J. Showalter, Nai-Wei Kuo, Cynthia M. Dupureur, and Michael E. Colvin analyzed the data; all authors assisted in writing manuscript.

Conflicts of Interest: The authors declare no conflict of interest.

Abbreviations

vCCI	Viral CC Chemokine Inhibitor; also called 35K or vCCI/35K
vMIP-II	Viral macrophage inflammatory protein II
E. coli	*Escherichia coli*
NMR	Nuclear magnetic resonance
HSQC	Heteronuclear single quantum coherence
NaOP	Sodium phosphate
HHV-8	Human herpesvirus 8, Kaposi's sarcoma-associated herpesvirus
MIP-1β	Macrophage inflammatory protein β, also known as CCL4
CCL4	CC chemokine ligand 4, also known as MIP-1β
IPTG	Isopropyl β-D-1-thiogalactopyranoside
DSS	4,4-dimethyl-4-silapentane-1-sulfonic acid
β-ME	β-mercaptoethanol
RMSD	Root mean squared deviation
RMSF	Root mean squared fluctuation (for specific residues)
MD	Molecular dynamics

References

1. Graham, K.A.; Lalani, A.S.; Macen, J.L.; Ness, T.L.; Barry, M.; Liu, L.-Y.; Lucas, A.; Clark-Lewis, I.; Moyer, R.W.; Mcfadden, G. The T1/35kDa family of poxvirus-secreted proteins bind chemokines and modulate leukocyte influx into virus-infected tissues. *Virology* **1997**, *229*, 12–24. [CrossRef] [PubMed]
2. Griffith, J.W.; Sokol, C.L.; Luster, A.D. Chemokines and chemokine receptors: Positioning cells for host defense and immunity. *Annu. Rev. Immunol.* **2014**, *32*, 659–702. [CrossRef] [PubMed]
3. Heidarieh, H.; Hernáez, B.; Alcamí, A. Immune modulation by virus-encoded secreted chemokine binding proteins. *Virus Res.* **2015**, *209*, 67–75. [CrossRef] [PubMed]
4. Lalani, A.S.; Graham, K.; Mossman, K.; Rajarathnam, K.; Clark-Lewis, I.; Kelvin, D.; McFadden, G. The purified myxoma virus γ interferon receptor homolog M-T7 interacts with the heparin-binding domains of chemokines. *J. Virol.* **1997**, *71*, 4356–4363. [PubMed]

5. Hughes, D.J.; Kipar, A.; Leeming, G.H.; Bennet, E.; Howarth, D.; Commerson, J.A.; Papoula-Pereira, R.; Flanagan, B.F.; Sample, J.T.; Stewart, J.P. Chemokine Binding Protein M3 of Murine Gammaherpesvirus 68 Modulates the Host Response to Infection in a Natural Host. *PLoS Pathog.* **2011**, *7*, e1001321. [CrossRef] [PubMed]
6. Alexander, J.M.; Nelson, C.A.; Van Berkel, V.; Lau, E.K.; Studts, J.M.; Brett, T.J.; Speck, S.H.; Handel, T.M.; Virgin, H.W. Structural basis of chemokine sequestration by a herpesvirus decoy receptor. *Cell* **2002**, *111*, 343–356. [CrossRef]
7. Webb, L.M.C.; Smith, V.P.; Alcami, A. The gammaherpesvirus chemokine binding protein can inhibit the interaction of chemokines with glycosaminoglycans. *FASEB J.* **2004**, *18*, 571–573. [CrossRef] [PubMed]
8. Alexander-Brett, J.M.; Fremont, D.H. Dual GPCR and GAG mimicry by the M3 chemokine decoy receptor. *J. Exp. Med.* **2007**, *204*, 3157–3172. [CrossRef] [PubMed]
9. Alejo, A.; Ruiz-Argüello, M.B.; Ho, Y.; Smith, V.P.; Saraiva, M.; Alcami, A. A chemokine-binding domain in the tumor necrosis factor receptor from variola (smallpox) virus. *Proc. Natl. Acad. Sci. USA* **2006**, *103*, 5995–6000. [CrossRef] [PubMed]
10. Burns, J.M.; Dairaghi, D.J.; Deitz, M.; Tsang, M.; Schall, T.J. Comprehensive mapping of poxvirus vCCI chemokine-binding protein. Expanded range of ligand interactions and unusual dissociation kinetics. *J. Biol. Chem.* **2002**, *277*, 2785–2789. [CrossRef] [PubMed]
11. Kuo, N.-W.; Gao, Y.-G.; Schill, M.S.; Isern, N.; Dupureur, C.M.; LiWang, P.J. Structural insights into the interaction between a potent anti-inflammatory protein, viral CC chemokine inhibitor (vCCI), and the human CC chemokine, eotaxin-1. *J. Biol. Chem.* **2014**, *289*, 6592–6603. [CrossRef] [PubMed]
12. Carfí, A.; Smith, C.A.; Smolak, P.J.; McGrew, J.; Wiley, D.C. Structure of a soluble secreted chemokine inhibitor vCCI (p35) from cowpox virus. *Proc. Natl. Acad. Sci. USA* **1999**, *96*, 12379–12383. [CrossRef] [PubMed]
13. Zhang, L.; DeRider, M.; McCornack, M.A.; Jao, S.C.; Isern, N.; Ness, T.; Moyer, R.; LiWang, P.J. Solution structure of the complex between poxvirus-encoded CC chemokine inhibitor vCCI and human MIP-1β. *Proc. Natl. Acad. Sci. USA* **2006**, *103*, 13985–13990. [CrossRef] [PubMed]
14. Arnold, P.L.; Fremont, D.H. Structural Determinants of chemokine binding by an ectromelia virus-encoded decoy receptor. *J. Virol.* **2006**, *80*, 7439–7449. [CrossRef] [PubMed]
15. White, G.E.; Mcneill, E.; Christou, I.; Channon, K.M.; Greaves, D.R. Site-directed mutagenesis of the CC chemokine binding protein 35K-Fc reveals residues essential for activity and mutations that increase the potency of CC chemokine blockade. *Mol. Pharmacol.* **2011**, *80*, 328–336. [CrossRef] [PubMed]
16. Beck, C.G.; Studer, C.; Zuber, J.F.; Demange, B.J.; Manning, U.; Urfer, R. The viral CC chemokine-binding protein vCCI inhibits monocyte chemoattractant protein-1 activity by masking its CCR2B-binding site. *J. Biol. Chem.* **2001**, *276*, 43270–43276. [CrossRef] [PubMed]
17. Seet, B.T.; Singh, R.; Paavola, C.; Lau, E.K.; Handel, T.M.; McFadden, G. Molecular determinants for CC-chemokine recognition by a poxvirus CC-chemokine inhibitor. *Proc. Natl. Acad. Sci. USA* **2001**, *98*, 9008–9013. [CrossRef] [PubMed]
18. Kledal, T.N.; Rosenkilde, M.M.; Coulin, F.; Simmons, G.; Johnsen, A.H.; Alouani, S.; Power, C.A.; Luttichau, H.R.; Gerstoft, J.; Clapham, P.R.; et al. A broad-spectrum chemokine antagonist encoded by Kaposi's sarcoma-associated herpesvirus. *Science* **1997**, *277*, 1656–1659. [CrossRef] [PubMed]
19. Sozzani, S.; Luini, W.; Bianchi, G.; Allavena, P.; Wells, T.N.C.; Napolitano, M.; Bernardini, G.; Vecchi, A.; D'Ambrosio, D.; Mazzeo, D.; et al. The viral chemokine macrophage inflammatory protein-II is a selective Th2 chemoattractant. *Blood* **1998**, *92*, 4036–4039. [PubMed]
20. Weber, K.S.; Gröne, H.J.; Röcken, M.; Klier, C.; Gu, S.; Wank, R.; Proudfoot, A.E.; Nelson, P.J.; Weber, C. Selective recruitment of Th2-type cells and evasion from a cytotoxic immune response mediated by viral macrophage inhibitory protein-II. *Eur. J. Immunol.* **2001**, *31*, 2458–2466. [CrossRef]
21. Liwang, A.C.; Wang, Z.X.; Sun, Y.; Peiper, S.C.; Liwang, P.J. The solution structure of the anti-HIV chemokine vMIP-II. *Protein Sci.* **1999**, *8*, 2270–2280. [CrossRef] [PubMed]
22. Zhao, B.; Liwang, P.J. Characterization of the interactions of vMIP-II, and a dimeric variant of vMIP-II, with glycosaminoglycans. *Biochemistry* **2010**, *49*, 7012–7022. [CrossRef] [PubMed]
23. Takami, S.; Minami, M.; Nagata, I.; Namura, S.; Satoh, M. Chemokine receptor antagonist peptide, viral MIP-II, protects the brain against focal cerebral ischemia in mice. *J. Cereb. Blood Flow Metab.* **2001**, 1430–1435. [CrossRef] [PubMed]

24. Ghirnikar, R.S.; Lee, Y.L.; Eng, L.F. Chemokine antagonist infusion promotes axonal sparing after spinal cord contusion injury in rat. *J. Neurosci. Res.* **2001**, *64*, 582–589. [CrossRef] [PubMed]

25. Bedke, J.; Stojanovic, T.; Kiss, E.; Behnes, C.-L.; Proudfoot, A.E.; Gröne, H.-J. Viral macrophage inflammatory protein-II improves acute rejection in allogeneic rat kidney transplants. *World J. Urol.* **2010**, *28*, 537–542. [CrossRef] [PubMed]

26. Zhang, L. Structural Study of the Interaction between Poxvirus-Encoded CC Chemokine Inhibitor VCCI and Human MIP-1β. Ph.D. Thesis, Texas A&M University, College Station, TX, USA, May 2008.

27. DeRider, M.L.; Zhang, L.; LiWang, P.J. Resonance assignments and secondary structure of vCCI, a 26 kDa CC chemokine inhibitor from rabbitpox virus. *J. Biomol. NMR* **2006**, *36*, 22. [CrossRef] [PubMed]

28. Pettersen, E.F.; Goddard, T.D.; Huang, C.C.; Couch, G.S.; Greenblatt, D.M.; Meng, E.C.; Ferrin, T.E. UCSF Chimera—A visualization system for exploratory research and analysis. *J. Comput. Chem.* **2004**, *25*, 1605–1612. [CrossRef] [PubMed]

29. PDBePISA (Proteins, Interfaces, Structures and Assemblies). Available online: http://www.ebi.ac.uk/pdbe/pisa/ (accessed on 12 July 2017).

30. Krissinel, E.; Henrick, K. Inference of macromolecular assemblies from crystalline state. *J. Mol. Biol.* **2007**, *372*, 774–797. [CrossRef] [PubMed]

31. Krissinel, E. Crystal Contacts as Nature's Docking Solutions. *J. Comput. Chem.* **2009**, *28*, 73–86. [CrossRef] [PubMed]

32. Taylor, P.C.; Feldmann, M. Anti-TNF biologic agents: Still the therapy of choice for rheumatoid arthritis. *Nat. Rev. Rheumatol.* **2009**, *5*, 578–582. [CrossRef] [PubMed]

33. Yi, X.; Manickam, D.S.; Brynskikh, A.; Kabanov, A.V. Agile delivery of protein therapeutics to CNS. *J. Control. Release* **2014**, *190*, 637–663. [CrossRef] [PubMed]

34. Boomker, J.M.; De Leij, L.F.M.H.; The, T.H.; Harmsen, M.C. Viral chemokine-modulatory proteins: Tools and targets. *Cytokine Growth Factor Rev.* **2005**, *16*, 91–103. [CrossRef] [PubMed]

35. Alcami, A.; Viejo-Borbolla, A. Identification and characterization of virus-encoded chemokine binding proteins. *Methods Enzymol.* **2009**, *460*, 173–191. [PubMed]

36. Adcock, S.A.; McCammon, J.A. Molecular dynamics: Survey of methods for simulating the activity of proteins. *Chem. Rev.* **2006**, *106*, 1589–1615. [CrossRef] [PubMed]

37. Shaw, D.E.; Maragakis, P.; Lindorff-Larsen, K.; Piana, S.; Shan, Y.; Wriggers, W. Atomic-level characterization of the structural dynamics of proteins. *Science* **2010**, *330*, 341–347. [CrossRef] [PubMed]

38. Dill, K.A.; MacCallum, J.L. The protein-folding problem, 50 years on. *Science* **2012**, *338*, 1042–1046. [CrossRef] [PubMed]

39. Chang, Y.-G.; Kuo, N.-W.; Tseng, R.; LiWang, A. Flexibility of the C-terminal, or CII, ring of KaiC governs the rhythm of the circadian clock of cyanobacteria. *Proc. Natl. Acad. Sci. USA* **2011**, *108*, 14431–14436. [CrossRef] [PubMed]

40. Wishart, D.S.; Bigam, C.G.; Yao, J.; Abildgaard, F.; Dyson, H.J.; Oldfield, E.; Markley, J.L.; Sykes, B.D. ^{1}H, ^{13}C and ^{15}N chemical shift referencing in biomolecular NMR. *J. Biomolec. NMR* **1995**, *6*, 135–140. [CrossRef]

41. Delaglio, F.; Grzesiek, S.; Vuister, G.W.; Zhu, G.; Pfeifer, J.; Bax, A. NMRPipe: A multidimensional spectral processing system based on UNIX pipes. *J. Biomol. NMR* **1995**, *6*, 277–293. [CrossRef] [PubMed]

42. Garrett, D.S.; Powers, R.; Gronenborn, A.M.; Clore, G.M. A common sense approach to peak picking in two-, three-, and four-dimensional spectra using automatic computer analysis of contour diagrams. *J. Magn. Reson.* **1991**, *95*, 214–220. [CrossRef]

43. Garrett, D.S.; Seok, Y.J.; Peterkofsky, A.; Clore, G.M.; Gronenborn, A.M. Identification by NMR of the binding surface for the histidine- containing phosphocarrier protein HPr on the N-terminal domain of enzyme I of the Escherichia coli phosphotransferase system. *Biochemistry* **1997**, *36*, 4393–4398. [CrossRef] [PubMed]

44. Conlan, L.H.; Dupureur, C.M. Dissecting the metal ion dependence of DNA binding by *Pvu*II endonuclease. *Biochemistry* **2002**, *41*, 1335–1342. [CrossRef] [PubMed]

45. Reid, S.L.; Parry, D.; Liu, H.H.; Connolly, B.A. Binding and recognition of GATATC target sequences by the *Eco*RV restriction endonuclease: A study using fluorescent oligonucleotides and fluorescence polarization. *Biochemistry* **2001**, *40*, 2484–2494. [CrossRef] [PubMed]

46. Abraham, M.J.; Murtola, T.; Schulz, R.; Pall, S.; Smith, J.C.; Hess, B.; Lindah, E. Gromacs: High performance molecular simulations through multi-level parallelism from laptops to supercomputers. *SoftwareX* **2015**, *1*, 19–25. [CrossRef]

47. Pronk, S.; Pall, S.; Schulz, R.; Larsson, P.; Bjelkmar, P.; Apostolov, R.; Shirts, M.R.; Smith, J.C.; Kasson, P.M.; van Der Spoel, D.; et al. GROMACS 4.5: A high-throughput and highly parallel open source molecular simulation toolkit. *Bioinformatics* **2013**, *29*, 845–854. [CrossRef] [PubMed]

48. Hess, B.; Kutzner, C.; van der Spoel, D.; Lindahl, E. GROMACS 4: Algorithms for highly efficient, load balanced, and scalable molecular simulations. *J. Chem. Theory Comput.* **2008**, *4*, 435–447. [CrossRef] [PubMed]

49. Hess, B.; Bekker, H.; Berendsen, H.J.C.; Fraaije, J.G.E.M. LINCS: A linear constraint solver for molecular simulations. *J. Comput. Chem.* **1997**, *18*, 1463–1472. [CrossRef]

50. Bussi, G.; Donadio, D.; Parrinello, M. Canonical sampling through velocity rescaling. *J. Chem. Phys.* **2007**, *126*, 1–7. [CrossRef] [PubMed]

51. Parrinello, M.; Rahman, A. Polymorphic transitions in single crystals: A new molecular dynamics method. *J. Appl. Phys.* **1981**, *52*, 7182–7190. [CrossRef]

52. Lindorff-Larsen, K.; Piana, S.; Palmo, K.; Maragakis, P.; Klepeis, J.L.; Dror, R.O.; Shaw, D.E. Improved side-chain torsion potentials for the Amber ff99SB protein force field. *Proteins Struct. Funct. Bioinforma* **2010**, *78*, 1950–1958. [CrossRef] [PubMed]

53. Jorgensen, W.L.; Chandrasekhar, J.; Madura, J.D.; Impey, R.W.; Klein, M.L. Comparison of simple potential functions for simulating liquid water. *J. Chem. Phys.* **1983**, *79*, 926. [CrossRef]

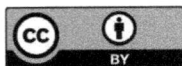

International Journal of
Molecular Sciences

MDPI

Article

Possible Roles of CC- and CXC-Chemokines in Regulating Bovine Endometrial Function during Early Pregnancy

Ryosuke Sakumoto [1,*], Ken-Go Hayashi [1], Shiori Fujii [1], Hiroko Kanahara [1], Misa Hosoe [2], Tadashi Furusawa [2] and Keiichiro Kizaki [3]

[1] Division of Animal Breeding and Reproduction Research, Institute of Livestock and Grassland Science, National Agriculture and Food Research Organization (NARO), Ibaraki 305-0901, Japan; hayaken@affrc.go.jp (K.-G.H.); s.love.sweets.03@gmail.com (S.F.); kanahara@affrc.go.jp (H.K.)
[2] Division of Animal Sciences, Institute of Agrobiological Sciences, National Agriculture and Food Research Organization (NARO), Ibaraki 305-8602, Japan; hosoe@affrc.go.jp (M.H.); tfuru@affrc.go.jp (T.F.)
[3] Laboratory of Veterinary Physiology, Iwate University, Iwate 020-8550, Japan; kizaki@iwate-u.ac.jp
[*] Correspondence: sakumoto@affrc.go.jp; Tel.: +81-29-838-8633

Academic Editor: Martin J. Stone
Received: 14 February 2017; Accepted: 27 March 2017; Published: 31 March 2017

Abstract: The aim of the present study was to determine the possible roles of chemokines in regulating bovine endometrial function during early pregnancy. The expression of six chemokines, including CCL2, CCL8, CCL11, CCL14, CCL16, and CXCL10, was higher in the endometrium at 15 and 18 days of pregnancy than at the same days in non-pregnant animals. Immunohistochemical staining showed that chemokine receptors (CCR1, CCR2, CCR3, and CXCR3) were expressed in the epithelial cells and glandular epithelial cells of the bovine endometrium as well as in the fetal trophoblast obtained from a cow on day 18 of pregnancy. The addition of interferon-τ (IFNT) to an endometrial tissue culture system increased CCL8 and CXCL10 expression in the tissues, but did not affect CCL2, CCL11, and CCL16 expression. CCL14 expression by these tissues was inhibited by IFNT. CCL16, but not other chemokines, clearly stimulated interferon-stimulated gene 15 (ISG15) and myxovirus-resistance gene 1 (MX1) expression in these tissues. Cyclooxygenase 2 (COX2) expression decreased after stimulation with CCL8 and CCL14, and oxytocin receptor (OTR) expression was decreased by CCL2, CCL8, CCL14, and CXCL10. Collectively, the expression of chemokine genes is increased in the endometrium during early pregnancy. These genes may contribute to the regulation of endometrial function by inhibiting COX2 and OTR expression, subsequently decreasing prostaglandin production and preventing luteolysis in cows.

Keywords: cow; endometrium; chemokines; tissue culture; pregnancy

1. Introduction

The establishment of pregnancy is the result of successful communication between the conceptus and the maternal endometrium. When animals become pregnant, the corpus luteum (CL) remains functional and the dynamics of prostaglandin (PG) F2α secretion from uterus in early pregnancy changes from that in the comparable stages of the estrous cycle [1–3]. At the time of recognition of pregnancy, the bovine conceptus produces interferon-τ (IFNT) to prevent luteolysis, which is induced by a pulsatile release of PGF2α from the uterus [2,3]. IFNT plays various roles in ruminants, such as uterine receptivity to implantation and differentiation of the conceptus [2–4]. Extensive research during the last decade, including global transcriptome studies, demonstrated the enrichment of immune-related genes, including interferon-stimulated genes (ISGs), in the endometrium of a pregnant cow compared to non-pregnant or cyclic heifers [5–11]. However, the physiological roles of these pregnancy-dependently regulated genes in the mechanism of maternal recognition are not yet fully understood. Understanding the role of the fetal-maternal interaction during early pregnancy might help to determine a way to improve reproductive efficiency and alleviate deficiencies.

Therefore, in the present study, we evaluated global gene expression patterns in the endometrium of pregnant and non-pregnant cows using a custom-made, 15 K bovine oligo DNA microarray analysis. Since the expression of messenger RNA of six chemokines, including CCL2, CCL8, CCL11, CCL14, CCL16, and CXCL10, drastically increased in the endometrium during early pregnancy, the effects of IFNT and fetal trophoblast-derived total protein on the expression of chemokine genes were subsequently evaluated. Furthermore, the effects of these chemokines and pregnancy-related substances, including IFNT, tumor necrosis factor-α (TNF) and leukemia inhibitory factor (LIF), on the expression of interferon-stimulated gene 15 (ISG15), myxovirus-resistance gene 1 (MX1), cyclooxygenase 2 (COX2), oxytocin receptor (OTR), and estrogen receptor α (ESR1) by cultured endometrial tissues were studied to assess the physiological roles of chemokines in regulating endometrial function during early pregnancy in cows.

2. Results

2.1. Expression of Chemokines and Their Receptors in the Bovine Endometrium during Early Pregnancy

Microarray analysis detected 344 and 1336 differentially expressed genes in the bovine endometrium at 15 and 18 days of pregnancy compared with the same days in non-pregnant cows (>2-fold change; $p < 0.05$). The expression of six chemokines, including CCL2, CCL8, CCL11, CCL14, CCL16, and CXCL10, was higher in the endometrium during early pregnancy than in the non-pregnant stage (Table 1).

Table 1. Comparison of mRNA levels for selected chemokines in the endometrium of pregnant vs. non-pregnant cows as determined by microarray analysis (Fold > 2.0; $p < 0.05$).

Genes	Day 15 (344 Genes)	Day 18 (1336 Genes)
CCL2 (MCP-1)	3.58	-
CCL8 (MCP-2)	4.91	12.9
CCL11 (Eotaxin)	-	61.1
CCL14 (HCC-1)	2.67	-
CCL16 (HCC-4)	2.55	-
CXCL10 (IP-10)	2.10	21.1

Messenger RNA expression of these chemokines was confirmed by real-time PCR. Transcripts of CCL2, CCL8, CCL14, CCL16, and CXCL10 were more abundant in the endometrium at day 15 of pregnancy than at day 15 in non-pregnant cows (Figure 1; $p < 0.05$). Moreover, the expression of CCL8, CCL11, and CXCL10 mRNA was higher in the endometrium at day 18 of pregnancy than at day 18 in non-pregnant cows (Figure 1; $p < 0.05$). Although messenger RNAs of chemokine receptors (CCR1, CCR2, CCR3, and CXCR3) were detected in the bovine endometrium during both the estrous cycle and pregnancy, there were no significant changes in the expression of these receptors between the estrous cycle and pregnancy.

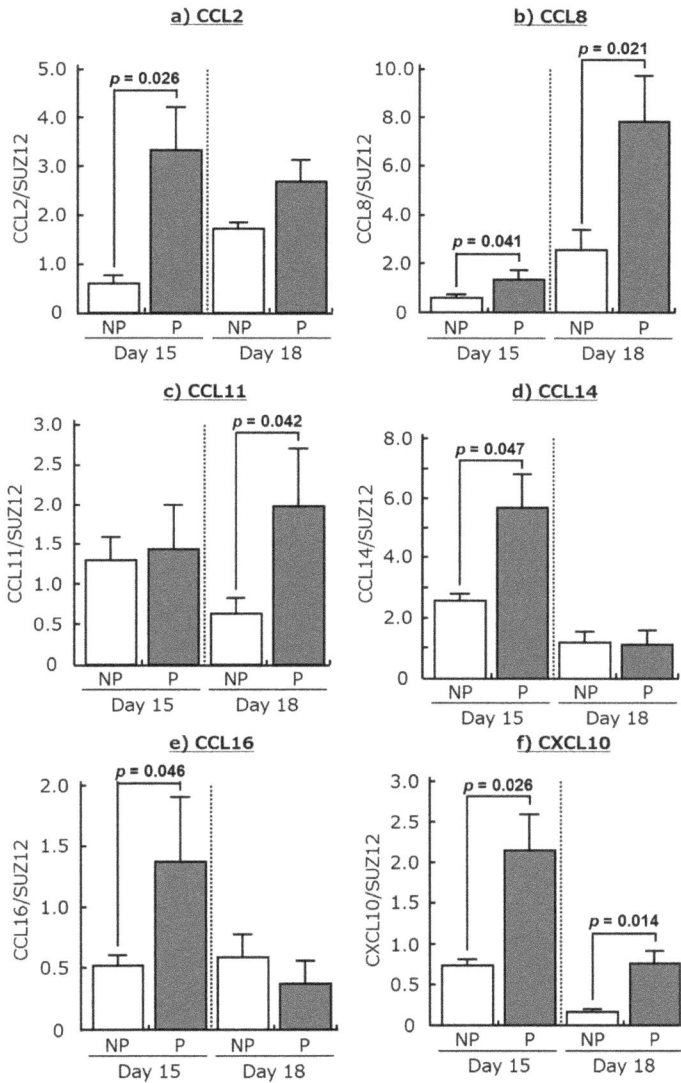

Figure 1. Changes in relative amounts of mRNA for (**a**) CCL2, (**b**) CCL8, (**c**) CCL11, (**d**) CCL14, (**e**) CCL16, and (**f**) CXCL10 in the endometrium at days 15 and 18 of non-pregnant cows (NP) and pregnant cows (P). Data are means ± SEM of four cows per stage and are expressed as relative ratios of the mRNAs to SUZ12 polycomb repressive complex 2 subunit (SUZ12). *p*-Values show significant differences between NP and P.

Immunohistochemical staining showed that CCR1 (binds to CCL8, CCL14, and CCL16), CCR2 (binds to CCL2, CCL8, and CCL16), CCR3 (binds to CCL11), and CXCR3 (binds to CXCL10) were expressed in the epithelial and glandular epithelial cells of the endometrium as well as in the fetal trophoblast obtained from day 18 of pregnancy (Figure 2).

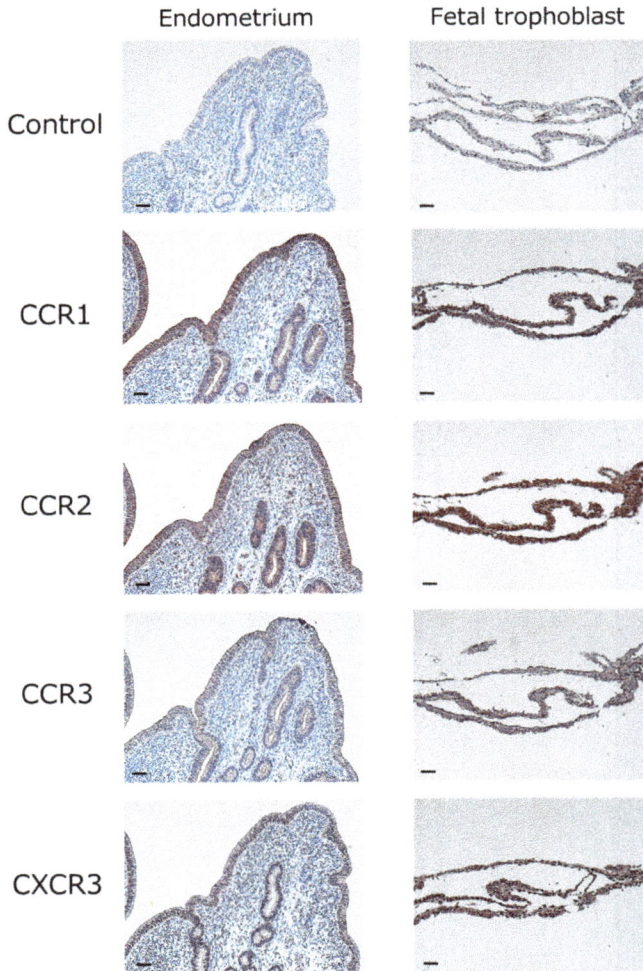

Figure 2. Localization of CCR1 (binds to CCL8, CCL14, and CCL16), CCR2 (binds to CCL2, CCL8, and CCL16), CCR3 (binds to CCL11), and CXCR3 (binds to CXCL10) in the bovine endometrium and fetal trophoblast obtained from cows in their 18th day of pregnancy. Intensive immunoreactivity was observed in endometrial epithelial cells, glandular epithelial cells, or fetal trophoblast. No positive immunoreactivity was observed in the negative control (Control). Scale bar = 50 µm.

2.2. Effects of IFNT and FMP on Chemokine Expression in Cultured Endometrial Tissues

The addition of IFNT increased CCL8 and CXCL10 expression in cultured endometrial tissue (Figure 3b,f; $p < 0.01$), but it did not affect CCL2, CCL11, and CCL16 expression. CCL14 expression in this tissue was inhibited by IFNT (Figure 3d; $p < 0.05$). In addition, the supernatant derived from homogenized fetal trophoblast (FMP) of day 18 of pregnancy stimulated CCL8 and CXCL10 expression in the endometrial tissues (Figure 3b,f; $p < 0.05$).

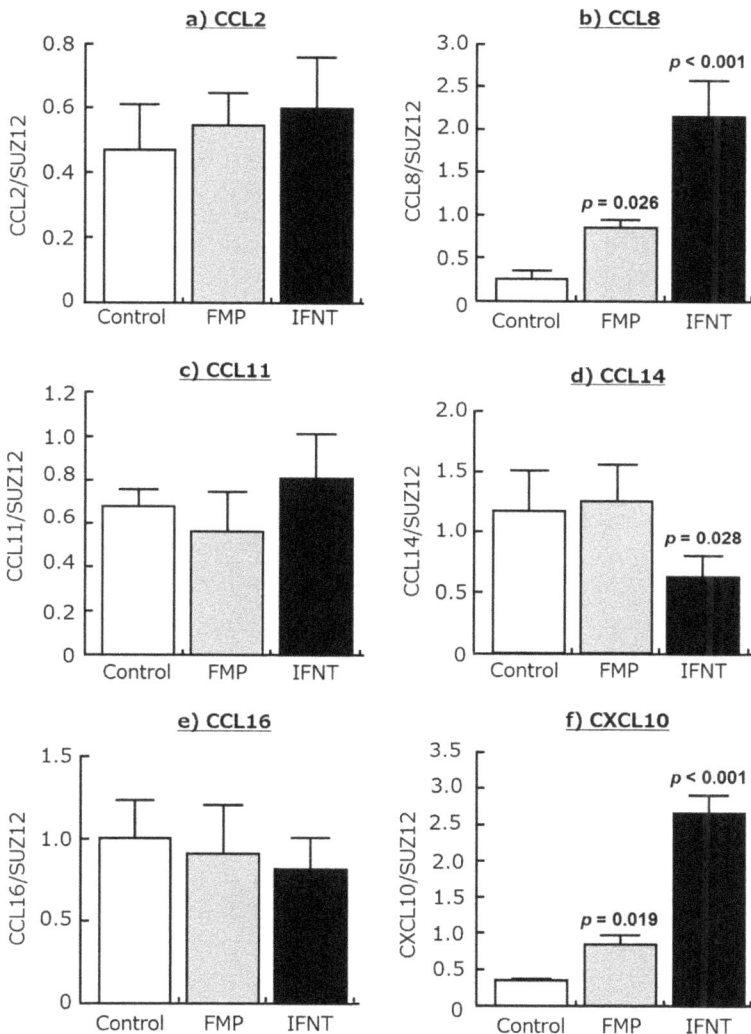

Figure 3. Effects of the supernatant derived from homogenized fetal trophoblast (FMP; 200 ng/mL) and interferon-τ (IFNT; 100 ng/mL) on the mRNA expression of (**a**) CCL2, (**b**) CCL8, (**c**) CCL11, (**d**) CCL14, (**e**) CCL16, and (**f**) CXCL10 in cultured bovine endometrial tissues. Homogenization buffer was added at the control group. Data are means ± SEM of five cows and are expressed as relative ratios of the mRNAs to SUZ12. *p*-Values show significant differences between treated group and control group.

2.3. Effects of Chemokines, IFNT, FMP, TNF, and LIF on ISG15, MX1, COX2, OTR, and ESR1 Expression in Cultured Endometrial Tissues

CCL16 clearly stimulated both ISG15 and MX1 expression in the cultured endometrial tissues ($p < 0.001$), whereas the other chemokines had no effect (Figure 4a,b). COX2 expression decreased after the stimulation of CCL8 and CCL14 (Figure 4c; $p < 0.05$ or lower), and OTR expression was decreased by CCL2, CCL8, CCL14, and CXCL10 (Figure 4d; $p < 0.05$ or lower). In contrast, ESR1 mRNA expression was not affected by all tested chemokines (Figure 4e).

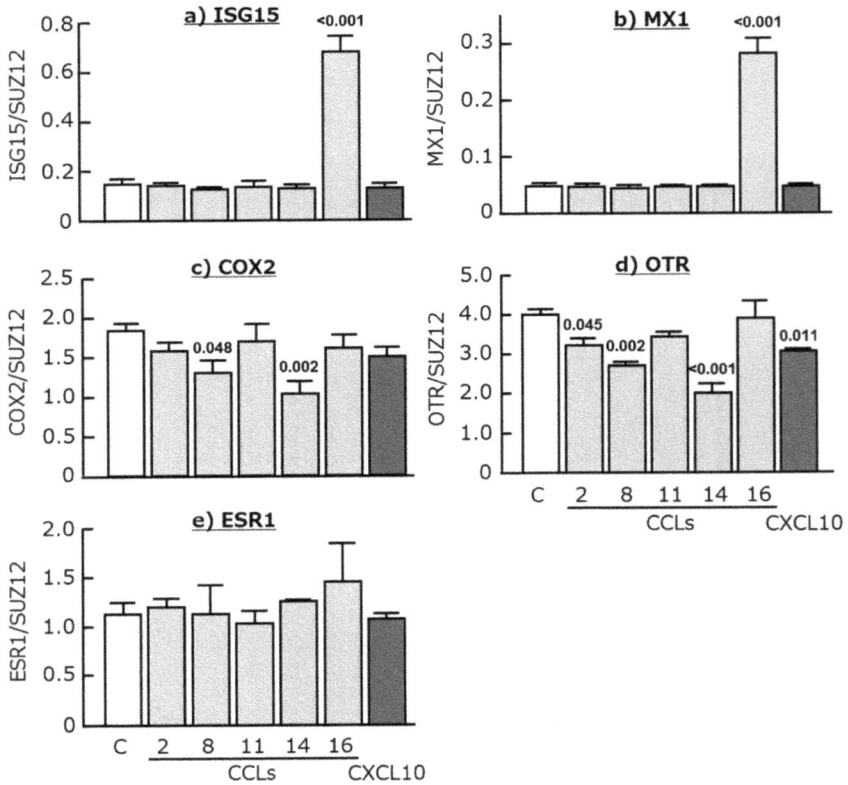

Figure 4. Effects of CCL2, CCL8, CCL11, CCL14, CCL16, and CXCL10 (50 ng/mL each) on the mRNA expression of (**a**) interferon-stimulated gene 15 (ISG15), (**b**) myxovirus-resistance gene 1 (MX1), (**c**) cyclooxygenase 2 (COX2), (**d**) oxytocin receptor (OTR), and (**e**) estrogen receptor α (ESR1) in cultured bovine endometrial tissues. Data are means ± SEM of five cows and are expressed as relative ratios of the mRNAs to SUZ12. p-Values show significant differences between treated group and control group.

The addition of IFNT and FMP increased the expression of ISG15 and MX1, and decreased the expression of COX2 and OTR, in cultured endometrial tissues (Figure 5a–d; $p < 0.05$ or lower) As expected, TNF stimulated COX2 expression and decreased OTR and ESR1 expression in these tissues (Figure 5c–e; $p < 0.05$). Interestingly, it also stimulated the expression of both ISG15 and MX1 (Figure 5a,b; $p < 0.05$). Moreover, LIF decreased the expression of COX2 and OTR in endometrial tissues (Figure 5c,d; $p < 0.05$), but did not affect ISG15, MX1, and ESR1 expression.

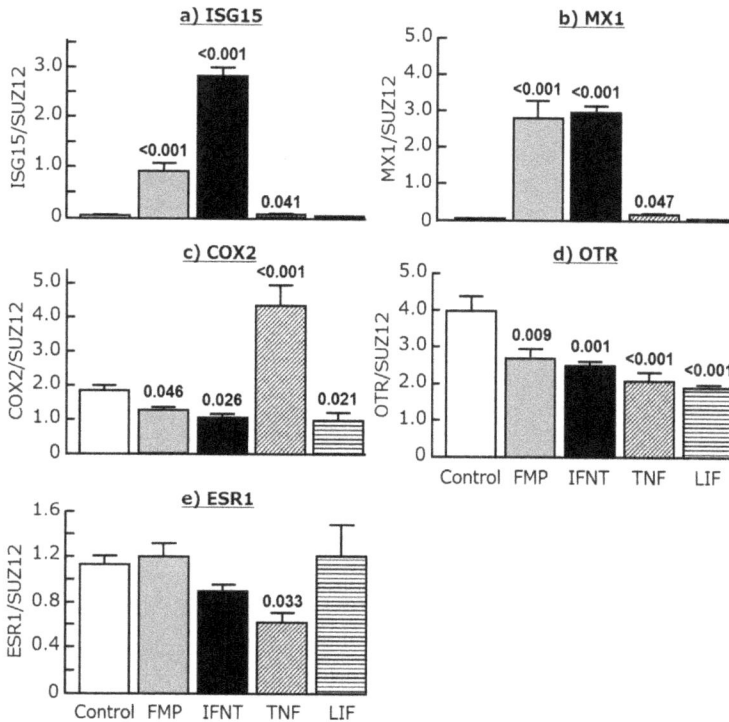

Figure 5. Effects of the supernatant derived from homogenized fetal trophoblast (FMP; 200 ng/mL), interferon-τ (IFNT; 100 ng/mL), tumor necrosis factor α (TNF; 50 ng/mL), and leukemia inhibitory factor (LIF; 50 ng/mL) on the mRNA expression of (**a**) ISG15, (**b**) MX1, (**c**) COX2, (**d**) OTR, and (**e**) ESR1 in cultured bovine endometrial tissues. Data are means ± SEM of five cows and are expressed as relative ratios of the mRNAs to SUZ12. *p*-Values show significant differences between treated group and control group.

3. Discussion

The results of the current study demonstrated that gene expression in the bovine endometrium during early pregnancy differs from that in the endometrium during the estrous cycle. In particular, gene expression of six chemokines was apparently high in the endometrium on days 15 and 18 in pregnant cows in comparison to the non-pregnant cows. In this study, we focused on the endometrial gene expressions on days 15 and 18 of pregnancy since IFNT production from trophoblast drastically increases around days 14–15 [12], and elongated conceptus is implanted to endometrial epithelial cells immediately after (on days 18–19) in cattle [5]. Messenger RNA expression of CCL8 and CXCL10 was higher in the endometrium during both day 15 and 18 of pregnancy, but the expression of CCL2, CCL14, and CCL16 were high in the endometrium of day 15 of pregnancy. CCL11 expression in the endometrium was high in the endometrium during only day 18 of pregnancy, suggesting that stage dependent changes of the expression of these chemokines have multiple roles in regulating maternal-conceptus communication. Moreover, CCL8 and CXCL10 were increased by stimulation with IFNT and FMP using an in vitro culture system. The binding sites of chemokines were present in the endometrial epithelial and glandular epithelial cells. All tested chemokines, except for CCL11, attenuated the expression of genes coding for pregnancy-related substances in the cultured endometrial tissues. These observations lead us to hypothesize that chemokines play an important role in regulating bovine endometrial function during early pregnancy.

Immune cells, the main sources and targets of chemokines, are present in bovine endometrium throughout the estrous cycle, and the number of immune cells increases around the late luteal stage [13]. Eosinophils secrete both CCL2 (known as MCP-1) and CCL8 (MCP-2) and the number of eosinophils increase within the uterus during early pregnancy in ewes [14]. Both CCL2 and CCL8 act through CCR2 found on monocytes and memory T cells [15]. In addition, CCL8 also binds to CCR1 found primarily on T cells, monocytes, and eosinophils [15]. Here, we demonstrated that both CCR1 and CCR2 are present in endometrial epithelial cells, and that the expression of CCL8 was increased by IFNT and FMP, suggesting that CCL2 and CCL8 could affect endometrial function during the early gestation period. Indeed, the present study demonstrated that CCL2 decreases COX2 expression and CCL8 decreases both the expression of COX2 and OTR in cultured endometrial tissues. Since oxytocin (OT) stimulates endometrial PG production by activating COX2 in endometrial cells [16], CCL2 and CCL8 may subsequently contribute to inhibit PGF2α production to establish pregnancy in cows.

CXCL10, also known as IP-10, is found in monocytes that are localized in the subepithelial stroma of ovine endometrium, and its expression is stimulated by IFNT and interferon-γ [17]. The expression level of CXCL10 in the endometrium is higher in pregnancy than in the non-pregnant stage in goats [18]. In cows, CXCL10 expression in the endometrium was high in pregnancy and its mRNA expression was stimulated by both FMP and IFNT in the present study. Furthermore, CXCR3, which is the binding site of CXCL10, was expressed in the bovine endometrium and fetal trophoblast on day 18 of pregnancy. CXCL10 inhibits OTR expression in cultured endometrial tissues. A previous study demonstrated that CXCL10 could induce the recruitment of numerous leukocytes, lymphocytes, and/or monocytes to the ovine uterus and enhance the ability to attach to day 17 trophoblasts and day 20 chorionic membranes [19]. CXCL10 also induces caprine trophoblast adhesion [20] and chemotaxis in human trophoblast cell lines [21]. These findings suggest that CXCL10 might affect not only PG production from the endometrium, but also conceptus elongation at an early stage of pregnancy in cows.

In the present study, since CCL14 (also known as HCC-1) expression increased in the endometrium of pregnant cows, we expected that CCL14 expression of the cultured endometrial tissues would have been increased by stimulation with FMP or IFNT. However, FMP had no effect and IFNT adversely inhibited CCL14 expression. We could not find an appropriate explanation for this apparently contradictory phenomenon. Since chemokine production is regulated by many factors, including cytokines, growth factors, and steroids [17,22,23], other factor(s) may have powerful effects on the stimulation of CCL14 production in the endometrium of early pregnant cows. For example, although IFNT inhibited CCL14 expression in these tissues, FMP showed no effect in this study. Hence, some substances other than IFNT in FMP might indirectly stimulate CCL14 production in cultured endometrial tissues, causing the inhibitory effects of IFNT on CCL14 expression to be masked. In humans, CCL14 is produced maximally by the endometrium at the time of embryo implantation and during early pregnancy, predominantly by decidualized stroma and epithelial cells [24], and its receptor (CCR1) is present on invasive extravillous trophoblasts [25]. In addition, the migration of trophoblasts is stimulated by CCL14 [25]. Since CCR1 protein was expressed in the fetal trophoblast as well as in endometrial epithelial cells in this study, CCL14 may induce the promotion of trophoblast migration in cows. In this study, CCL14 reduced COX2 and OTR expression in cultured endometrial tissues, suggesting that CCL14 decreases PG production in the bovine uterus. Taken together, although further studies regarding the physiological impact of CCL14 in regulating endometrial function are required, CCL14 may be an important factor in maternal-fetal communication in cows.

Little information is available about the involvement of CCL11 in bovine reproduction. CCL11, also known as eotaxin-1, increased in the endometrium on day 18 of pregnancy in this study. Since the binding sites of CCL11 (CCR3) are expressed in bovine and human [26] endometrial epithelial cells, we expected that this chemokine would act as a paracrine factor in the endometrium after day 18 of pregnancy. However, CCL11 expression was not affected by FMP and IFNT, and CCL11 did not affect the expression of any gene in cultured endometrial tissues. A previous study demonstrated that CCL11 induces angiogenic responses by human CCR3-positive endothelial cells [27], and that estradiol-17β (E2) acts through CCL11 to recruit eosinophils to the uterine stroma during the estrous cycle in mice, but that these cells do not have a function in regulating either the duration of the estrous cycle or the fertility of mice [28]. In addition, CCL11 regulates extravillous trophoblast migration, invasion, and adhesion, highlighting a potential regulatory role for these chemokines during uterine decidual spiral arteriole remodeling in the first trimester of human pregnancy [29]. Thus, CCL11 may act on the trophoblast-conceptus via CCR3 rather than on endometrial cells in pregnant cows.

The precise roles of CCL16 in the bovine endometrium are currently unknown, but there is considerable information regarding its functions in immunological disease and cancer in humans. CCL16 mRNA was elevated in women with endometriosis, and immunoreactive CCL16 was predominantly demonstrated in the endometrium [30]. CCL16 increases antigen presentation of macrophages, enhances T-cell cytotoxicity, and stimulates the production of a number of inflammatory-type cytokines (interleukin-1β, TNF, interleukin-12) [31]. CCL16 and its receptors were identified in preterm placenta [32]. In addition, CCL16 induces endothelial cell motility, which is pivotal in vessel formation by stimulating the release of proinflammatory and proangiogenic chemokines [33,34]. In this study, CCL16 receptors (CCR1, CCR2) were expressed in the endometrial epithelial cells, and CCL16 drastically stimulated the expression of ISG15 and MX1 in cultured endometrial tissues. These effects are comparable with those of FMP and IFNT. Although a further study is needed to clarify the role of CCL16 in regulating bovine endometrial function in detail, it may positively influence angiogenesis and anti-viral activity by up-regulating ISG15 and MX1 expression at the time of maternal recognition in cows.

IFNT, the pregnancy recognition hormone in ruminants, is produced by mononuclear trophectoderm cells of conceptuses at a critical time to prevent regression of the CL function. One mechanism by which IFNT inhibits luteolysis is the down-regulation of OTR, which prevents OT-stimulated PGF secretion [35]. As expected, IFNT clearly stimulated ISG15 and MX1 expression but inhibited COX2 and OTR expression by the cultured endometrial tissues, suggesting that in vitro culture systems can support previous data regarding the biological effects of IFNT. On the other hand, TNF is well recognized as a potent luteolytic factor in many mammalian species, including cows. TNF and TNF receptors are present in the bovine endometrium, and TNF stimulates PGF production only in the bovine endometrial stromal cells by increasing COX2 mRNA in cattle [36–38]. IFNT reduced TNF-induced PGF synthesis directly by attenuating COX2 gene expression in bovine endometrial stromal cells in a dose-dependent manner [38]. Indeed, TNF stimulated COX2 and inhibited the expression of OTR and ESR1 in endometrial tissues in the present study. In contrast, TNF significantly stimulated the expression of both ISG15 and MX1 in endometrial tissues, similar to INFT, which is a known anti-luteolytic agent. Since TNF acts through TNF receptor type I/type II via various intracellular signaling pathways, including nuclear factor-kappa B/activator protein-1 and mitogen-activated protein kinase [39], TNF may contribute directly or indirectly to anti-viral activity within the uterus. LIF mRNA expression is observed in the endometrium of both humans and mice and its concentration increases in mid- and late secretory phases [40]. LIF is regarded as an important factor in both murine and human embryo implantation or decidualization. LIF-deficient female mice are infertile due to the failure of implantation [41]. Since LIF reduced COX2 and OTR expression in cultured endometrial tissues in this study, LIF may play an important role in establishing pregnancy in the process of maternal recognition in cows as well as in humans and rodents.

4. Materials and Methods

4.1. Collection of the Bovine Uterus and Fetal Trophoblast

Bovine uteri were obtained from Japanese Black cows at the institute ranch within 10–30 min of exsanguination. For the microarray analysis and immunohistochemistry, tissue samples were collected from cows on days 15 and 18 after artificial insemination (n = 4 animals/stage). The day of artificial insemination was designated as day 1. The uterine horn with ipsilateral of the CL was obtained and immediately cut open to see the endometrium. The presence or absence of fetal trophoblast was checked macroscopically to determine whether the cows were pregnant or not. The caruncular endometrial tissues (<0.5 cm^3) were collected and submerged in RNAlater (Qiagen GmbH, Hilden, Germany) or in 10% neutral formalin and stored until use.

Supernatants derived from homogenized fetal trophoblast on day 18 of pregnancy (FMP) were collected as described previously [42]. Briefly, the fetal trophoblast was transferred into 2.5 mL of ice-cold homogenized buffer (300 mM sucrose, 25 mM Tris-HCl, 2 mM EDTA; pH 7.4) containing a proteinase inhibitor tablet (cOmplete Ultra tablet EDTA-free, Roche Diagnostics, Tokyo, Japan), and was homogenized in an ice bath with a rotor-stator homogenizer (TissueRuptor; Qiagen) using three 30 s bursts at maximum speed with 20 s intervals of cooling between each burst. The homogenate was subsequently centrifuged at 23,500× g for 30 min at 4 °C. The supernatant was collected and total protein concentration was measured using a commercial protein assay kit (DC Protein Assay Kit, 500-0111JA, BIO-RAD Laboratories Co., Ltd., Tokyo, Japan).

All procedures for animal experiments were carried out in accordance with guidelines approved by the Animal Ethics Committee of the National Institute of Agrobiological Sciences on 1 April 2014 (#H18-036-3).

4.2. Microarray Analysis

A custom-made 15 K bovine oligo DNA microarray was used for the microarray analysis, which was performed according to previous reports [43,44]. After verifying the quality of the RNA with a NanoDrop ND-1000 spectrophotometer (NanoDrop Technology Inc., Wilmington, DE, USA), and an Experion RNA StdSens kit (700-7104JA, BIO-RAD Laboratories), we performed one-color microarray analysis. RNA integrity was confirmed, and all samples had an A260/280 ratio greater than 1.8 and an RNA integrity number greater than 8.5. The oligomicroarray produced by Agilent Technologies (Palo Alto, CA, USA) was used in this study. Sixty-mer nucleotide probes for the customized microarray were synthesized on a glass slide. cDNA synthesis, Cy3-labeled cRNA preparation, hybridization, and the washing and scanning of the array slides were performed according to the Agilent one color microarray-based gene expression analysis protocol. Briefly, 400 ng of total RNA from each sample were reverse-transcribed into cDNA using the Quick Amp Labeling Kit (Agilent Technologies) with an oligo dT-based primer, and then Cy3-labelled cRNA was prepared by in vitro transcription. Labeled cRNA was purified with an RNeasy Mini Kit, and the concentration and Cy3 dye incorporation (pmol Cy3/μg cRNA) were measured with a spectrophotometer. Labeled cRNA (600 ng) was fragmented and hybridized using the Gene Expression Hybridization Kit (Agilent Technologies), according to the manufacturer's instructions. The arrays were washed using a Gene Expression Wash Pack Kit and scanned using an Agilent Microarray Scanner. Feature Extraction ver. 9.5 was used for image analysis and data extraction. The microarray data from each sample were imported into GeneSpring 12 (Agilent Technologies) for use in the software's normalization algorithm and for candidate gene detection. Normalization was performed by dividing each measurement of each array by the median of all measurements in that array (per chip normalization). The Gene Expression Omnibus (GEO, available online: http://www.ncbi.nlm.nih.gov/geo/query/acc.cgi) accession numbers are as follows: GPL9284 for the platform, GSM2455260 to GSM2455274 for the samples, and GSE93580 for the series.

4.3. Real-Time PCR

Total RNA isolation and subsequent reverse transcription and real-time PCR steps were carried out as previously described [45]. The primers encoding the bovine sequences were chosen using an online software package (available online: http://primer3.ut.ee/) and synthesized as listed in Table 2. The primer length (18–25 bp) and GC contents of each primer (50–60%) were selected to avoid primer dimer formation.

Table 2. Primers used in real-time PCR.

Genes	Sequence (5'-3')	GenBank Accession Number	Size (bp)
CCL2	Forward: TGCAGACCCCAAGCAGAAAT Reverse: AGAGGGCAGTTAGGGAAAGC	NM_174006	144
CCL8	Forward: AACATGAAGGTCTCCGCTGG Reverse: GCAGCAGGTGATTGGGGTAG	NM_174007	108
CCL11	Forward: TCACGAGCAGCAAATGTCCT Reverse: CATGGCATTCTGGACCCACT	NM_205773	101
CCL14	Forward: ACTAAATTTCCCCGCTCGCT Reverse: TGGCCAAACTTCTGCAGAGT	NM_001046585	121
CCL16	Forward: GCCCACTGAGAGGATGAAGG Reverse: TACTTCAGGCAGCAGTTGGG	XM_002695627	129
CXCL10	Forward: CTCGAACACGGAAAGAGGCA Reverse: TCCACGGACAATTAGGGCTT	NM_001046551	117
ISG15	Forward: GCAGACCAGTTCTGGCTGTCT Reverse: CCAGCGGGTGCTCATCAT	NM_174366	58
MX1	Forward: GAGGTGGACCCCCAAGGA Reverse: CCACCAGATCGGGCTTTGT	NM_173940	58
COX2	Forward: TGTGAAAGGGAGGAAAGAGC Reverse: GGCAAAGAATGCAAACATCA	AF004944	115
OTR	Forward: TGTGCTGGACGCCATTCTT Reverse: GGAGCATGGCGATGATGAAAG	NM_174134	93
ESR1	Forward: CAGGCACATGAGCAACAAAG Reverse: TCCAGCAGCAGGTCGTAGAG	NM_001001443	84
SUZ12	Forward: GAACACCTATCACACACATTCTTGT Reverse: TAGAGGCGGTTGTGTCCACT	NM_001205587	130

Gene expression was measured by real-time PCR using an Mx3000P Real time PCR analyzing system (Agilent Technologies) and a QuantiFast SYBR Green PCR kit (204054, Qiagen) starting with 500 ng of reverse-transcribed total RNA. PCR was performed under the following conditions: (first step) 95 °C for 5 min; 45 cycles of 95 °C for 15 s, 60 °C for 30 s, and (second step) 95 °C for 60 s; then 60 °C for 30 s. The reaction was then held at 25 °C. Each PCR was followed by obtaining melting curves to ensure single product amplification. As standard curves, serial dilutions of appropriate cDNA were used for gene quantification. The expression ratio of each gene to SUZ12 polycomb repressive complex 2 subunit (SUZ12) mRNA, which has been demonstrated to be suitable for normalization in bovine endometrial tissue [46], was calculated to adjust for any variations in the PCR reaction. Use of the Mx3000P real-time PCR analyzing system at elevated temperatures resulted in reliable and sensitive quantification of the RT-PCR products with high linearity (Pearson correlation coefficient $r > 0.96$). To exclude any contaminating genomic DNA, all experiments included controls that lacked the reverse transcription enzyme. As a negative control, water was used instead of RNA for the PCR to exclude any contamination from buffers and tubes.

4.4. Immunohistochemistry

Immunohistochemistry for CCR1, CCR2, CCR3, and CXCR3 in the bovine endometrium and fetal trophoblast on day 18 of pregnancy was performed using the automated Ventana HX System Discovery with a DabMapKit (Roche Diagnostics), as described previously [47]. The 5 μm-thick sections from paraffin-embedded tissue were incubated at room temperature with rabbit polyclonal anti-human CCR1 antibody (ab140756, Abcam PLC, Cambridge, UK; dilution 1:200), rabbit polyclonal anti-human CCR2 antibody (NBP1-48337, Novus Biologicals LLC, Littleton, CO, USA; dilution 1:100), rabbit polyclonal anti-human CCR3 antibody (251536, Abbiotec LLC, San Diego, CA, USA; dilution 1:50), or rabbit polyclonal anti-mouse CXCR3 antibody (orb5924, Biorbyt Ltd., Cambridge, UK; dilution 1:50) for 12 h. The signals were detected using anti-rabbit IgG-Biotin conjugate (Sigma-Aldrich Co., LLC,

St. Louis, MO, USA) diluted 1:100 for 1 h, and then counterstained with hematoxylin. Negative controls were performed using normal rabbit IgG (NBP2-24891, Novus Biologicals) diluted at concentrations equivalent to the primary antibodies. The sections were observed with a Leica DMRE HC microscope (Leica Microsystems K.K., Tokyo, Japan) and photographed with a Nikon Digital Sight DS-Fi1-L2 (Nikon Instruments Co., Tokyo, Japan).

4.5. Endometrial Tissue Culture

For the tissue culture study, endometrial tissue samples were collected from cows on days 10–12 of the estrous cycle (n = 5 animals). The endometrial tissues from the bovine uterus were separated using a modification of procedures described previously [36,42]. The uterine lumen was washed three times with 30–50 mL of sterile physiological saline supplemented with 100 IU/mL penicillin, 100 µg/mL streptomycin, and 0.1% BSA (735078, Roche Diagnostics). The uterine horn was cut transversely with scissors into several segments, which were slit to expose the endometrial surface. Caruncular endometrial strips were dissected from the myometrial layer with a scalpel and washed once in 50 mL of sterile saline-containing antibiotics. The endometrial strips were then cut into small pieces (2 mm^3). The tissues (approximately 20–30 mg wt) were pre-incubated in Dulbecco's Modified Eagle's medium (DMEM; D1152, Sigma-Aldrich Co.) supplemented with 0.1% BSA. After pre-incubating for 4 h, the endometrial tissues were placed in culture medium (DMEM/Ham's F-12; 1:1 (v/v); D8900, Sigma-Aldrich Co.) supplemented with 10% (v/v) calf serum (C6278, Sigma-Aldrich Co.), 20 IU/mL penicillin, 20 µg/mL streptomycin, and 0.05 µg/mL amphotericin B (516104, EMD Millipore Corp. Billerica, MA, USA), and cultured at 37.5 °C in a humidified atmosphere of 5% CO_2 in air. Cultured endometrial tissues were further incubated in the medium with recombinant proteins as follows: bovine CCL2 (RP0027B, Kingfisher Biotech., Inc. St. Paul, MN, USA), human CCL8 (281-CP, R&D Systems, Inc. Minneapolis, MN, USA), bovine CCL11 (RP0071B, Kingfisher Biotech.), human CCL14 (1578-HC, R&D Systems), human CCL16 (TP723266, OriGene Technologies, Inc., Rockville, MD, USA), bovine CXCL10 (RP0079B, Kingfisher Biotech.), bovine tumor necrosis factor-α (TNF; 2279-BT, R&D Systems), human leukemia inhibitory factor (LIF; TP723270, OriGene Technologies), bovine IFNT (1.1 × 10^5 U/mg, generated from HEK293 cells as described previously; Takahashi et al., 2017 [48]) or supernatant derived from homogenized fetal trophoblast on day 18 of pregnancy (FMP). After incubation for 18 h, the endometrial tissue and supernatant were collected and stored at −80 °C until use.

To determine the responsibility of cultured endometrial tissue, the concentrations of PGE2 and PGF2α in the culture media after stimulation with TNF were examined using commercial ELISA kits (PGE2; 500141, PGF2α; 516011, Cayman Chemical Co., Ann Arbor, MI, USA). Both the PGE2 (299.7% ± 7.4%) and PGF2α (185.2% ± 16%) concentrations were significantly increased by the addition of TNF.

4.6. Statistical Analyses

Microarray data were analyzed statistically with an unpaired Student's *t*-test and summarized using GeneSpring 12 (Agilent Technologies). The differences of mRNA expression in the endometrium between the non-pregnant and pregnant group (each day 15 and 18) were analyzed statistically with an unpaired Student's *t*-test. In tissue culture experiments, the difference of mRNA expression in the endometrial tissues between control group and treated group was analyzed using one-way ANOVA with Dunnett's Multiple Comparison post hoc test with the KaleidaGraph 3.6 (Synergy Software, Reading, PA, USA) software package. All Experimental data for real-time PCR are presented as the mean ± SEM. A *p*-value < 0.05 was considered statistically significant.

5. Conclusions

In conclusion, chemokines that are increased in the endometrium of early pregnant cows, including CCL2, CCL8, CCL11, CCL14, CCL16, and CXCL10, may regulate PG production and antiviral activity in the uterus at the time of maternal recognition, together with IFNT, TNF, or LIF (Figure 6).

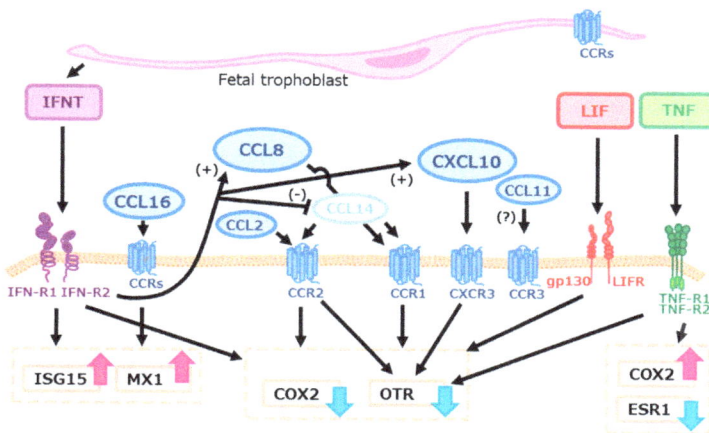

Figure 6. Hypothetical model for inhibition of luteolysis by IFNT and chemokines. Although this model is not concerned with the effects of steroids or growth factors, IFNT, CCL2, CCL8, CCL16, CXCL10, and LIF may block TNF-stimulated-COX2 expression in bovine endometrial cells, leading to the reduction of TNF-induced PGF2α output from the cells. Furthermore, IFNT and CCL16 may stimulate anti-viral activity by up-regulating ISG15 and MX1 expression at the time of maternal recognition in cows. Red and blue arrows show stimulatory and inhibitory actions of each substance, respectively. IFNT may stimulate both CCL8 and CXCL10 production and inhibit CCL14 production from bovine endometrium. Effects of CCL11 on bovine endometrial function are still unclear, although its receptor (CCR3) is expressed in the endometrial epithelial cells.

Acknowledgments: This research was supported by Grants-in-Aid for the Research Program on Innovative Technologies for Animal Breeding, Reproduction, and Vaccine Development (REP1001) from the Ministry of Agriculture, Forestry and Fisheries of Japan. The authors thank the staff of the Livestock Operations Unit 1, Tsukuba Technical Support Center, National Agriculture and Food Research Organization (NARO) for their skilled technical assistance.

Author Contributions: Ryosuke Sakumoto participated in the design of the study, carried out all experiments, and drafted the manuscript; Ken-Go Hayashi and Misa Hosoe collected the materials and helped to carry out quantitative real-time PCR; Shiori Fujii and Hiroko Kanahara carried out immunohistochemistry and quantitative real-time PCR; Tadashi Furusawa participated in the design of the study and helped to draft the manuscript; Keiichiro Kizaki carried out microarray and microarray data analysis. All authors read and approved the final manuscript.

Conflicts of Interest: The authors declare no conflict of interest.

Abbreviations

IFNT	interferon τ
COX2	cyclooxygenase 2
OTR	oxytocin receptor
ESR1	estrogen receptor α
CL	corpus luteum
PG	prostaglandin
TNF	tumor necrosis factor α
LIF	leukemia inhibitory factor
FMP	supernatant derived from homogenized fetal trophoblast
MCP	monocyte chemoattractant protein
MIP	macrophage inflammatory protein
E2	estradiol-17β

References

1. Thatcher, W.W.; Bartol, F.F.; Knickerbocker, J.J.; Curl, J.S.; Wolfenson, D.; Bazer, F.W.; Roberts, R.M. Maternal recognition of pregnancy in cattle. *J. Dairy Sci.* **1984**, *67*, 2797–2811. [CrossRef]
2. Bazer, F.W. Mediators of maternal recognition of pregnancy in mammals. *Proc. Soc. Exp. Biol. Med.* **1992**, *199*, 373–384. [CrossRef] [PubMed]
3. Demmers, K.J.; Derecka, K.; Flint, A. Trophoblast interferon and pregnancy. *Reproduction* **2001**, *121*, 41–49. [CrossRef] [PubMed]
4. Bazer, F.W.; Spencer, T.E.; Ott, T.L. Interferon tau: A novel pregnancy recognition signal. *Am. J. Reprod. Immunol.* **1997**, *37*, 412–420. [CrossRef] [PubMed]
5. Bauersachs, S.; Ulbrich, S.E.; Gross, K.; Schmidt, S.E.; Meyer, H.H.; Wenigerkind, H.; Vermehren, M.; Sinowatz, F.; Blum, H.; Wolf, E. Embryo-induced transcriptome changes in bovine endometrium reveal species-specific and common molecular markers of uterine receptivity. *Reproduction* **2006**, *132*, 319–331. [CrossRef] [PubMed]
6. Oliveira, J.F.; Henkes, L.E.; Ashley, R.L.; Purcell, S.H.; Smirnova, N.P.; Veeramachaneni, D.N.; Anthony, R.V.; Hansen, T.R. Expression of interferon (IFN)-stimulated genes in extrauterine tissues during early pregnancy in sheep is the consequence of endocrine IFN-τ release from the uterine vein. *Endocrinology* **2008**, *149*, 1252–1259. [CrossRef] [PubMed]
7. Forde, N.; Carter, F.; Spencer, T.E.; Bazer, F.W.; Sandra, O.; Mansouri-Attia, N.; Okumu, L.A.; McGettigan, P.A.; Mehta, J.P.; McBride, R.; et al. Conceptus-induced changes in the endometrial transcriptome: How soon does the cow know she is pregnant? *Biol. Reprod.* **2011**, *85*, 144–156. [CrossRef] [PubMed]
8. Bauersachs, S.; Ulbrich, S.E.; Reichenbach, H.D.; Reichenbach, M.; Büttner, M.; Meyer, H.H.; Spencer, T.E.; Minten, M.; Sax, G.; Winter, G.; et al. Comparison of the effects of early pregnancy with human interferon, alpha 2 (IFNA2), on gene expression in bovine endometrium. *Biol. Reprod.* **2012**, *86*, 1–15. [CrossRef] [PubMed]
9. Cerri, R.L.; Thompson, I.M.; Kim, I.H.; Ealy, A.D.; Hansen, P.J.; Staples, C.R.; Li, J.L.; Santos, J.E.; Thatcher, W.W. Effects of lactation and pregnancy on gene expression of endometrium of Holstein cows at day 17 of the estrous cycle or pregnancy. *J. Dairy Sci.* **2012**, *95*, 5657–5675. [CrossRef] [PubMed]
10. Forde, N.; Lonergan, P. Transcriptomic analysis of the bovine endometrium: What is required to establish uterine receptivity to implantation in cattle? *J. Reprod. Dev.* **2012**, *58*, 189–195. [CrossRef] [PubMed]
11. Oliveira, L.J.; Mansourri-Attia, N.; Fahey, A.G.; Browne, J.; Forde, N.; Roche, J.F.; Lonergan, P.; Fair, T. Characterization of the Th profile of the bovine endometrium during the oestrous cycle and early pregnancy. *PLoS ONE* **2013**, *8*, e75571. [CrossRef] [PubMed]
12. Ealy, A.D.; Yang, Q.E. Control of interferon-tau expression during early pregnancy in ruminants. *Am. J. Reprod. Immunol.* **2009**, *61*, 95–106. [CrossRef] [PubMed]
13. Cobb, S.P.; Watson, E.D. Immunohistochemical study of immune cells in the bovine endometrium at different stages of the oestrous cycle. *Res. Vet. Sci.* **1995**, *59*, 238–241. [CrossRef]
14. Asselin, E.; Johnson, G.A.; Spencer, T.E.; Bazer, F.W. Monocyte chemotactic protein-1 and -2 messenger ribonucleic acids in the ovine uterus: Regulation by pregnancy, progesterone, and interferon-τ. *Biol. Reprod.* **2001**, *64*, 992–1000. [CrossRef] [PubMed]
15. Balestrieri, M.L.; Balestrieri, A.; Mancini, F.P.; Napoli, C. Understanding the immunoangiostatic CXC chemokine network. *Cardiovasc. Res.* **2008**, *78*, 250–256. [CrossRef] [PubMed]
16. Asselin, E.; Drolet, P.; Fortier, M.A. Cellular mechanisms involved during oxytocin-induced prostaglandin F2α production in endometrial epithelial cells in vitro: Role of cyclooxygenase-2. *Endocrinology* **1997**, *138*, 4798–4805. [PubMed]
17. Nagaoka, K.; Sakai, A.; Nojima, H.; Suda, Y.; Yokomizo, Y.; Imakawa, K.; Sakai, S.; Christenson, R.K. A chemokine, interferon (IFN)-γ-inducible protein 10 kDa, is stimulated by IFN-τ and recruits immune cells in ovine endometrium. *Biol. Reprod.* **2003**, *68*, 1413–1421. [CrossRef] [PubMed]
18. Imakawa, K.; Nagaoka, K.; Nojima, H.; Hara, Y.; Christenson, R.K. Changes in immune cell distribution and IL-10 production are regulated through endometrial IP-10 expression in the goat uterus. *Am. J. Reprod. Immunol.* **2005**, *53*, 54–64. [CrossRef] [PubMed]

19. Imakawa, K.; Imai, M.; Sakai, A.; Suzuki, M.; Nagaoka, K.; Sakai, S.; Lee, S.R.; Chang, K.T.; Echternkamp, S.E.; Christenson, R.K. Regulation of conceptus adhesion by endometrial CXC chemokines during the implantation period in sheep. *Mol. Reprod. Dev.* **2006**, *73*, 850–858. [CrossRef] [PubMed]

20. Nagaoka, K.; Nojima, H.; Watanabe, F.; Chang, K.T.; Christenson, R.K.; Sakai, S.; Imakawa, K. Regulation of blastocyst migration, apposition, and initial adhesion by a chemokine, interferon γ-inducible protein 10 kDa (IP-10), during early gestation. *J. Biol. Chem.* **2003**, *278*, 29048–29056. [CrossRef] [PubMed]

21. Dominguez, F.; Martínez, S.; Quiñonero, A.; Loro, F.; Horcajadas, J.A.; Pellicer, A.; Simón, C. CXCL10 and IL-6 induce chemotaxis in human trophoblast cell lines. *Mol. Hum. Reprod.* **2008**, *14*, 423–430. [CrossRef] [PubMed]

22. Simon, C.; Caballero-Campo, P.; Garcia-Velasco, J.A.; Pellicer, A. Potential implications of chemokines in reproductive function: An attractive idea. *J. Reprod. Immunol.* **1998**, *38*, 169–193. [CrossRef]

23. Hannan, N.J.; Salamonsen, L.A. Role of chemokines in the endometrium and in embryo implantation. *Curr. Opin. Obstet. Gynecol.* **2007**, *19*, 266–272. [CrossRef] [PubMed]

24. Hannan, N.J.; Jones, R.L.; Critchley, H.O.; Kovacs, G.J.; Rogers, P.A.; Affandi, B.; Salamonsen, L.A. Coexpression of fractalkine and its receptor in normal human endometrium and in endometrium from users of progestin-only contraception supports a role for fractalkine in leukocyte recruitment and endometrial remodeling. *J. Clin. Endocrinol. Metab.* **2004**, *89*, 6119–6129. [CrossRef] [PubMed]

25. Hannan, N.J.; Jones, R.L.; White, C.A.; Salamonsen, L.A. The chemokines, CX3CL1, CCL14, and CCL4, promote human trophoblast migration at the feto-maternal interface. *Biol. Reprod.* **2006**, *74*, 896–904. [CrossRef] [PubMed]

26. Zang, J.; Lathbury, L.J.; Salamonsen, L.A. Expression of the chemokine eotaxin and its receptor, CCR3, in human endometrium. *Biol. Reprod.* **2000**, *62*, 404–411. [CrossRef]

27. Salcedo, R.; Young, H.A.; Lourdes Ponce, M.; Ward, J.M.; Kleinman, H.K.; Murphy, W.J.; Oppenheim, J.J. Eotaxin (CCL11) induces in vivo angiogenic responses by human CCR3$^+$ endothelial cells. *J. Immunol.* **2001**, *166*, 7571–7578. [CrossRef] [PubMed]

28. Gouon-Evans, V.; Pollard, J.W. Eotaxin is required for eosinophil homing into the stroma of the pubertal and cycling uterus. *Endocrinology* **2001**, *142*, 4515–4521. [CrossRef] [PubMed]

29. Chau, S.E.; Murthi, P.; Wong, M.H.; Whitley, G.S.; Brennecke, S.P.; Keogh, R.J. Control of extravillous trophoblast function by the eotaxins CCL11, CCL24 and CCL26. *Hum. Reprod.* **2013**, *28*, 1497–1507. [CrossRef] [PubMed]

30. Chand, A.L.; Murray, A.S.; Jones, R.L.; Hannan, N.J.; Salamonsen, L.A.; Rombauts, L. Laser capture microdissection and cDNA array analysis of endometrium identify CCL16 and CCL21 as epithelial-derived inflammatory mediators associated with endometriosis. *Reprod. Biol. Endocrinol.* **2007**, *5*, 18. [CrossRef] [PubMed]

31. Cappello, P.; Caorsi, C.; Bosticardo, M.; de Angelis, S.; Novelli, F.; Forni, G.; Giovarelli, M. CCL16/LEC powerfully triggers effector and antigen-presenting functions of macrophages and enhances T cell cytotoxicity. *J. Leukoc. Biol.* **2004**, *75*, 135–142. [CrossRef] [PubMed]

32. Mäkikallio, K.; Kaukola, T.; Tuimala, J.; Kingsmore, S.F.; Hallman, M.; Ojaniemi, M. Umbilical artery chemokine CCL16 is associated with preterm preeclampsia and fetal growth restriction. *Cytokine* **2012**, *60*, 377–384. [CrossRef] [PubMed]

33. Bussolino, F.; Mantovani, A.; Persico, G. Molecular mechanisms of blood vessel formation. *Trends Biochem. Sci.* **1997**, *22*, 251–256. [CrossRef]

34. Strasly, M.; Doronzo, G.; Cappello, P.; Valdembri, D.; Arese, M.; Mitola, S.; Moore, P.; Alessandri, G.; Giovarelli, M.; Bussolino, F. CCL16 activates an angiogenic program in vascular endothelial cells. *Blood* **2004**, *103*, 40–49. [CrossRef] [PubMed]

35. Lafrance, M.; Goff, A.K. Effect of pregnancy in oxytocin-induced release of prostaglandin F2α in heifers. *Biol. Reprod.* **1985**, *33*, 1113–1119. [CrossRef] [PubMed]

36. Miyamoto, Y.; Skarzynski, D.J.; Okuda, K. Is tumor necrosis factor α a trigger for the initiation of endometrial prostaglandin F2α release at luteolysis in cattle? *Biol. Reprod.* **2000**, *62*, 1109–1115. [CrossRef] [PubMed]

37. Skarzynski, D.J.; Miyamoto, Y.; Okuda, K. Production of prostaglandin F2α by cultured bovine endometrial cells in response to tumor necrosis factor-α: Cell type specificity and intracellular mechanisms. *Biol. Reprod.* **2000**, *62*, 1116–1120. [CrossRef] [PubMed]

38. Okuda, K.; Kasahara, Y.; Murakami, S.; Takahashi, H.; Woclawek-Potocka, I.; Skarzynski, D.J. Interferon-τ blocks the stimulatory effect of tumor necrosis factor-α on prostaglandin F2α synthesis by bovine endometrial stromal cells. *Biol. Reprod.* **2004**, *70*, 191–197. [CrossRef] [PubMed]

39. Okuda, K.; Sakumoto, R. Multiple roles of TNF super family members in corpus luteum function. *Reprod. Bio . Endocrinol.* **2003**, *1*, 95. [CrossRef] [PubMed]

40. Mor, G.; Cardenas, I.; Abrahams, V.; Guller, S. Inflammation and pregnancy: The role of the immune system at the implantation site. *Ann. N. Y. Acad. Sci.* **2011**, *1221*, 80–87. [CrossRef] [PubMed]

41. Shuya, L.L.; Menkhorst, E.M.; Yap, J.; Li, P.; Lane, N.; Dimitriadis, E. Leukemia inhibitory factor enhances endometrial stromal cell decidualization in humans and mice. *PLoS ONE* **2011**, *6*, e25288. [CrossRef] [PubMed]

42. Sakumoto, R.; Hayashi, K.G.; Takahashi, T. Different expression of PGE synthase, PGF receptor, TNF, Fas and oxytocin in the bovine corpus luteum of the estrous cycle and pregnancy. *Reprod. Biol.* **2014**, *14*, 115–121. [CrossRef] [PubMed]

43. Kizaki, K.; Shichijo-Kizaki, A.; Furusawa, T.; Takahashi, T.; Hosoe, M.; Hashizume, K. Differential neutrophil gene expression in early bovine pregnancy. *Reprod. Biol. Endocrinol.* **2013**, *11*, 6. [CrossRef] [PubMed]

44. Sakumoto, R.; Hayashi, K.G.; Hosoe, M.; Iga, K.; Kizaki, K.; Okuda, K. Gene expression profiles in the bovine corpus luteum (CL) during the estrous cycle and pregnancy: Possible roles of chemokines in regulating CL function during pregnancy. *J. Reprod. Dev.* **2015**, *61*, 42–48. [CrossRef] [PubMed]

45. Sakumoto, R.; Komatsu, T.; Kasuya, E.; Saito, T.; Okuda, K. Expression of mRNAs for interleukin-4, interleukin-6 and their receptors in porcine corpus luteum during the estrous cycle. *Domest. Anim. Endocrinol.* **2006**, *31*, 246–257. [CrossRef] [PubMed]

46. Walker, C.G.; Meier, S.; Mitchell, M.D.; Roche, J.R.; Littlejohn, M. Evaluation of real-time PCR endogenous control genes for analysis of gene expression in bovine endometrium. *BMC Mol. Biol.* **2009**, *10*, 100. [CrossRef] [PubMed]

47. Ushizawa, K.; Takahashi, T.; Hosoe, M.; Kizaki, K.; Hashizume, K. Characterization and expression analysis of SOLD1, a novel member of the retrotransposon-derived Ly-6 superfamily, in bovine placental villi. *PLoS ONE* **2009**, *4*, e5814. [CrossRef] [PubMed]

48. Takahashi, T.; Sakumoto, R.; Hayashi, K.G.; Hosoe, M.; Shirai, J.; Hashizume, K. Generation of recombinant bovine interferon tau in the human embryonic kidney cell line and its biological activity. *Anim. Sci. J.* **2017**, in press.

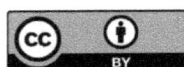

MDPI AG

St. Alban-Anlage 66

4052 Basel, Switzerland

Tel. +41 61 683 77 34

Fax +41 61 302 89 18

http://www.mdpi.com

International Journal of Molecular Sciences Editorial Office

E-mail: ijms@mdpi.com

http://www.mdpi.com/journal/ijms

www.ingramcontent.com/pod-product-compliance
Lightning Source LLC
Chambersburg PA
CBHW051840210326
41597CB00033B/5721